Emerging Issues in Family and Individual Resilience

Series Editors
Amanda W. Harrist
Joseph G. Grzywacz

More information about this series at http://www.springer.com/series/13415

Ginger L. Welch • Amanda W. Harrist
Editors

Family Resilience and Chronic Illness

Interdisciplinary and Translational Perspectives

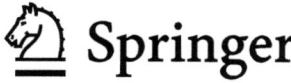 Springer

Editors
Ginger L. Welch
College of Human Sciences
Oklahoma State University
Stillwater, OK, USA

Amanda W. Harrist
Oklahoma State University
Stillwater, OK, USA

ISSN 2366-6072   ISSN 2366-6080   (electronic)
Emerging Issues in Family and Individual Resilience
ISBN 978-3-319-26031-0   ISBN 978-3-319-26033-4   (eBook)
DOI 10.1007/978-3-319-26033-4

Library of Congress Control Number: 2016933861

© Springer International Publishing Switzerland 2017
This work is subject to copyright. All rights are reserved by the Publisher, whether the whole or part of the material is concerned, specifically the rights of translation, reprinting, reuse of illustrations, recitation, broadcasting, reproduction on microfilms or in any other physical way, and transmission or information storage and retrieval, electronic adaptation, computer software, or by similar or dissimilar methodology now known or hereafter developed.
The use of general descriptive names, registered names, trademarks, service marks, etc. in this publication does not imply, even in the absence of a specific statement, that such names are exempt from the relevant protective laws and regulations and therefore free for general use.
The publisher, the authors and the editors are safe to assume that the advice and information in this book are believed to be true and accurate at the date of publication. Neither the publisher nor the authors or the editors give a warranty, express or implied, with respect to the material contained herein or for any errors or omissions that may have been made.

Printed on acid-free paper

This Springer imprint is published by Springer Nature
The registered company is Springer International Publishing AG Switzerland

*In memory of Steve,
whose strength, optimism, humor, and grace allowed
our family to be resilient in the face of so many challenges.
We will keep our promise to be happy. A.W.H.*

*For Hayden and Kathy, whose lives
inspired parts of this volume,
and to Addy, who inspires me always. G.W.*

Preface

"To work and to love," those are the foundations of life, so said Freud, and as many new human service professionals enter the field, they are prepared to help their clients build resources, manage strong emotions, and learn to cope in order to establish a career and successful relationships with others. Underlying much of what a typical clinician is taught, however, is the essence that patients can learn to control their lives. What many clients, and we ourselves, fail to recognize is the impact of a chronic health crisis… one that has been described as the ultimate pulling-the-rug-out-from-under experience. To work, to care for others, and to care for ourselves under healthy circumstances provides a challenge; however, when our illusions of chronic wellness are threatened, either for ourselves or someone we care for, we can become consumed with the path "back" to wellness. When a condition does not easily lend itself to returning to our old normal, a "new normal" way of being, of co-existing with a diagnosis and pursuing a path to wellness, becomes the goal. Such is the goal of living with chronic illness. In this volume, we have brought together experts in the meaning of chronic illness, its origins, prevention, treatment, and consequences across the lifespan. Contributors include physicians, nurses, psychologists, and researchers, as well as child development specialists, child protection workers, educators, counselors, ethicists, and others. It is intended to be a three-dimensional view of chronic illness, encompassing the person with the chronic condition, his or her family, the medical team, and the experience of having a chronic illness over time. This volume, while providing information about diagnoses and psychosocial interventions, is not about disease. It is about living resiliently… surviving and thriving, if you will… in the face of a chronic diagnosis.

As each chapter addresses an illness along the lifespan spectrum, it also reaches into the past of the disease process, illuminating yesterday's missteps and successes; provides a snapshot of modern-day functioning; and offers a glimpse into the future, often as we would like to see it. However, the future will unfold most likely in the hands of the students and emerging professionals reading this book. We provide you our collective vision of the future based on our own research and experiences. We want the next generation to understand the role of multiple chronic conditions in lived experience. Chronic illness as "real" life needs to come center stage in research and practice. Our clients and patients are not only the mothers of preterm babies but also mothers with breast cancer; not only teens with cystic fibrosis but also children of divorce struggling with obesity; not only grandfathers with heart conditions but also widowers who are caring for grandchildren with sickle cell. In the future, we need not only 504 Plans to protect children's education, but real, livable work and insurance plans to protect those who love and work and are touched by a chronic illness. We need something to stand in the gap between work and disability. As we pen this, we can acknowledge our own best laid plans, protected by education, financial prudence, and sacrifice, and we also acknowledge the relentless march of aging, the inherent risk of being alive, and the fear that today's joy will be replaced by unpredictable suffering tomorrow. There are no protections, spiritual, financial, or otherwise, that spare us. We look to you as the next generation to integrate the medical, the psychological, the political, and the ethical. We don't envy you the task ahead, but we do believe you'll get there.

Finally, we want the human service trainees who use this book to know that chronic illness is not for the faint of heart. As you choose to take on the momentous task of working alongside those touched by chronic illness, we ask that you have the awareness that you are, for now, making a choice. You elect to become entangled with those of us who are unwillingly engaged in the family dynamics that chronic illness entails. And if you choose so, we hope that this book will help you make that conscious decision to engage ethically, respectfully, and meaningfully with consideration for the whole person in his or her whole context. We hope that you will be inspired to choose to work in an integrated medical setting where you can make a real difference; we hope that you can change a broken system that treats only the medical or the psychological or the interpersonal. We hope that you are inspired to pursue mindfulness, wholeness, and peace in all circumstances, and to recognize that all families, regardless of diagnosis, deserve to be resilient, even in circumstances beyond their control.

Stillwater, OK, USA
Ginger L. Welch, Ph.D.
Amanda W. Harrist, Ph.D.

Acknowledgements

This volume is the result of the contributions of countless individuals, families, and institutions who worked together over the last 2 years not only to conceptualize a series of books, but to write and edit endless drafts, design and organize a conference at which to present ideas about chronic illness and family resilience, and to continue to believe in the importance of family resilience across the lifespan. First, to Jennifer Hadley at Springer, you are both endlessly enthusiastic and unfailingly patient. Thank you for your support. Thank you to Robert Larzelere for conceptualizing the series and approaching Jennifer at NCFR. To everyone who drove the long miles, made the phone calls, sent the emails, managed registration, and pulled together a powerful Chautauqua, we thank you. Canada Parrish, Elizabeth Files, Katelyn McAdams, Jillian Caldwell, Ragan Jessell, Julie Barnard, and Judi Horn, we couldn't have done this without you. Many thanks also to Dean Stephan Wilson, Dr. Jennifer Hays-Grudo, Dr. Michael Merten, Dr. Christine Johnson, and Jarrod Noftsger for allowing us to access these amazing talents. Thank you to Shelby Snyder and the Mayo Hotel of Tulsa for hosting our group so elegantly and for taking such good care of our out-of-town guests. Special thanks go to Drs. Amy Tate, Karina Shreffler, and Catherine Curtis for their early reviews and comments on this collection and to Dr. Debbie Guilfoyle, Dr. Michael Criss, and Kelley Scott for acting as reviewers and discussants at the 2014 Chautauqua. We are indebted to the community professionals and families who were willing to contribute to the breakout boxes that provide practical application and advice to professionals in each chapter. Dr. Jamie Alexander, Dr. Alex Bishop, Sherre Davidson, Dr. Scott Gelfand, Dr. Janice Hermann, Cyd Roberts, Laura Shellhammer, Alyssa Siler, and the case management team at Life Senior Services: Thank you for your expertise on chronic conditions and resilience, both in this text and in life. Finally, we acknowledge the generous support of Oklahoma State University, the College of Human Sciences, and the Center on Family Resilience which helped bring the issues of chronic illness and family resilience from vision to volume.

Contents

1 **Using a Life-World Approach to Understand Family Resilience** 1
Catherine A. Chesla and Victoria Leonard

2 **The Experience of Preterm Birth: Helping Families Survive and Thrive**.. 19
Patricia Williams, Raja Nandyal, Eleanor Hutson, and Ginger L. Welch

3 **Enhancing Coping and Resilience Among Families of Individuals with Sickle Cell Disease**.. 39
Sunnye Mayes and Ashley Baker

4 **Translational Research and Clinical Applications in the Management of Cystic Fibrosis**.. 63
Alexandra L. Quittner, Christina J. Nicolais, Estefany Saez-Flores, and Ruth Bernstein

5 **Improving Physician Self-Efficacy and Reducing Provider Bias: A Family Science Approach to Pediatric Obesity Treatment** 91
Sally Eagleton, Colony S. Fugate, and Michael J. Merten

6 **Facing Changes Together: Teamwork and Family Resilience During Transition of Pediatric Solid Organ Transplant Patients to Adult Care** 115
Noel Jacobs, Marilyn Sampilo, Dianne Samad, and Judith O'Connor

7 **Fighting for the Forgotten: Risk and Resilience of Children and Families Involved with the Foster Care System**........................... 133
Deborah Shropshire, Amanda Williams, Lauren Burge, and Larissa Hines

8 **Strengthening Families Facing Breast Cancer: Emerging Trends and Clinical Recommendations**............................... 153
Merle Keitel, Alexandra Lamm, and Alyson Moadel-Robblee

9 Fostering Resilience Among Older Adults Living with Osteoporosis and Osteoarthritis 179
Brenda J. Smith and Whitney A. Bailey

10 The Unfolding of Unique Problems in Later Life Families 197
Lee Hyer, Christine M. Mullen, and Krystal Jackson

Index 225

About the Editors

Ginger Welch received her Ph.D. in Counseling Psychology at Oklahoma State University. She is currently a Clinical Associate Professor and Internship Coordinator for the Human Development and Family Science Department at OSU. Her research interests include child clinical issues such as child maltreatment fatalities, child neglect, and infant assessment as well as pediatric psychology issues including prematurity and sickle cell disease.

Amanda Harrist received her Ph.D. in Child Development at the University of Tennessee. She is currently Associate Director for Education and Translation at the Center for Family Resilience at Oklahoma State University, where she is also a Professor of Human Development and Family Science. Her research is focused on understanding psychosocial risk and protective processes in children's social contexts, particularly the parent-child relationship and peer relations at school.

Joseph Grzywacz received his Ph.D. in Child and Family Studies from the University of Wisconsin-Madison. He is an NCFR Fellow, past Director for OSU's Center for Family Resilience, and is currently the Norejane Hendrickson Professor and Chair of the Department of Family and Child Science at Florida State University. His area of expertise is as an interdisciplinary social scientist in health, family, and work.

Contributors

Whitney A. Bailey Department of Human Development and Family Science, Stillwater, OK, USA

Ashley Baker Department of Pediatrics, University of Oklahoma Health Sciences Center, Section of Pediatric Hematology/Oncology, Oklahoma City, OK, USA

Ruth Bernstein Department of Psychology, University of Miami, Coral Gables, FL, USA

Lauren Burge University of Oklahoma College of Medicine, Oklahoma City, OK, USA

Catherine A. Chesla Family Health Care Nursing, University of California San Francisco, San Francisco, CA, USA

Sally Eagleton Department of Human Development and Family Science, Oklahoma State University, Stillwater, OK, USA

Colony S. Fugate Center for Health Sciences, Oklahoma State University, Stillwater, OK, USA

Larissa Hines University of Oklahoma College of Medicine, Oklahoma City, OK, USA

Eleanor Hutson Oklahoma Infant Transition Program, University of Oklahoma Health Sciences Center, Oklahoma City, OK, USA

Lee Hyer Mercer University Medical School & Georgia Neurosurgical Institute, Macon, GA, USA

Krystal Jackson Georgia Neurosurgical Institute, Macon, GA, USA

Noel Jacobs University of Oklahoma Health Sciences Center, Oklahoma City, OK, USA

Merle Keitel Counseling & Counseling Psychology, Fordham University, NY, USA

Alexandra Lamm Fordham University, Bronx, NY, USA

Victoria Leonard Western States Pediatric Environmental Health Specialty Unit, University of California San Francisco, San Francisco, CA, USA

Sunnye Mayes Department of Pediatrics, University of Oklahoma Health Sciences Center, Section of Pediatric Hematology/Oncology, Oklahoma City, OK, USA

Michael J. Merten Department of Human Development and Family Science, Oklahoma State University, Stillwater, OK, USA

Center for Family Resilience, Oklahoma State University, Stillwater, OK, USA

Alyson Moadel-Robblee Albert Einstein College of Medicine, Bronx, NY, USA

Christine M. Mullen Georgia Neurosurgical Institute, Macon, GA, USA

Raja Nandyal Neonatal-Perinatal Medicine Section, University of Oklahoma Health Sciences Center, Oklahoma City, OK, USA

Christina J. Nicolais Department of Psychology, University of Miami, Coral Gables, FL, USA

Judith O'Connor University of Oklahoma Health Sciences Center, Oklahoma City, OK, USA

Alexandra L. Quittner Department of Psychology and Pediatrics, University of Miami, Coral Gables, FL, USA

Estefany Saez-Flores Department of Psychology, University of Miami, Coral Gables, FL, USA

Dianne Samad University of Oklahoma Health Sciences Center, Oklahoma City, OK, USA

Marilyn Sampilo University of Oklahoma Health Sciences Center, Oklahoma City, OK, USA

Deborah Shropshire Oklahoma Department of Human Services, University of Oklahoma College of Medicine, Oklahoma City, OK, USA

Brenda J. Smith Department of Nutriitional Sciences, Oklahoma State University, Stillwater, OK, USA

Ginger L. Welch Department of Human Development and Family Science, Oklahoma State University, Stillwater, OK, USA

Patricia Williams Neonatal-Perinatal Medicine Section, University of Oklahoma Health Sciences Center, Oklahoma City, OK, USA

Amanda Williams University of Southern Mississippi, Hattiesburg, MS, USA

Chapter 1
Using a Life-World Approach to Understand Family Resilience

Catherine A. Chesla and Victoria Leonard

Approaching family resilience from a phenomenological life-world perspective offers opportunities to learn from families how they respond to, and evolve, family habits and care practices in the face of health challenges. Here, we will explore aspects of family life-world in relation to the challenges of living with chronic illnesses in families, drawing on our own and others' research. We will illustrate how using interpretive methods to study families who are thrown into the condition of living with chronic illness in a family member allows the researcher to learn how families change their orientations to illness, to health practices, and to everyday life. Habits and practices that families develop for managing the illness condition, and for reconfiguring priorities in the face of illness, figure importantly in the development of family resilience. The creativity and courage that families demonstrate as they adapt their lives to accommodate their chronically ill member can be breathtaking. In order to understand resilience in families coping with chronic illness, we certainly should structure into our research an opening through which to hear their narratives, which are grounded in particular experiences and suffering.

In this chapter, we hope to do three things: first, to lay out some definitions of the interpretive approach to resilience that we are promoting; second, to review some of the philosophical precepts that suggest that using a narrative or life-world approach to family responses to chronic illness fills a gap that a predominantly theory-driven approach leaves behind; and third, we hope to demonstrate, using empirical research,

---

C.A. Chesla, R.N., Ph.D. (✉)
Family Health Care Nursing, University of California San Francisco,
2 Koret Way, UCSF Box 0606, San Francisco, CA 94143, USA
e-mail: kit.chesla@ucsf.edu

V. Leonard, R.N., Ph.D.
Western States Pediatric Environmental Health Specialty Unit, University of California San Francisco, San Francisco, CA 94143, USA
e-mail: victoria.leonard@ucsf.edu

© Springer International Publishing Switzerland 2017
G.L. Welch, A.W. Harrist (eds.), *Family Resilience and Chronic Illness*,
Emerging Issues in Family and Individual Resilience,
DOI 10.1007/978-3-319-26033-4_1

examples of what shows up in family narratives of care of chronically ill members that are not captured by current resilience theories.

Life-world is "the world as immediately or directly experienced in the subjectivity of everyday life" (Life-world, 2014). Life-world comprises our everyday reality and is distinguished from the world as known via objective science. Family life-worlds comprise shared, taken for granted, background understandings of the everyday world that members share and unquestionably accept as real. For the purposes of this discussion, family resilience is defined within an interpretive framework as the family's capacity to adapt to a health challenge in a manner that is in synchrony with its background concerns and practices. Family resilience involves the holistic acceptance of a challenge into a new or altered set of family habits, practices, and concerns.

1.1 How the Study of Life-World Contributes to Resilience Theory

Family resilience theory helps scientists distinguish and identify elements in family life that are central to resilience and to identify the sorts of relations that exist among those constituent parts. Certainly efforts at theorizing family resilience have added tremendously to our capacity to identify objects in family lives that are deserving of exploration and description. For example, in the Family Adjustment and Adaptation Response model, Patterson (1988, 2002) theorizes that a balance of demands and capabilities may result in a healthier family outcome in the face of a significant stress, like chronic illness.

Formal theory, by definition, leaves behind the concrete commitments and concerns that constitute family life. Because resilience theory is constructed of context-free, independent concepts, which are then proposed to be interrelated by the theorist via rules of logic (White & Klein, 2008), the complex interrelationships and connectedness of aspects of everyday life are excluded. To capture these requires a move away from formal theorizing toward a narrative approach to understanding. The general problematic of formal theory is summarized by Dreyfus as follows. "While everyday understanding is implicit, concrete, local, holistic and partial, theories, by contrast, are explicit, abstract, universal and range over elements organized into a new total whole" (Dreyfus, 1994, p. viii).

Elements in a formal theory are decontextualized, abstracted from everyday life, and isolable from one another. In theorizing, concepts or ideas about the world are clearly defined so that they are distinct from other concepts in the theory and from the context in which they arose. Theory building involves the reordering of relations between concepts via laws or rules rather than via everyday practical understanding (White & Klein, 2008). Theory building is a rational, cognitive process that adds tremendously to the sharpness of our *conceptions* about the world. However, we want to argue that family life-worlds cannot be reduced to these isolable elements without also losing access to the relational and contingent meanings and practices that fundamentally constitute family life. "If human beings were simply rational animals ... then it might be possible to reduce the world to theories about having a world and how to keep it" (Dreyfus, 1994, p. ix). We, along with others, argue that the diversity of human experience cannot be adequately contained in theories, because human experience is holistic, and embodies practical, engaged skills that only make sense in the contexts in which they arise (Benner, 1994; Dreyfus, 1994; Flyvbjerg, 2001). Even a complete, well worked out theory, such as family resilience, eclipses the concerns that construct family action, and drains the experience of its meaning to the family.

What novel understandings might arise by approaching resilience via careful consideration of families' life-worlds via narrative inquiry of their relations, concerns, and practices? We begin to answer this question by highlighting the phenomenological concepts that support a narrative approach to studying family resilience. In explaining family life-world, we draw on the writings of Benner, Dreyfus, Heidegger, and others to explain interpretive phenomenology (IP) with families (Benner, 1994; Dreyfus, 1991; Heidegger, 1962). Heideggerian philosophical concepts that serve as an underpinning for interpretive investigations have been described in other writings (Benner, 1994; Leonard, 1994; van Manen, 1997) but the relevance to families, as opposed to individuals (Chesla, 1995), deserves further exploration.

In contrast with the predominant philosophical understanding of human beings as individuals possessing unique minds that perceive and translate the 'external' world to internal, individual consciousness, Heidegger (1962) posits that humans instead emerge from and are fully practically engaged in a world that stands full of possibility and constraints for different patterns of human involvement. Worldhood, according to Heidegger, precedes any particular individual and provides the background habits, practices, self-understandings, and concerns that constitute human possibilities for a particular time in history. Worldhood is not to be understood as the physical environment. Rather, it is the interlocking totality of human practices and understandings that stand behind and make possible everyday life (Dreyfus, 1991). Chairs are meaningful as things to sit upon and are understood in nuanced ways because human activities involve desk chairs for classrooms versus dining room chairs for sharing a meal versus bleachers for watching a ballgame.

In families, the understanding of chairs or tables or silverware, or of more abstract relations such as motherhood, are first understood preconceptually. One learns, via living in a family, how elements in a home (tables, chairs, silverware) or family relations (mother versus uncle) fit together. Building on this background understanding of how the world works and fits together allows humans to live and work together.

Families are the central social institution from which humans come to understand themselves, their place in the world, and the historically and culturally available ways of acting. Drawing on culturally and historically available patterns of self-understanding and action, families instill general societal, as well as family-specific, habits, practices, and concerns (Dreyfus, 1991).

For example, all families have to address the nutritional needs of family members. For some families, this consists of an irregular pattern of purchasing fast or carryout foods that are consumed by individuals according to their own schedules and habits. In other families, there is a planned approach to family meals, where an adult provisions the household, prepares the meal, and shares it with other family members in a patterned and predictable way. In the latter, further variability is possible. A meal presented with love and attention to the special tastes of family members, and accompanied by conversation about each member's well-being, can be contrasted with a meal prepared begrudgingly because the children have to eat, and shared in an atmosphere of irritability, indifference, or silence. Each of these patterns provides children with a holistic understanding of how families "are" and how they as individuals in a family are regarded. It is this pervasive background tone and pattern of family life, taken for granted and absorbed through many interactions over time, which set up an initial background understanding of the world. It is why, when beginning to visit friends' households for dinner or overnight stays, children can be surprised or taken aback by how different other families' lives can be. The differences they experience and the beliefs that are upset by visiting a friend's family are implicit, local, and most often preconscious.

Heidegger suggests that human beings exist primarily and predominantly in engaged practical activity (Dreyfus, 1991; Heidegger, 1962). Humans have an effortless, nonreflective, direct grasp of worldhood and of themselves in the world. This engagement does not require reflection or self-consciousness, and is instead lived through. Consider driving to work or preparing a meal. Seldom does one reflect on or think about an activity, but instead one enacts the driving or cooking, without resorting to reflection. Via direct engagement in activities that have significance and value, and relying on background understandings acquired from family and other societal institutions, humans create new action. Such actions are both self- and world-defining and are founded upon existing worldhood that precedes the individual.

Situational possibilities *and* limits available to individual family members for coping with chronic illness in themselves or a family member issue from the habits and practices, language, self-understandings, and concerns that families elaborate over time, which are themselves shaped by the economic, social, and historic circumstances in which they are elaborated. The tone and tenor of family life largely sets up the possibilities available for individual family members' lives. For example, a family who predominantly views the world as threatening or noxious is likely to produce an individual frightened of novel encounters with the social and physical world. Such fear is a preconscious embodied response, based on multiple experiences over time, observing and learning from the attunement of family members to the world (Dreyfus, 1991). Rather than assessing a situation and deliberately and consciously responding with fear, a novel situation simply shows up as harmful. The predominant background understanding instilled by the family over time and across situations dominates the individual's preconscious grasp of any situation. While the background understandings may dominate how one moves into new situations, it does not *determine* movement. Human agency allows for reinterpreting situations and their possibilities. Heidegger's ideas would suggest that being raised in a household with physical conflicts and abuse can lead to spontaneous withdrawal from intimate human relations.

However, if the abuser is removed from the household, then humans are capable of reinterpreting the situation and their responses over time. In fact, it is often an important role of the clinician to help patients and their families find possibilities in their situation that they hadn't recognized.

Since human beings are thrown into a preexisting world, and that world constitutes who they are, they are not radically free to become anyone or anything they choose to be. Rather, human beings take shape and are defined by their unfolding lives. Each individual and family has situated possibilities for who they are and who they can become. Certain paths are open to them because of their background and family traditions. Additionally, certain paths are simply not accessible to them: they neither show up as possible nor even enter their field of vision (Benner, 1994; Dreyfus, 1991).

For example, for a son who personally identifies with his father's capabilities as a leader, an active member of the community, a coach, and a physically active construction contractor, the father's concrete involvements set the stage for what he himself might be. When that father is diagnosed with dementia, the son's experience of his father's, as well as his own, possibilities is shaken (Phinney, Dahlke, & Purves, 2013).

Another notion of being human that is relevant to understanding family resilience is that humans are beings for whom things matter, and this caring for and about people and things constitute human beings in particular ways. In his beautiful language Heidegger states, "Each one of us is what he pursues and cares for. In everyday terms, we understand ourselves and our existence by way of the activities we pursue and the things we take care of" (quoted in Leonard, 1994, p. 49). Habits of caring for one another (in childhood, in everyday interactions, in illness) disclose important self-understandings that arise in family relations. Parents caring for a child with colic would not choose to have their days punctuated by the wailing of an infant in pain. But the possibilities for parenting are structured by the child's physiology and by the remedies they can find, in their family traditions, in consult with other parents and health care providers, and in medical sources. Colic allows a parent to be with and care for their child in unique ways that general infant care does not. It challenges parents' wits, resources, and capacity to withstand the infant's suffering. And it opens a space or a clearing for the parent to *become* the parent that the child needs them to be because, for most parents, it *matters* what kind of parent they become. This "mattering" sets up the situation. The hundreds of ways that parents learn to respond to their particular child in each particular set of circumstances open up new ways for them to evolve their parenting skills and practices, and their identities as parents.

Embodiment or the capacity of human bodies to operate knowledgeably in the world is another notion that is frequently passed over in human science. Probably the most important aspect of embodiment for family investigations is the habitual skilled body that understands the culturally and socially embedded ways of physically managing within the world (Benner & Wrubel, 1989). Families transmit societal and cultural habits and practices that allow one to survive and thrive in the world. Families also share particular familial embodied characteristics and physical ways of being. How embodiment figures in family resilience has never been articulated but is deserving of our attention. It is likely that members of families share bodily skills, like balance, calmness, or patterns of muscular tension as well as bodily characteristics such as bad knees or risk for heart disease. Observing and mimicking family members' bodily skills, and family understandings of knees and hearts, likely sets up the range of options that each generation brings to their everyday situations. We highlight this aspect of human existence because in family science embodiment is so completely overlooked; Gudmundsdottir's (2009) example of family coping with bereavement, reviewed later in this chapter, suggests that this might be an important area for future investigation and understanding.

1.2 Interpreting Family Responses to the Challenges of Chronic Illness

These Heideggerian background understandings of family life compel us to examine family resilience from the ground up, especially via observations and narrative investigations with families directly involved in situations of care (Kesselring, Chesla, & Leonard, 2010). Making visible the creative, resourceful responses of families who are called to care for an ill member introduces fresh understandings of family life that are passed over by current conceptualizations of family resilience. These responses also offer paradigms of how we might work with other families who struggle in their caregiving. By attending directly to the life-world concerns of family members and their practices of care, new understandings of what the current age both supports and impedes in family resilience can be articulated.

We hope to demonstrate, by drawing on published empirical research, that attention to the life-world of families can illuminate significant processes of resiliently responding to chronic illness challenges.

We will review research that examines family responses to multiple chronic illnesses including dementia, schizophrenia, and the sudden death of a child. This review does not systematically explore any particular theme, or life stage, but rather draws on studies that employed an interpretive phenomenological approach to understanding how families holistically responded to the varied challenges of chronic illness. Each project explored the family life-world by observing or conducting intensive, narrative interviews over time with those affected. It is the nature of interpretive phenomenology to spend significant amounts of time to try to understand the family from their own perspective. This requires substantial time spent with families in order to understand their worlds from the "inside."

A common question that guides these investigations is, "What are the varieties of ways in which families take up, respond to, or care for a family member with a chronic condition?" The projects frequently identify multiple patterns of family response that were observed in the sample. These patterns are understood to represent the range of possibilities for how families might respond to the chronic illness given the current state of treatment, support for families, insurance coverage, and so on. Additionally, there is an understanding that each chronic illness has its own unique set of demands that it places on family life, demands that create possibilities and limits for how families respond.

1.2.1 Resilience in Family Caring Practices with Schizophrenia

Parents' caring practices with emerging adults with schizophrenia are reviewed first. In this investigation, Chesla (Chesla, 1988, 1989, 1991) spent time in 14 families' homes conducting narrative interviews with the mother, father, and person with schizophrenia (PWS) individually once a month for three months. In addition, half the families were observed for an average of 25 hours over an average of eight visits. This intense investigation of family habits and practices in living with and caring for a family member with schizophrenia afforded a rich understanding of the patterns that families developed in response to this multifaceted illness. These patterns included engaged care, conflicted care, managed care, and distanced care.

Parents who provided engaged care viewed caregiving to be an extension of parenting and provided responsive, intuitive, and thoughtful care of the PWS, regardless of symptoms. A paradigm case, or a strong instance of this form of care, was a couple who welcomed their son in their own home, despite his serious symptomatology. All aspects of the son's behavior, including his delusions and obsession with knives, were understood to be part of his disease process. In addition, this couple provided loving, accepting care throughout 15 years of the disease.

Like this couple, engaged care parents attempted to structure their interactions so that they could understand their child's perspective. They wanted to know what their child was thinking, both to understand the PWS's perspective, and to have a sense of the risks that the child might be facing. Engaged care parents aimed to encourage in the child a sense of competence and self-esteem. As much as possible in their dealings with the community, these parents worked to protect their child's sense of self-worth. Additionally, while they grasped the severity of the disease, they believed that the child was suffering with his or her symptoms, and thus they worked to protect the child from additional suffering in the family or community. Symptoms such as anhedonia or low energy were additionally understood to be part of the disease or its treatment, rather than willful behavior. Remarkably, engaged care parents expressed joy, satisfaction, and acceptance of their care responsibilities. The difficulty that arose in this form of care was setting limits on the child. In their view, schizophrenia already caused suffering and many parental actions were structured by a concern to prevent further discomfort. This identification of engaged care arose from narratives related by parents who provided this form of care. Although the specifics of their care might have been quite different, there was a "family resemblance" in the ways in which they approached their child.

Father: We have one of these instant hot water taps for the kitchen sink. The darn thing sticks. My wife says, "He is fixing the hot water faucet." (Laughs.) Like it's going to be a disaster. We had a feeling he was going to really screw this up. He didn't fix it, but rather than telling him, "leave it alone," to me it is worth even buying a new hot water faucet than to discourage him. (Chesla, 1991, p. 456)

This story illuminates an instance of protecting the child's self-esteem, even if it meant disrupting the household and added cost. A second narrative from the same paradigm case illuminates the parents' capacity to accept the child, even during extremely difficult phases of the illness. The PWS had become increasingly paranoid for several weeks prior to the incident. The parents locked their bedroom door for the first time in their married life. During the night they awoke to hear their son tearing apart his room. They called the police and waited in their locked bedroom until police arrived to take the PWS to a hospital. Unfortunately the son escaped into deep woods behind their home. After spending the night elsewhere, the parents went to search for their son, primarily to prevent him from harming someone else before he could be detained. In the aftermath, their concern was to keep their son safe and to hide evidence of his psychotic behavior.

Mother: (I just coped by) putting the room back in order and getting things so that when he did come back it would be a livable room again and he wouldn't have to look at what he had done. Part of my motive was so he wouldn't be embarrassed about it. (Chesla, 1988, p. 145)

Engaged care parents found parallels between caregiving and parenting itself, although they were often asked to cope with extreme situations.

Mother: I think (caregiving) is like motherhood you know? You just do these things without even thinking about them.... We have been so interested in the kids. They've been the most important things in our life and everything else was really secondary... It's what I'm called to do right now. (Chesla, 1991, p. 455)

Multiple parents who provided engaged care explicitly identified some good that had arisen out of their child's diagnosis.

Mother: It's been devastating, on the whole family. It's a terrible thing; I wouldn't want anybody to have to go through with an illness like that... If there was any way to avoid it. But it's done some wonderful things in our lives, too. It's brought out love that maybe just would have been buried. We've become a more giving, loving family, who's not afraid to show it. (Chesla, 1988, p. 153)

Other mothers identified the responsibilities of caregiving as providing an opportunity for realizing their own power. Rather than following their husbands' decisions, they found they had a stronger basis for stating their own position. One single mother joked that she was so strengthened by caring for her son that even the tax man couldn't frighten her.

Resilience, as we define it, is a pattern of family response to chronic illness that allows family members to maintain their values and concerns and find meaning in their caregiving, while at the same time responding effectively to the demands of the illness. It is best understood as a continuum, and as being changeable over time depending upon the situation. Schizophrenia is a good chronic illness in which to examine family resilience because of its variability and the ongoing, novel challenges it presents. Engaged care parents were highly resilient because they had found new ways of relating to the child with schizophrenia, and patterns of living that felt acceptable; they achieved new patterns of relating to and caring for the child that allowed them to feel 'at home,' satisfied, and rewarded in their efforts. These parents evolved new ways to stay involved in their children's care, to respect their independence, and to protect their identity in a community context that stigmatized mental illness.

A second form of parental care was labeled conflicted care because parents expressed persistent conflicts between doing what was needed for the PWS and meeting their own needs. One father had worked extremely hard in order to be able to retire early and travel the world. His dream was thwarted because his son's illness was so destabilizing that he and his wife did not feel safe leaving him alone at home for an extended time. This father characterized care as:

> Father: Kind of a pain in the ass because even though you want life to continue as normal, and you still try, it definitely changes your life.
> F: It's annoying as hell, but you've got to do it. (Chesla, 1988 p. 167)

Another father who provided conflicted care told a story about a Sunday morning when his son offered to do him a favor. Pleased, the father asked him to wash the family car. Over the next several hours the son prepared himself to wash the car by washing himself, putting on special clothes, and gathering the materials needed. He then spent several additional hours meticulously vacuuming and washing the car. Rather than experiencing gratitude at his son's efforts the father was furious about how he went about cleaning the car.

> I feel he should not get a sense of satisfaction out of having washed the car under those conditions because that's not helping him. I think what's important is the *way* you do anything. If you're going to do it under those conditions you don't begin to deserve congratulations. (Chesla, 1988, p. 178)

Contrast these two fathers' responses to their sons' efforts to fix the hot water tap or wash the car. In the former, there was happiness that the son made an effort, and the father would not interrupt the possibility of his son's accomplishment, even if the tap had to be replaced. In the latter, the father felt he was capitulating to the illness if he gave the slightest praise to his son for obsessively washing the car.

For parents in conflicted care, concern for oneself conflicted with concern for the child. Overall these parents were the *most* distressed group; they were emotionally unsettled, "seething" at their situation. In their concern for their children, these parents felt they had to take action, but all action was unsatisfying because it didn't change the situation. At the same time, their sense of responsibility and concern for the child did not allow them to emotionally disengage or physically distance themselves from the PWS.

Regarding their relationship with their child, conflicted care parents expressed limited awareness of the child's symptom experience, fearfulness, or suffering. And this was the only group of parents who interpreted the symptoms of the disease to be manipulation.

> M: I'm angry at the fact that we all have to deal with this and cope with all this crap of our son's antics. He is really paranoid.

And

> M: He's very manipulative mind-wise, very manipulative. Very self-centered. (Chesla, 1991, p. 458)

Parents who were conflicted in their care were less resilient than those engaged in care. Whether the discomfort arose from misunderstanding the illness, from not being able to give up on the emancipation of the PWS, or from their own lost dreams, these parents were unhappy and unsettled. They had lost their familiar patterns of relating to their children because of the diagnosis, and had not recovered or discovered a satisfactory way of living with, and being with, their ill child.

In a third form of care, labeled managed care, parents took on schizophrenia as a challenge amenable to training or treatment. They explicitly defined their role as being that of a trainer, nurse, or therapist.

> M: Since I really consider that the role I'm playing now is that of a psychiatric technician, I have to have a certain number of hours off. (Chesla, 1991, p. 459)

Parents who provided managed care of the PWS had clear objectives for what they wanted their child to accomplish, and strategies to help the child reach that goal. To this end, one mother set up multiple "therapies" such as pet therapy, music therapy, cooking, and shopping therapies. She said of this approach:

> M: I tried to figure out all the ways that I could work with him with all of those *enormous* disabilities, and still do something that would be creative and that he wouldn't realize was therapy. (Chesla, 1991, p. 460)

This mother's structured efforts to bring her child back to a higher level of functioning were both imaginative and exhausting. She took him to the opera, which he enjoyed, so that he would have to get dressed in formal clothes. She hired additional caregivers to get him involved in physical activities and social interaction. And her son did improve, to the extent that he was able to complete high school and attend community college.

One of the difficulties of managed care was that parents' actions were guided by external goals, frequently their own, rather than by goals or desires of the child. The same mother, a paradigm case for managed care, learned that her son's grades at the community college were declining. She investigated, without her son's knowledge or permission. She wrote a note to his college instructors explaining her son's history of schizophrenia and asked them to fill out a "behavioral checklist" so that she could see how he was functioning at school. In her eagerness to help her son, she took over for him and revealed his disease to significant people in his life, people with whom he had not disclosed his illness and with whom he was passing as normal. Such incidents were repeated because these parents structured their care based on external goals rather than on those based on the suffering of, or concerns expressed by, the child (Chesla, 1991).

Parents who provided managed care for their child were resilient in finding new patterns of living with and accepting the schizophrenia; they took the symptoms of the disease to be a challenge, and threw themselves quite wholeheartedly into meeting the challenge. Their efforts were novel, creative, and drew on the parents' acknowledged capabilities. These parents were proud of their efforts and their success in moving the child toward an explicit goal. Two elements of managed care, however, raise questions about resilience. First, parents lacked curiosity about the child's wishes and experiences and, second, parent's efforts felt like "work" and therefore they felt worn out by their caregiving.

A final form of parental care of emerging adults with schizophrenia was distanced care. All of the parents who provided distanced care were fathers who relied upon their wives to do primary care of the PWS. These fathers were aware of the child's symptoms and experience, but their awareness was less refined, less engaged, and thus missed nuances and minor changes in the child's fluctuating illness. It's difficult to know how they might have engaged in care had their wives not been available to take responsibility for hands-on care. However, these fathers seemed content with the division of labor. This form of care was not without its risks, however. Because their appreciation of the situation was more distant, they were not able to participate in the small moments of improved symptoms, nor in the uplifts and satisfactions described by parents who provided other forms of care (Chesla, 1988). Fathers who were involved in distanced care were all married to spouses who provided engaged care. This pattern of family roles appeared acceptable to everyone involved, and thus could be considered resilient.

Although all of these forms of parental care of a PWS could be considered at least marginally resilient, they were not equally so. Certainly, if we identify with the person with schizophrenia, there are forms of care that we would more or less prefer. So what do these differences in approaching care of the child illuminate about resilience?

All forms of caregiving described here revolved around continued engagement with the child. Although this engagement was at times fraught, and parents (particularly in conflicted care) felt dejected or angry at the situation in which they found themselves, they remained involved in the child's life. Even in distanced care, fathers checked in with their wives for intermittent reports on the child's status. Thus, all forms identified had elements of resilience. If we had cast the net wider and used different recruitment strategies, we undoubtedly would have found instances where the PWS was abandoned by or extruded from family relations. So one aspect of family response that supported the PWS was continued involvement.

The challenges of schizophrenia care appeared to some parents to be opportunities for personal growth. Although they would never have wished the condition on themselves or anyone else, they observed that the demands of caring for their child brought them to a new and preferred stage of adult development.

Most parents demonstrated creativity and flexibility in their self-definitions and practices for responding to the PWS's illness demands. For some, caregiving was an unquestioned, if unexpected, extension of parenting, while others identified more with professional caregiving roles like nurses or therapists. With distanced care, responsibilities were delegated to another family member, and intimate personal engagement was let go.

Conflicted care raises the most substantial questions about resilience in the face of schizophrenia. Anger, emotional upset, inability to distance from the child's symptoms, and unwillingness to leave the situation alone comprised these parents' responses. These parents could not get over the illness demands that were placed on their lives. They remained angry that their child had become ill, and frequently angry at their child for his or her symptoms. It is difficult to think of this situation as healthy or settled for either the parent or the child.

Treating the PWS with dignity and recognizing a degree of autonomy, even when the PWS was quite ill, was more apparent in engaged care than in other forms of care. If our goal as health care providers is to assist individuals and families to experience meaningful, dignified, interdependent activities, and to reduce the stress of caregiving, then engaged care practices are preferable to conflicted or managed care. Intervention studies are needed to explore whether health care providers might be able to work with parents of PWS to help them move away from conflicted or managed care toward engaged care. Situated coaching, which would require attunement to the possibilities and constraints in families' situations, and to the meanings and practices that exist, could promote resilience in families caring for a PWS.

1.2.2 Family Resilience in Dementia

Phinney has repeatedly examined close family relationships of persons diagnosed with dementia. A recent report (Phinney et al., 2013) examined family processes in response to the recent diagnosis of dementia in husbands and fathers. The authors argue that family life-world in this phase of the illness has received insufficient attention and that the literature assumes that patients with this diagnosis live parallel but unlinked or disengaged lives within their families. In their intensive examination of two similar cases of late middle-aged men newly diagnosed with dementia, they found, instead, that persons with dementia (PWD) were deeply embedded in family life. At diagnosis and early in the disease, an individual's identity was colored by the limitations imposed by dementia, but so too were the identities of family surrounding the PWD. Children, for example, found themselves disturbed by their father's diminished engagement with activities that previously defined him, such as helping his children or neighbors with house repairs. This withdrawal was upsetting because "the father they have always known is not really here," and thus, "who are they in relation to this man?" (p. 365).

Resilience in the face of dementia requires flexibility of roles and responsibilities. Children of men with dementia began protecting their father from neighbors' requests for help in household tasks but also struggled with maintaining his public 'face' as a capable adult.

Family identity may be implicated in the early diagnosis of dementia of a member (Phinney et al., 2013). Habits and practices of family life are, of necessity, challenged or changed by the diagnosis of dementia in a family leader. What Phinney and colleagues discovered is that this shift imposes both possibilities and constraints. For example, in one family, the husband/father's difficulty in maintaining his rose gardening was experienced by his wife as both a loss, and an opportunity for learning. There was a loss in that the ill individual could no longer garden independently, and his role evolved from sharing gardening with his wife, to primarily giving advice and assistance. His wife enjoyed learning from him about roses, and for a while it was something they could do together. In transferring this responsibility from the individual to the couple, the family maintained continuity with their self-identity as being able to meet challenges with shared hard work. We want to argue such a nuanced interpretation is unlikely to be appreciated in a formal theory of resilience. The fitting together of the family's concerns, the evolution of his wife's role vis-à-vis her husband's roses over time, and the sadness plus contentment at their current state could, we posit, only be captured in narrative.

1.2.3 Family Resilience in Sudden Death

Gudmundsdottir (Gudmundsdottir, 2009) demonstrates the importance of attending to *embodiment* as an element in family members' responses to a critical event. Although her project focused on parental responses to sudden death of a child, rather than chronic illness, it nonetheless demonstrates how the body is passed over in grief. In their narratives about their everyday responses to the sudden loss of a child, parents described stories of intense bodily pain or aches. In a similar way we suspect that family members' bodily responses to hearing the news of a life-threatening diagnosis in a child or family member arise but pass unnoticed. Bodily reactions to caring for an ill member are correspondingly largely ignored, unless that care involves physical strain on the caregiver. Two examples from Gudmundsdottir's descriptions of parents' bodily responses to loss are provided. The first is the experience of a mother's loss that accompanied the sudden death of a 3½- month-old daughter from histiocytosis.

> It feels like [the baby is] just snatched from you. And it's an incredible feeling, as if your arms have been chopped off. ... Maybe I would feel different if I had already gone out to work, and I was used to having a few hours of separation. I would have at least known what separation was like. ... But because I was so used to holding her in my arms, and when she died it felt as if a part of my body had gone too, with the baby. (p. 260)

This mother consciously realizes that her arms are fully intact, and yet her bodily experience is that her arms are missing and useless when the mothering that engaged her before the child's death is no longer needed. This mother's experience of physical loss diminished with time and with the subsequent birth of a second daughter yet was an intense part of her suffering in the immediate aftermath of the death.

In the second instance, a father described his bodily sensation three years after the loss of his 4-month-old daughter to SIDS. He experienced heaviness or a "gnawing sensation, you know. You feel it in your heart, I think" (p. 264). This father specifically differentiated the physical manifestation of his grief from psychological pain, from which he believed he had recovered. Rather he frequently experienced his pain as physical pressure or a weight, which was always present but intensified when he thought of his daughter. He believed that this heaviness would always be a part of his life.

Embodied responses to difficult family experiences are an overlooked, and under attended, aspect of experience. So little is understood about whole body responses to difficult situations that we really don't know the extent and import of these responses. Perhaps family members experience in their arms, or their stomach, grief that is beyond words. However, attending to the body, and family members' bodily experiences regarding the losses experienced in chronic illness and family caregiving, provides an important window onto the whole of their experience. With further investigation, interventions can be developed to assist family members to recognize and understand the meaning of their bodily expressions, and ease their painful or discomforting reactions to their situations.

1.3 Discussion and Implications

On balance, using life-world or narrative approaches to understanding family responses to chronic illness adds depth and richness to our understanding of family processes, helps identify new family patterns of response that have not been identified in existing resilience theories, and provides accessible paradigm cases of family patterns of response. Paradigm cases are also a powerful teaching tool for clinical educators. Examining family lives directly, through observation or through their narratives, will add to our body of knowledge about the range of responses that families have to different chronic illness conditions. While some of the patterns observed in families coping with different conditions may already be alluded to in theoretical constructions about family resilience, undoubtedly new ideas will emerge.

One principle of this kind of research is that the researcher must commit to a curious, nonjudgmental stance toward the subject. Not all researchers are able to adopt the kind of at once participatory and observing stance over time that it requires. For those who can manage the balancing act of this kind of work, what emerges is a nuanced and fascinating grasp of families' coping in which there is no predefined good or bad family response. Rather than looking for 'positive coping' the objective is to focus on what is possible for families *given the situations they are in*. There is a commitment to articulating the situated possibilities of a range of families in similar situations of care, taking into account the context in which they live (Kesselring et al., 2010). The life-world approach suggested by Heidegger is compassionate, because families are understood to be constrained in their possibilities for both understanding themselves and for responding to life challenges. Additionally, there is a deep commitment to understanding families from their own perspectives by dwelling with, observing, and listening to their narratives.

That said, there are better or worse ways for families to respond to and care for an ill member that can be identified. In the example of schizophrenia, different patterns of family response were assessed as more or less resilient when resilience is defined as the family's capacity to adapt to a health challenge in a manner that is in synchrony with its background concerns and practices. Depending upon whose point of view is taken, both conflicted care and managed care give pause. For parents, conflicted care was clearly upsetting and unsettling. Determining ways to ease their direct involvement in care, or to deepen their understanding of their child's illness experience and their understanding of the meaning of symptoms, might have helped those parents to have a more comfortable pattern of living. Conversely, from the perspective of the PWS, the managed care approach raises concerns about whether the dignity, identity, and capabilities of the PWS are acknowledged and affirmed (Box 1.1).

> **Breakout Box 1.1 Implications for Policy**
> The authors argue from an interpretive phenomenology point of view that medical practitioners need to take into account a family's "habits, practices, and concerns" without imposing their own set of assumptions onto the family. This challenge is complicated by the fact that physicians and other medical personnel are committed to a variety of moral principles that motivate a number of difficult questions, including: respect for patient autonomy ("What does the patient *truly* want?"), acting in the best interest of the patient ("What is the best medical outcome, and is this consistent with what the patient wants?"), and using medical resources wisely and justly ("How many resources should be devoted to this specific patient?"). These principles are sometimes at odds and, to further complicate the situation, physicians are sometimes unaware that these principles are in conflict. Consequently, they may arrive at a decision without being consciously aware that this decision may not respect one (or more) of the principles.
>
> That is why it is important to have people from different backgrounds make ethics decisions together. I have been a member of an urban hospital's Ethics Board for years, and I am still impressed with my colleagues; the doctors, nurses, and social workers have been amazing in their openness to considering an individual family's needs and cultural values. I heard about one case in which the family followed Santería (and animal sacrifice was a ritual). In accordance with the family's requests, the hospital allowed a squirrel to be sacrificed in an operating room, separate from the sterile field. The ethical conundrum that arises, of course, is where do you draw the line between cultural sensitivity and practices considered contrary to societal standards?
> —Scott D. Gelfand, Ph.D., J.D., Associate Professor of Philosophy, Ethics Center Director

Approaching family resilience from a life-world perspective has multiple implications for clinical practice. Clinical use of family narratives can assist health professionals in orienting families who are new to the challenges of a chronic illness, normalizing family responses within an observed range of responses, and illustrating possible new patterns of family adjustment for families struggling with their situations.

Clinicians can assist families who are struggling with a newly diagnosed member by offering narratives of similar situations that other families have faced, and examples of how other families have responded. We argue that stories of families' patterns of response are more accessible and likely more comforting than are formal theories about their situation. Family stories, collected in empirical life-world research, or via the clinician's caseloads, can often serve as a touchstone about what other families are facing and how they have responded.

The skills needed for conducting life-world research are wholly applicable in doing family clinical work. Listening with care and attending to the family's concerns and narratives of distress open up each family's experience from their own perspective. A nonjudgmental stance, appropriate in any clinical encounter, is particularly relevant when exploring with family members their honest, relational responses to the ill member and their experience of illness symptoms. Interpreting family responses in general, but generous terms (e.g., "that must have been really challenging to realize your father was no longer able to drive") are similar in clinical and research work, with the exception of the central goal of the work. For clinicians, the aim is to assist the family to adapt to their circumstances, while in research the aim is simply to understand. In fact, however, families frequently remark that they have never been asked about their situations in the same way as they are asked in an interpretive interview, and that they find the review healing.

Normalizing the responses of families to extreme events can be facilitated by providing narratives of families in similar situations. Transitional periods, such as diagnosis or relapse in particular, might be more easily traversed by providing family members with stories of other concrete instances of families who have successfully weathered such periods, and how. Narratives of family patterns of response that differ significantly from what a family sees as being possible for itself might provide new, pragmatic approaches that they can consider. Given their different backgrounds and differences in relations with the chronically ill member, no two families are going to respond in exactly the same way, but narratives of others' patterns of response may provide a spur to positive change.

Finally, paradigm cases of family resilience provide powerful exemplars for clinical teaching. A particularized and nuanced story can provide the novice clinician with access to the illness experience that formal theory just can't provide. As new clinicians juggle clinical encounters that are increasingly abbreviated, the use of carefully researched stories is a critical piece of clinical education that allows them to enter a clinical situation with a more fleshed out grasp of what the patient and family might be dealing with, and what is possible with careful listening and attunement.

Discussion Questions

1. Consider your own or a patient's experience in struggling with care of a chronically ill family member. What aspects of the situation seem most important to you? Do key theories of family resilience appear to capture this concern of yours?
2. Consider the four different patterns of family care that were identified in parents caring for a person with schizophrenia. Do these patterns seem believable and/or familiar? Do these patterns fit within the concepts of third-wave family resilience theory?

References

Benner, P. (1994). The tradition and skill of interpretive phenomenology in studying health, illness and caring practices. In P. Benner (Ed.), *Interpretive phenomenology: Embodiment, caring and ethics in health and nursing* (pp. 99–127). Thousand Oaks, CA: Sage.
Benner, P., & Wrubel, J. (1989). *The primacy of caring; Stress and coping in health and illness*. Menlo Park, CA: Addison-Wesley.
Chesla, C. A. (1988). *Parents' caring practices and coping with schizophrenic offspring, an interpretive study*. University of California, San Francisco, San Francisco, CA.
Chesla, C. A. (1989). Parents' illness models of schizophrenia. *Archives of Psychiatric Nursing, 3*, 218–225.
Chesla, C. A. (1991). Parents' caring practices with schizophrenic offspring. *Qualitative Health Research, 1*, 446–468.
Chesla, C. A. (1995). Hermeneutic phenomenology: An approach to understanding families. *Journal of Family Nursing, 1*, 63–78.
Dreyfus, H. L. (1991). *Being-in-the-world: A commentary on Heidegger's Being and Time*. Cambridge, MA: MIT Press.
Dreyfus, H. (1994). Preface. In P. Benner (Ed.), *Interpretive phenomenology: Embodiment, caring and ethics in health and nursing* (pp. vii–xi). Thousand Oaks, CA: Sage.
Flyvbjerg, B. (2001). *Making social science matter*. Cambridge, England: Cambridge University Press.
Gudmundsdottir, M. (2009). Embodied grief: Bereaved parents' narratives of their suffering bodies. *OMEGA, 58*, 253–269.
Heidegger, M. (1962). *Being and time*. New York, NY: Harper & Row (K. Macquarrie & E. Robinson, Trans.).
Kesselring, A., Chesla, C., & Leonard, V. (2010). Why study caring practices? In G. Chan, K. Brykczynski, R. Malone, & P. Benner (Eds.), *Interpretive phenomenology in health care research* (pp. 3–22). Indiannapolis, IN: Sigma Theta Tau International.
Leonard, V. (1994). A Heideggerian phenomenologic perspective on the concept of a person. In P. Benner (Ed.), *Interpretive phenomenology* (pp. 43–64). Thousand Oaks, CA: Sage.
Life-world (2014). *Encyclopædia britannica*.
Patterson, J. M. (1988). Families experiencing stress: I. The family adjustment and adaptation response model: II. Applying the FAAR model to health-related issues for intervention and research. *Family Systems Medicine, 6*, 202–237.
Patterson, J. M. (2002). Integrating family resilience and family stress theory. *Journal of Marriage and the Family, 64*, 349–360.
Phinney, A., Dahlke, S., & Purves, B. (2013). Shifting patterns of everyday activity in early dementia: Experiences of men and their families. *Journal of Family Nursing, 19*, 348–374.
van Manen, M. (1997). *Researching lived experience: Human science for an action sensitive pedagogy* (2nd ed.). London, Ont.: Althouse Press.
White, J. M., & Klein, D. M. (2008). *Family theories* (3rd ed.). Los Angeles, CA: Sage.

Chapter 2
The Experience of Preterm Birth: Helping Families Survive and Thrive

Patricia Williams, Raja Nandyal, Eleanor Hutson, and Ginger L. Welch

Despite public health efforts and advances in health care over the past decade, the birth rate of premature infants has been relatively steady and remains a significant health issue in the United States. According to data from the Center for Disease Control and Prevention (CDC), a half million infants are born at less than 37 weeks gestation each year, accounting for approximately 11.5% of live born infants (Martin, Hamilton, Osterman, Curtain, & Matthews, 2013). Of those, about 76,000 are classified as very preterm, being born at less than 32 weeks gestation (Martin et al., 2013). Infants who are born prematurely have an increased risk of requiring medical interventions and having to be admitted to a Neonatal Intensive Care Unit (NICU). They may require extensive medical treatment including oxygen, ventilator support, central line placement, intravenous nutrition, antibiotics, and other medications to support vital functions such as blood pressure and respiration. Additionally, infant deaths due to prematurity occur in approximately 103.8 per 100,000 live births (Martin et al., 2013). Rates of survival generally increase with increasing birth weight and gestational age (Stoll et al., 2010). Rates of neurodevelopmentally intact survival are correlated with single gestation pregnancy, larger

---

P. Williams, M.D. (✉) • R. Nandyal, M.D.
Neonatal-Perinatal Medicine Section, University of Oklahoma Health Sciences Center,
1200 Everett Dr, 7th Floor N Pavillion, ETNP 7357, Oklahoma City, OK, USA
e-mail: patricia-k-williams@ouhsc.edu

E. Hutson, R.N.
Oklahoma Infant Transition Program, University of Oklahoma Health Sciences Center,
Oklahoma City, OK, USA
e-mail: raja-nandyal@ouhsc.edu; bunny-hutson@ouhsc.edu

G.L. Welch, Ph.D.
Department of Human Development and Family Science, Oklahoma State University,
Stillwater, OK, USA
e-mail: gwelch@okstate.edu

© Springer International Publishing Switzerland 2017
G.L. Welch, A.W. Harrist (eds.), *Family Resilience and Chronic Illness*,
Emerging Issues in Family and Individual Resilience,
DOI 10.1007/978-3-319-26033-4_2

birth weight, older gestational age, female gender, and the antenatal administration of corticosteroids (Tyson, Parikh, Langer, Green, & Higgins, 2008). Families who are facing the early arrival of a newborn start down a path of uncertainty regarding their infant's survival as well as a lengthy list of possible short-term and long-term complications.

2.1 Medical Issues Related to Premature Birth

Surviving premature infants are at risk for several common yet serious complications which can lead to medical and developmental issues. Among the most common are issues with the respiratory system, problems with feeding and growth, and neurological difficulties. Premature infants are at risk for respiratory problems due to having underdeveloped lungs at birth. This, combined with the need for ventilator support and/or oxygen and exposure to inflammatory mediators, results in the disruption of normal lung development which can lead to chronic lung disease (CLD) or bronchopulmonary dysplasia (BPD). Affected infants may require home oxygen and cardiopulmonary monitors as well as long-term medications. In addition, they are at increased risk of respiratory infections after discharge home. Some infants may require long-term ventilator support, needing placement of a tracheostomy for airway abnormalities such as subglottic stenosis, tracheomalacia, or pulmonary hypertension.

Feeding and growth issues are also very common in the NICU. Many preterm infants are discharged home to their families at less than the tenth percentile on growth charts measuring weight, length, and head circumference. Premature infants in the NICU face many challenges to achieving typical growth and growth patterns, including intolerance of enteral milk feeds, intestinal infections such as necrotizing enterocolitis (NEC) paired with high metabolic requirements due to cardiorespiratory and temperature regulation demands. In addition, many of these infants have significant difficulties learning to breast- or bottle-feed and are at risk for oral aversion or aspiration. In some cases, infants may require placement of a gastrostomy tube in order to ensure adequate nutrition to support growth.

While respiratory and feeding issues are the most common complications of prematurity, families have reported the greatest anxiety regarding potential complications that can occur in the developing brain. Structural changes in the gray and white matter of the brain can occur as a result of bleeding such as intraventricular hemorrhage (IVH), intraparenchymal hemorrhage (IPH), and periventricular leukomalacia (PVL). These changes can lead to long-term problems for the infant such as cerebral palsy, intellectual disabilities (formerly mental retardation), and issues with learning, behavior, and executive functioning. Neurosensory systems can also be impacted by prematurity. Vision loss can occur as a result of retinopathy of prematurity (ROP) due to abnormal growth of blood vessels in the retina. Infants are at risk for hearing loss due to exposure to ototoxic medications, inflammatory mediators, and environmental exposures. During the NICU stay, premature infants will undergo repeated head ultrasounds, eye exams, and hearing tests to screen for these conditions and monitor for any concerning deviations from the typical progression of development. Even after discharge home from the NICU, the infant will continue to need regular examinations to assess their development, vision, and hearing through primary care medical homes to provide early detection and early intervention for any delays or deficits.

One additional significant medical challenge that families face as they support their infant through an NICU stay and beyond is the fact that it is very difficult to accurately predict which infants will develop any or all of these complications. Most adults perceive medical science as exact, and in the context of lifesaving care for their infant, expect that science will be able to accurately forecast the medical and developmental path for their baby. While percentages from multinational scientific studies can be quoted to families regarding the likelihood of occurrence in the patient population as a whole, it is impossible to know for certain that an individual baby will develop a specific complication and to what degree of severity. Statistically, for example, we can look at a 700 g (1lb, 9oz) 26-week premature infant and find literature to support that this infant has an 85% chance of survival, a 42% chance of developing BPD/CLD, a 79% likelihood of growth at less than the tenth percentile, a 13% chance of having a severe IVH (with a 60% chance of those going on to develop CP), a 14% chance of developing severe ROP with a 20% chance of visual impairment, and an 8% likelihood of hearing impairment (Stoll et al., 2010). This dizzying array of confusing and sometimes contradictory statistics is simply not meaningful for a family who just wants to know, "Will my baby be ok?" Current best practices in ethical care of premature infants require that health care providers inform families about the various risks facing their babies, as well as the need for careful monitoring of the infant for the potential development of these and other complications. However, this type of disclosure can lead to additional anxiety for families as they worry whether or not their child will be impacted by one or more serious diagnoses. Parents can experience anticipatory mourning, both for the loss of the expected birth experience as well as the newborn they thought they would have. They may feel anxiety in not knowing if their child will survive and, if so, whether or not he or she may suffer multiple long-term health and developmental problems. In order to facilitate the best possible outcomes for the infant and the family, health care providers must be equipped to fully support families through every step of the process, from preterm birth, to the NICU stay, through the discharge to home and follow-up visits.

2.2 The NICU Experience for the Family

Families' experiences following the birth of a premature infant are often markedly different than the anticipated birth experience. In the 40 weeks of a full-term pregnancy, many parents prepare for their baby's birth by readying their home, purchasing or borrowing clothes and other supplies, or perhaps even interviewing pediatricians. A hospital bag for mom might be packed, relatives are put on alert for the due date, and a newborn-sized "going home" outfit is selected. However, when babies are born early, parents and extended family often find themselves unprepared emotionally, physically, and cognitively for the "preemie" world into which they have been thrust. The first visit to the NICU nursery can easily leave the most informed parents awed and frightened by the unfamiliar medical equipment now in place to support their infant's life. Instead of finding themselves in a private room, holding their baby and perhaps surrounded by extended family discussing who the baby looks like, parents are instead greeted by the new faces of multiple medical caregivers and the sounds, bright lights, and activity inherent to the NICU. These experiences are, of course, in addition to the mother's own medical experience of giving birth and her necessary recovery. It is little wonder, then, that, giving birth to a preterm infant is a stressful life event that places parents at an increased risk for psychological distress in addition to the medical threats present for the baby.

2.2.1 The Infant NICU Experience

Infants born during the third trimester of pregnancy are undergoing a period of critical brain development and neuronal connectivity that is best carried out in the womb. Infant's brains are overly sensitive to external stimulation to which they would not have been exposed in the womb and they lack inhibitory controls (Als, 1986). In the womb, the fetus grows and develops in a fluid, quiet, calm, dimly lit, biologically and evolutionarily expected environment with few disturbances. At a full 40 weeks gestation, the newborn is prepared to interact with the world and make the necessary social–emotional connections that assure his or her survival (Als, 1982). Preterm birth, however, exposes infants to the completely different environment of the NICU with its lifesaving, albeit intrusive, medical interventions. This premature or "displaced" fetus is not prepared to function in a world of air, flat surfaces, unfamiliar touch, and overwhelming sensory input. The sounds, light, and activity in the NICU, as well as caregiving interventions, are intrinsically uncomfortable and often painful. At birth, the premature infant becomes a fully functioning person at his or her developmental stage and has a difficult time managing the demands of the physiological functions of blood pressure, breathing, temperature regulation, and digestion in order to survive, as well as to tolerate necessary caregiving activities. The combination of a critically developing brain and maternal separation has been shown to correlate with negative effects on infant development (Feldman, Rosenthal, & Eidelman, 2013).

2.2.2 The Parent NICU Experience

The mothers of premature infants have been found to demonstrate signs of anxiety as well as reported feelings of alienation from their maternal roles when faced with an inability to care directly for their acutely ill newborn in the NICU (Miles,

Holditch, Schwartz, & Scher, 2007). Parents often wonder what their role will be in the life of their baby with so many experts providing lifesaving care in such an overwhelming environment. Everyday caregiving activities, such as changing a diaper, holding the baby, and sharing the baby with other family and friends may not be possible for a day or longer. Parents may feel displaced, overwhelmed, and stressed. Members of the medical caregiving team are key factors in helping parents regain their parenting roles. Parents generally want to learn how to interact with their fragile baby but may need encouragement. Specific steps in helping parents begin that first relationship with their baby may include teaching them how to hold the baby's hand, cradle the baby with warm and gentle hands, change the diaper, and help the nurse change the baby's position on the bedding; whispering to the baby; and participating in decisions about the level of their participation. Feelings of helplessness may be complicated for mothers by tendencies to engage in high levels of self-blame for pregnancies that end in preterm birth (Powell & Wilson, 2000). While there are many risk factors for preterm delivery that can be prevented via behavior change, such as smoking or alcohol use, the majority of premature infants born each year are to mothers who did "everything right" with no known risk factors. Support and reassurance communicated to these mothers by health care providers may be critically important in order to engage mothers early on in baby-care activities.

Both mothers and fathers of preterm infants report high stress levels concerning their parenting roles (Martricardi, Agostino, Fedeli, & Motorosso, 2013). However, stress levels are reduced when mothers are taught about their infant's behavioral cues and ways to interact with, touch, and comfort their infant (Martricardi et al., 2013). Additional beneficial strategies for coping with the NICU experience included participation in their infant's care, getting away from the NICU, gathering information, involvement of family and friends, and engagement with other NICU parents (Smith, SteelFisher, Salhi, & Shen, 2012). Parental self-confidence has been found to improve when parents are allowed to participate in diaper changes and feedings for their infant. Parents identified the greatest sources of support as being in their own home, reconnecting with their partner, family, and other children; most cited the greatest emotional support coming from their partners.

2.2.3 *The Infant and Parent Relationship in the NICU*

For premature infants and their parents, there are many barriers that may interfere with early infant–parent attachment and the parents' emotional bond to the baby. These can include the technological nature of the lifesaving equipment in the NICU, the mother's chaotic delivery, physical separation of the infant and mother, being a parent to a sick baby, feeling uncertain of what to expect of their baby or experience while in the NICU, and the baby's continued illness. Factors outside of the NICU can contribute, as well, as worries mount for sibling care, parents feel the stress of separation from family support at home, there is limited or expensive transportation, the family lives a distance from the hospital, there is stress or expense associated with parental lodging outside of the hospital while the baby is in the NICU, and they must spend time away from paid work. While partnering with social service professionals within the hospital can address a host of external barriers, a comprehensive and high-quality NICU system will also work to address many of the internal barriers.

When medical care is provided within a developmental framework that supports the infant's strengths and minimizes infant vulnerabilities, infant experiences can be improved and their brains may wire in a developmentally typical way; this gentler care can lead to improved developmental, social, and medical outcomes. The Newborn Individualized Developmental Care and Assessment Program (NIDCAP) was developed by Dr. Heidelise Als in 1982 to give all NICU caregivers and families a framework from which to understand each infant. In the Synactive Theory of Infant Development, Als proposed the observation of infant behavioral subsystems (autonomic, motor, state, attention and interaction, self-regulation) to understand how each individual infant is managing him or herself, and what supports the infant may need to progress along the developmental path to more mature self-regulation (Als, 1982). Dr. Als described NIDCAP as a "comprehensive approach to care that is developmentally supportive and individualized to the infant's goals and level of stability" that offers supports to both family and professional caregivers. Several studies offer support for the NIDCAP model. Both medical and developmental improvements have been observed in infants who are cared for using the NIDCAP approach when compared to those infants cared for using more traditional practices (Als, 2003). In one study, which compared a group of premature infants receiving NIDCAP care with a similar group receiving standard care, those in the NIDCAP group "demonstrated that quality of experience before term may influence brain development significantly"(Als et al., 2004). The long-term effect of NIDCAP care for children at 8 years of age compared to control group children at the same age revealed clinically significant results on executive functioning, visual-motor integration, and activity in the frontal lobes (McAnulty et al., 2009).

NIDCAP involves teaching parents and staff to read infants' behavioral cues, making responsive changes in the environment to support rest and relaxation, and promoting tucked positions for comfort and proper muscle development. Subtle but important changes may be implemented including dimmed lights, quiet voices, and a calm environment. Additional efforts toward NIDCAP care include early and continuous parent involvement and care, early and regular skin-to-skin holding, consistent cradling support by parents during procedures, involvement of parents in decision making, and support for parent involvement on their infant's medical team. These parent experiences may assist the family to engage in many more "typical" opportunities for infant–parent interactions, leading to increased opportunities to optimize neonatal brain development. In NIDCAP, parents are viewed as the most important nurturers of their infant; the infant must come to trust the parent to provide that nurturance, protection, love, and comfort as the basis for attachment. Simultaneously, parents develop competency in their roles as caregivers, thus increasing their confidence and self-esteem. Information about infant needs is gathered through structured behavioral observations in the NICU as a way to understand the babies' behavioral cues. The resulting in-depth report paints a picture of an infant's individual needs, and goals and recommendations are made based on these unique needs. NICU staff are encouraged to modify their care in response to the individual needs of the infant.

Another empirically supported practice to enhance family experiences in the NICU is Kangaroo Care or Skin-to-Skin holding. Kangaroo Care is a way for parents to safely hold their often small and fragile infants which has been shown to improve attachment between infants and parents through close and intimate holding (Browne, 2003). In Kangaroo Care, parents hold their baby against their bare warm chest, cuddling together for long periods. Only the baby's parents can provide this special activity to facilitate deep relaxation and release of oxytocin, the pleasure hormone which facilitates mothers to produce more breast milk (Browne, 2004). This experience helps parents become familiar with the baby's comfort and stress cues as they make accommodations to support the baby's comfort and sleep. Babies held skin-to-skin experience sensations more reflective of their in utero experience with their mother's scent; warmth of parent's skin; and the sounds of parental heartbeat, breathing, and digestion. Kangaroo Care assists babies to settle into deep restful sleep, which is difficult to attain while lying in the incubator. After skin-to-skin holding, infants are better able to sleep, tolerate caregiving activities, and self-soothe (Browne, 2004).

In 2002, Feldman (Feldman et al., 2002) identified positive outcomes of Kangaroo Care on parental perceptions and behaviors, as well as on neonatal development. For a group of premature infants and their mothers who participated in one hour of Kangaroo Care each day for 14 days in the NICU, both short- and long-term benefits were identified. Participating mothers were found to have lower levels of depression and to perceive their infant as more "normal." Once at home, parents who had participated in NICU-based Kangaroo Care provided a more sensitive and appropriately stimulating environment. Mothers in the Care group were rated as more responsive, adaptive, and resourceful during infant interactions at 6 months of age, and infants in the Kangaroo Care group were more socially alert and scored higher on the Bayley Scales of Infant Development mental and motor domains. Findings revealed enhanced mother–child reciprocity, as well as improved child cognitive development and executive functions at 10 years of age (Feldman et al., 2013).

2.3 Building Resilience

Although no family ever truly returns to identical prebaby functioning after the birth of a child, the goal of family resilience in neonatology is to assist families to establish functional and healthy patterns that will allow them to reengage in their multiple roles including those as parents, partners, siblings, and employees, but now with a new member of the family. Resilience in this context may best be described as the malleability of a family to continue functioning after a significant life event, and not merely to return to previous functioning as if there had been no life event.

High-quality NICU functioning supports infant and family resilience through inclusion of the family at all levels of care. Attachment to a fragile or small infant may be difficult in the NICU, yet infant–parent attachment is essential for long-term infant and parent mental health. For mothers in particular, feelings of being an "outsider" in the NICU are common. However, when the infant and family are cared for with a developmental focus, mothers can transition from "outsider" to an engaged parent. Her focus can transition from the NICU at large to her baby. Empowering feelings of 'ownership' can transform her language from "their" baby to "my" baby. Tentative or initially passive interactions with her baby can become more active and participatory as her voice moves from silent to one of advocacy for her baby. NICU staff has the opportunity to facilitate this transition by partnering with parents in developmental ways (Heermann, 2005). This developmental focus has also been shown to benefit fathers.

Fathers, though perhaps less well represented in research, play an important role in the NICU. In a recent study by Arockiasamy, Holsti, and Albersheim (2008), it was found that the male partner or father is most likely to communicate with staff at admission, and then relay important medical information back to the mother who may herself be unable to come to the NICU immediately. While fathers in the study provided support for the mother, they often report perceived lack of support for themselves. Fathers reported visiting the NICU less regularly than mothers due to perceived lack of control over the situation and an inability to participate in decision making when the infant is critical. Many fathers identified the need to speak with their infant's physician as a way to receive support and expressed a desire to be included on discussions regarding their infant's caregiving plan with NICU staff and physicians. Reliable and consistent communication with the care team, including access to online information and receiving consistent updates regarding the infant's health, appears to be a significant factor in engaging fathers in the NICU (Arockiasamy et al., 2008).

2.3.1 Building Resilience While in the NICU

Parents can build their resilience by receiving help to recognize their strengths and those of their infant, by reflecting on what they may need in the moment, and by receiving encouragement to care for themselves (Beardslee, Avery, Ayoub, Watts, & Lester, 2010). Parents have been found to value relationships that are supportive of their experience, especially during engagement with other NICU parents. Opportunities to gather with NICU parent peers can provide perspective, practical information, and social avenues to visit about their babies, share photos, and discuss celebrations and successes as well as sadness and worries. All of these can help reduce parent stress. At the University of Oklahoma Children's Hospital, there are two groups whose purpose is to provide support to NICU parents: the Oklahoma Infant Transition Program (OITP) and the Family-Centered Developmental Care Committee. Together, these organizations sponsor several activities for parents who are caring for their baby in the NICU. Examples of activities designed to support parents and build connections include a catered weekly parent lunch, scrapbooking sessions, informational video presentations, and a closed Facebook site. The group environment is designed to be a safe one where parents can tell their birth stories, discuss babies' progress, share their own feelings, or discuss graduation to the care-by-parent area. Simply setting aside an afternoon each week for parents to scrapbook with other NICU families has been found to be a practical and stress-reducing strategy (Mouradian, 2013). The OITP supports this activity by taking a picture of the baby and providing a calm and quiet room with supplies; the hospital volunteer program provides scrapbooking supplies that sustain the program. At discharge, the family has created a scrapbook showing their baby's progress while in the NICU.

2.3.2 Building Resilience in Transition

One of the most common questions parents have after admission to the NICU is "When can my baby come home?" Premature infants must be able to demonstrate physiologic maturity in order to be ready to be discharged home with the family. The American Academy of Pediatrics has defined parameters which are followed by health care providers: The infant must be able to maintain his/her body temperature when clothed in an open crib, be able to breathe consistently and effectively on his/her own without significant episodes of dropping their heart rate or oxygen saturation levels (apnea-associated bradycardia and desaturations), and be able to effectively take oral feedings with consistently demonstrated adequate weight gain (Fetus & Newborn, 2008). The age at which premature infants reach these milestones varies significantly with the degree of prematurity at birth and the number of complications that the infant has experienced during his or her NICU stay. Most infants are ready to go home within a few weeks of their original due date.

For the family of a NICU graduate, hospital discharge is often a period of stress and dysfunction (Robison, Pirak, & Morrell, 2000). As the family prepares to take their infant home, they may struggle with continuing to view their infant as a "sick preemie," requiring constant vigilance. After many weeks or even months of seeing their baby in intensive care and having the support of nurses, doctors, and other health care providers immediately available, it can be lonely and scary for family to be in charge of their infant's care on their own, particularly if the child will be discharged home with chronic medical issues. Health care providers can assist parents in preparing for discharge by providing education, encouraging parental care while in the NICU, and assisting with structuring appropriate follow-up care regarding their child's anticipated social–emotional, medical, and developmental needs. Such an effective discharge requires an individualized yet comprehensive approach which includes assessment of the infant, the parents, and the family as a unit by a Multidisciplinary Neonatal Health Care team (MNHC team). Comprehensive discharge planning initiated early by the team may shorten the length of an infant's hospitalization and also may positively influence infant–parent bonding and parenting by decreasing the period of separation between the infant and the family.

Both the family and the MNHC team need to feel comfortable and confident in the education and training essential for the infant's transition to home and their community. Educational topics that should be covered prior to discharge include infection control by immunizations, hand washing and limiting exposures, car seat education, CPR classes, and when needed, caloric supplementation, medication administration, and appropriate use of equipment such as oxygen, monitors, or feeding pumps (Fetus & Newborn, 2008). Predischarge counseling should also include discussions about safe sleep practices, the effects of passive smoke, and the benefit of an 18 to 23 month interpregnancy interval to achieve optimal health outcomes (Nandyal, 2014). Additionally, many NICUs now provide "rooming in" suites, private rooms with beds for the baby and parents which allow them to stay all day and night to participate in their infant's care. These rooms help build parental skills and confidence in providing for their infant's needs prior to discharge home and assist in smoothing the transition to home. Predischarge assessment includes recognition of the newborn's current and future health needs, identifying existing risk factors and available family resources, and an evaluation of the family's ability to provide optimal care (Robison et al., 2000).

2.3.3 Transition to Community Providers

Currently, many smaller infants are discharged home from the NICU much earlier than they were in the past due to improved infant outcomes. To facilitate smoother medical and social transition, transition programs must act as safety nets for the NICU graduates, their families, and the primary care providers (PCP) whom the infants will see for regular care. In the first two weeks after discharge, the rate of rehospitalization among NICU graduates is higher than among healthy term infants (Escobar et al., 1999). Providing proper training to parents in the required skills and educating them about their infant's medical problems and their management may decrease the risk for rehospitalization. Each rehospitalization has the potential for further compromising the infant's heath and may further add stress to the family. In fact, when mothers perceive that professionals recognize their caregiving skills, provide information in ways they prefer, and are sensitive to their emotional needs, positive parent–professional relationships can develop or even improve. An individualized approach can give parents more confidence and can provide them with practical strategies for caring for their medically fragile infants and for interacting with NICU professionals (Bruns & McCollum, 2002).

Good communication is essential among professionals to facilitate smooth transition of care of such complex infants and their families from NICU to the community providers/PCPs. The pediatric population differs from the adult population in their absolute dependence on parents/caregivers. The NICU population has the additional disadvantage of having no prior relationship with a PCP at the time of discharge home from the hospital. Additionally, NICU graduates frequently have conditions PCPs are neither comfortable with nor knowledgeable about. Therefore, active interaction prior to discharge between an MNHC team and the community providers/PCPs is essential for NICU infants.

In addition to a child's PCP, a number of other professionals may be involved, either on the child's MNHC team or in the community. These may include the services of an infant mental health specialist, usually a licensed mental health professional with advanced training in infant development and parenting, who can assist with the emotional processes of relating to and caring for a premature infant; a personal or marital counselor to assist with the adjustment to parenthood and changing roles, or children's therapists who specialize in speech–language (SLP), occupational therapy (OT), physical therapy (PT), or child development (CD). Most of the latter services can be secured through early intervention or nurse home visiting programs (Box 2.1).

Breakout Box 2.1 Implications for Practice

The best training either of us ever received on how to stay family centered was the "fan" approach from the Fussy Baby Institute. We also agree that if there was one piece of advice from that approach that we could go back and whisper in our own ears as young clinicians, it would be "you don't have to rush." Babies arrive in their own time, sometimes very early. Families grieve, mourn, celebrate, resent, hover over, and rage over babies in their own time and in their own way. For everything we know about preterm infants, their outcomes, and their families at the group level, we have to respect the individual journey that each family takes. We never know what it is really like for them since preterm labor began, and we have to be brave enough to ask. To speak those words that strip us of our own façade of expertise: "Tell me what it is like to care for your baby." And then, the riskiest moment of all, to listen. To sit in silence. To allow tears to slip silently down the face of a grieving father, or sit empathetically as the willing target of an angry mother who can finally let loose. Ask and listen. Don't tell. Don't be in such a hurry to dispense advice and facts about milestones. Don't rush past the feelings. Don't assume that everything you did in a session last week has been neatly tucked away. Welcome it back. Slow down. Let the circuitous nature of parenting a fragile infant unfold. Don't rush. Going faster doesn't make it go away, but instead just makes it seem unimportant. Don't rush. The dream of having a baby includes the dream of being a family, with functional, happy parents, supportive loved ones, health, smiles, life… Slow down and respect those dreams. Don't rush. When you are working with the family of a preterm infant, you work in a world where a few 24-hour days can make the difference in organ development, survival, and growth. Don't rush.

—Sherre Davidson, M.S., CCPS, LPC, & Laura Shellhammer, M.S., CCPS.
Child Development Specialists

2.3.4 Home Visits

Home visits by Public Health Nurses (PHN) prior to discharge are also valuable for transition and home assessment. These visits can help the PHN in developing rapport with the parents and also help parents to know their resource personnel (Robison et al., 2000). Having that interaction prior to discharge can provide reassurance to the staff regarding the family's comfort level in an environment outside the NICU. Home visits also allow an opportunity for the NICU staff to convey to the PCPs what the expected level of expertise and time commitment required to provide specialized care to these complex infants will be. Home Visiting Programs (HVP) provide bridging and "safety nets" for the NICU graduate to the home environment by partnering with primary care providers and other community resources. In general, the goals of such programs include improving child health, reducing developmental delays, and optimizing utilization of scarce community resources. Home visitation programs are available in every state and the District of Columbia, and state-by-state information can be obtained at http://mchb.hrsa.gov/programs/homevisiting/states/index.html. With excellent research support behind maternal and infant visitation programs, including longitudinal evidence for cognitive, social, economic, and relational benefits, NICU programs should have ready information about enrollment opportunities.

2.3.5 Medical Home

The American Academy of Pediatrics (AAP) recommends that the medical care of infants, children, and adolescents should be accessible, continuous, comprehensive, family centered, coordinated, compassionate, and culturally effective (Committee, 2002). These characteristics define the "medical home" and are used to measure the quality of primary care (Hoilette, Blumkin, Baldwin, Fiscella, & Szilagyi, 2013).

There are model Medical Homes described in the literature with blueprints for the care of children with and without complex issues. The Building Healthy Children (BHC) collaborative is one example of a successful medical home program. The BHC offers a unique model of evidence-based home visiting services integrated into primary care serving families residing in Rochester, New York, an ethnically and racially diverse area (Paradis, Sandler, Manly, & Valentine, 2013). The goals of the program are to avoid child maltreatment, improve parent and child health, and enhance family functioning. Through home visitation, this program provides parenting education and therapy for parent–child trauma and maternal depression. Of the mothers that participated, 37% were victims of child abuse/neglect, 22% showed serious symptoms of depression, and 59% of their children were exposed to domestic violence. It has successfully integrated home visitation into the medical care of infants born to young, low-income mothers.

Efficient care coordination, consistent with medical home principles in improving medical outcomes, can reduce medical resource utilization and can improve parent satisfaction, especially for children with complex medical conditions. Training pediatric residents in the principles of care coordination as noted in the medical home concept is incorporated in the Medical Home Project at UCLA (Klitzner, Rabbitt, & Chang, 2010). It serves as a vehicle for training pediatric residents in the principles of the medical home. It also has the potential to decrease the use of emergency services.

For the medically underserved, primary care practices serve as the backbone of the US health care system. These practices include Community Health Centers (CHCs), public hospital clinics, county or city operated clinics, and free clinics, all of which serve a large number of racially and ethnically diverse patients, uninsured individuals, and Medicaid enrollees (Hoilette et al., 2013). CHCs also include 1200 Federally Qualified Health Centers (FQHCs) and about 100 FQHC-like organizations, in addition to city/county operated clinics and community health centers sponsored by charitable organizations such as churches. Although the majority of patients attending CHCs are adults, a large number of low income children are also served. Therefore, as health reform is realized in the United States, the reported quality of care provided by CHCs could further influence care delivered to a sizable portion of our nation's most vulnerable children. Currently, such safety net practices are challenged by caring for many patients with chronic diseases and complex social and mental health conditions. Their quality is affected by limited resources, difficulty in both recruiting and retaining providers, inadequate staffing, and often limited access to specialty referral services for mental, surgical, dental, vision care, and social work.

2.4 Child Maltreatment and Caregiving Burden for NICU Graduates

Neonatal medical problems such as premature birth, low birth weight, or physical disabilities are associated with higher rates of child maltreatment reports, especially child neglect. Other risk factors associated with child maltreatment include young, single, or nonbiological parents; parental lack of understanding of children's needs, child development, or parenting skills; poor parent–child relationships or negative interactions; parental thoughts or emotions that support maltreatment behaviors; family dysfunction or violence; parental history of abuse or neglect in the family of origin; substance abuse within the family; social isolation, poverty, or other socioeconomic disadvantages; and parental stress and distress (Moyer, 2013). The Oklahoma Caregiving Burden Index (OKCaBI) analyzed the data of 2463 NICU graduates born and treated in a level 4 NICU over a four-year period (Nandyal et al., 2013). Just over 20% of these graduates ($N=523$) were reported to the Department of Human Services (DHS) for concerns including general neglect (82%), medical neglect (14%), physical abuse (9%), and sexual abuse (7%) of children. The OKCaBI study, and others like it, underscore that child maltreatment is a significant public health problem that also affects NICU graduates. Experiencing childhood abuse is associated with negative impact on emotional, social, biological, and cognitive areas of development. Adverse childhood experiences, including maltreatment, have been associated with adult risk behaviors, negative health outcomes, and disease; these include increased rates of substance abuse, risky sexual practices, chronic disease, and cancer (Gonzalez & MacMillian, 2008). The ability to prevent child maltreatment through support of family resilience will help to reduce or prevent a range of negative long-term physical and mental health outcomes.

Nandyal et al. (2013) also studied the relationship between child maltreatment and the burden experienced by the caregivers of NICU grads. Five selected components of caregiving burden (need for home oxygen support, other respiratory support, multiple medications, feeding equipment, and multiple specialist referrals) were scored. Infants contributing to high caregiving burden were noted to be at an increased risk for referral to child protective services (CPS). The risk associated with caregiving burden was concentrated in the first year of life, and especially during the first month or two after discharge. Therefore, focusing preventive community services on the immediate post-discharge time window may be most beneficial. Another important finding was that patients with the same OKCaBI score, but a longer length of stay (LOS), appeared to have lower incidences of maltreatment. Patients with a LOS in the NICU of more than 50 days had statistically significant fewer maltreatment reports when compared to NICU graduates who had LOS of less than 50 days. While this association does not prove causality between LOS and CPS reports, there are several possible explanations for this difference. The authors suggest that additional time might have helped the families to master the necessary skills, address some of the psycho-socio-economic issues, and improve the infants' clinical status resulting in less demand for prolonged complex care. Another subanalysis of that study assessed the siblings of the study patients and their risk for child maltreatment reports. It concluded that NICU graduates with shorter follow-up intervals had lower incidence maltreatment reports than those with longer follow-up intervals when compared with the control group of siblings (Risch, Owora, Nandyal, Chaffin, & Bonner, 2014). One program that has demonstrated efficacy in preventing child maltreatment is the Nurse Family Partnership (NFP), which has undergone rigorous evaluation in three randomized controlled trials (Gonzalez & MacMillian, 2008). This program provides nurses to first-time socially disadvantaged mothers. It has demonstrated consistent reduction in reports of maltreatment and associated outcomes. Connecting families of NICU graduates to support programs such as these can help families cope with the stressors of parenting children who may have complex needs and may decrease the incidence of maltreatment in this population.

2.5 Developmental Outcomes

Early identification of developmental delays is essential to the ongoing care of the children as a part of the medical home concept. The developmental outcome of preterm infants is a result of complex interactions between the biological vulnerability of the infant and a number of environmental risk factors. Parental perceptions of their child's vulnerability, medical stability, and parental anxieties about their child's psychological, developmental, and health outcomes can potentiate the risk factors. However, medical risk factors alone are thought to be poor predictors of behavioral and developmental outcomes in high-risk children. De Ocampo, Macias, Saylor, and Katikaneni (2003), with a sample of 90 NICU graduates, noted child vulnerability to be a stronger correlate of child behavior than medical problems at birth, child age, child developmental quotient, family income, or maternal age. Parents whose children were perceived as more vulnerable were more likely to rate their children as having problems on the Child Behavior Checklist (CBCL) internalizing, externalizing, and total problem behavior scores.

Delayed or disordered development can be caused by specific medical conditions and may also indicate an increased risk of other medical complications, behavior disorders, or associated developmental disorders. While screening tools are not intended for diagnosis, the results of such tests should lead to a full assessment, diagnosis, and/or treatment, as needed. Identification of a developmental disorder and its underlying etiology may also affect a range of treatment planning, from medical treatment of the child to family planning for his or her parents (Council on Children with Disabilities, 2006). AAP recommends incorporation of developmental surveillance at every well-child visit, with prompt follow-up for any concerns. Additionally, standardized developmental screening tests should be administered at the 9-, 18-, and 30-month visits. Consultation with a child development specialist through a state early intervention program can assist with identification of an appropriate instrument; likewise, information about developmental screening and assessment tools can be downloaded through the Early Childhood Technical Assistance Center (ECTAC) at http://ectacenter.org/topics/earlyid/screeneval.asp. However, consultation is still recommended prior to selecting an instrument, as not all screeners provide the same level of information. One example of a highly successful, evidence-based practice that integrates developmental screening and services into primary care settings is Healthy Steps for Children, or Healthy Steps. Sustained gains from the program have been identified with benefits including increased patient satisfaction, decreased parental use of severe forms of discipline, and increased rates of receiving anticipatory guidance (Minkovitz et al., 2007). Healthy Steps information can be accessed at www.healthysteps.org, where support is available for integration into new or existing medical practices.

Although all developmental screening tools are designed to identify children with potentially delayed development, each one approaches the task in a different way. In general, screening tools should address developmental domains including fine and gross motor skills, language and communication, problem solving/adaptive behavior, and personal–social skills. Screening tools also must be culturally and linguistically sensitive (Council on Children with Disabilities, 2006). Screening tests should be both reliable and valid, with good sensitivity and specificity. When a child has a screening result that may indicate a developmental delay, developmental and medical evaluations to identify the specific developmental disorders and related medical problems are warranted. Children diagnosed with developmental disorders should be identified as children with special health care needs, and chronic condition management for these children should be initiated. For children with disabilities, Public Law 99-457 necessitates all states provide early intervention services. The states also should offer provisions for interdisciplinary educational services to all disabled toddlers, infants, and their families. Most NICU graduates qualify for and should be screened by Early Childhood Intervention (ECI) programs, and designated NICU personnel should be prepared to make a referral prior to NICU graduation. These programs are federally mandated state-funded programs that provide developmental services for free or at a reduced cost to high-risk patients in the home or school environment up to age three.

2.6 Chronic Conditions

Less than 1% of all children consume up to 33% of total pediatric health care costs. These children are known as Children with Medical Complexity (CMC). They have multiple specialty needs, technology dependence, and high health care utilization. An example of CMC would be a child with cerebral palsy and developmental delay who requires technology assistance for optimal nutrition and ventilation. Kuo et al. (2014) analyzed three, full-year data sets from the Medical Expenditure Panel Survey. Of 27,755 total study subjects (<17 years), 4851 had special needs and 541 were classified as CMC. Children with CMC require intensive caregiving from families and are at risk for recurrent hospital admissions (Kuo et al., 2014). However, the majority of CMC outpatient visits were for mental health issues. Compared to families without CSHCN (children with special heath care needs), those with CMC have lower satisfaction with health care, on average. The primary health care model seems to have neglected integration of mental health services despite evidence for improved outcomes. Streamlining supportive services, including home health, therapies, and prescription medications, may reduce inefficiencies and improve timely access to mental health with the goal to reduce mental health crises. The reforms should focus on integration of community-based services which provide appropriate levels of proactive preventive care and include resources to support mental and behavioral health (Kuo et al., 2014).

The challenges for the US health care system of high health care costs and poor health outcomes in individuals with multiple concurrent, chronic conditions have been well documented (Parekh, Kronick, & Tavenner, 2014). The 'Vision and Goals of the US Health and Human Services' Strategic Framework on Multiple Chronic Conditions states several goals which focus primarily on adult patient issues but can be applied to the pediatric population as well. These include changes to the foster health system, empowering individuals, equipping clinicians to identify best practices and tools, and enhancing research to increase the external validity of trials. Several steps have been recommended to improve patient outcomes and reduce costs. First, more delivery and payment models are needed to focus specifically on the populations with multiple chronic conditions that are at highest risk for poor outcomes and high costs. Second, evidence-based community prevention and wellness programs currently reaching hundreds of thousands of individuals should be expanded further. Finally, the multiple chronic conditions population needs to be an area of focus for research on patient-centered outcomes to inform the development of future clinical practice guidelines, best practices, and quality measures (Parekh et al., 2014).

2.7 Conclusions

A premature birth can set a family on an unexpected journey consisting of a lengthy NICU stay with an uncertain outcome, followed by the potential for a variety of long-term chronic medical, developmental, and emotional issues. Providing early support in the NICU through understanding infant behaviors, supporting family interactions, and addressing stressors can set families on the pathway for successful attachment and bonding with their high-risk infant. As discharge approaches, the role of the family becomes increasingly important as they prepare to assume the role of primary caregivers to their infant. Families will benefit from counseling, education, and training given by the health care professionals; assessment of home and community resources; communication between the MNHC team and the PCPs; and follow-up appointments with a transition clinic, home health team, PCP, and/or another model of Medical Home, appropriate subspecialists, and a neurodevelopmental clinic. Communication among all team members, especially including the family members, and adherence to a well-designed and individualized care plan, are essential. In the home environment, families continue to need support and access to resources as their child grows and develops. These needs may be met through publicly funded programs such as early intervention programs, hospital transition programs, private medical or counseling clinics, or personal support systems that may exist through family or NICU graduate parent groups. Supported families with adequate access to resources at birth, in the NICU, through the discharge process, and in the home environment, result in the best resilience outcome of a complex scenario—a thriving child and family.

Discussion Questions

1. This chapter touches on the roles of physicians, nurses, social workers, psychologists, and child development specialists when working with preterm infants and their families. Discuss the unique contributions of each of these specialties. How would you determine which families receive which of the social services, and why? Discuss the risk for duplication of services, as well as any gaps in services.
2. For children classified as CMC, the chapter references the fact that mental health has not yet become a standard part of the care plan in most NICUs or in NICU

follow-up. If you were charged with developing a cost-saving and efficient plan to insert social service visits into just one time period (maternal prenatal visits, NICU-based services during the infants stay, or NICU follow-up), which would you choose, and which services would be included? What data would you use to justify your selection?
3. Although preterm birth is associated with a number of risk factors such as maternal smoking, many preterm births have no identifiable cause. Discuss the balance between providing education about prevention of preterm birth and avoiding "mother blaming."
4. Imagine that you are working for an agency that facilitates adoptions. You are meeting with a family who is preparing to adopt an infant who was born at 27 weeks gestation and was classified as extremely low birth weight. As you ask about what they understand about premature infants, the parents state, "We know that it will take her about 2 years to catch up developmentally, so we're prepared for her to be a little bit behind for awhile." Knowing that prematurity comes with an inability to accurately predict outcomes, what would be your next step in interacting with this family? What would you most want them to know about preterm birth?

References

Als, H. (1982). Toward a synactive theory of development: Promise for the assessment and support of infant individuality. *Infant Mental Health Journal, 3*, 229–244.
Als, H. (1986). A synactive model of neonatal behavioral organization: Framework for the assessment of neurobehavioral development in the premature infant and support of infants and parents in the neonatal intensive care environment. *Physical and Occupational Therapy in Pediatrics, 6*, 3–55.
Als, H. (2003). A three-center randeomized, controlled trial of individualized developmental care for very low birth weight preterm infants: Medical, neurodevelopmental, parenting and caregiving effects. *Developmental and Behavioral Pediatrics, 24*, 399–408.
Als, H., Duffy, F., McAnulty, G., Rivkin, M., Vajapeyam, S., & Mulkern, R. (2004). Early experience alters brain function and structure. *Pediatrics, 113*, 846–857.
Arockiasamy, V., Holsti, L., & Albersheim, S. (2008). Father's experiences in the neonatal intensive care unit: A search for control. *Pediatrics, 121*, e215–e222.
Beardslee, W., Avery, M., Ayoub, C., Watts, C., & Lester, P. (2010). Building resilience: The power to cope with adversity. *Zero to Three, 31*, 50–51.
Browne, J. (2003). New perspectives on premature infants and their families. *Zero to Three, 24*, 4–12.
Browne, J. (2004). Early relationship environments: Physiology of skin-to-skin contact for parents and their preterm infant. *Clinical Perinatology, 31*, 289–298.
Bruns, D., & McCollum, J. (2002). Partnerships between mothers and professionals in the nicu: Caregiving, information exchange, and relationships. *Neonatal Network: The Journal of Neonatal Nursing, 21*, 15–23. doi:10.1891/0730-0832.21.7.15
Committee, Medical Home Initiatives for Children with Special Needs Project advisory. (2002). The medical home. *Pediatrics, 110*, 184–186.
Council on Children with Disabilities, Section on Developmental Behavioral Pediatrics, Bright Futures Steering Committee, Medical Home Initiatives for Children with Special Needs Project

Advisory Committee. (2006). Identifying infants and young children with developmental disorders in the medical home: An algorithm for developmental surveillance and screening. *Pediatrics, 118*, 405–420. doi:10.1542/peds.2006-1231

De Ocampo, A., Macias, M., Saylor, C., & Katikaneni, L. (2003). Caretaker perception of child vulnerability predicts behavior problems in NICU graduates. *Child Psychiatry and Human Development, 34*, 83–96.

Escobar, G., Joffe, S., Gardner, M., Armstrong, M. A., Folck, B., & Carpenter, D. (1999). Rehospitalization in the first two weeks after discharge from the neonatal intensive care unit. *Pediatrics, 104*, e2.

Feldman, R., Eidelman, A., Sirota, L., & Weller, A. (2002). Comparison of skin-to-skin (kangaroo care) and traditional care: Parenting outcomes and preterm infant development. *Pediatrics, 110*, 16–26.

Feldman, R., Rosenthal, Z., & Eidelman, A. (2013). Maternal-preterm skin-to-skin contact enhances child physiologic organization and cognitive control across the first 10 years of life. *Journal of Biological Psychiatry, 75*, 56–64.

Fetus, Committee on, & Newborn. (2008). Hospital discharge of the high-risk neonate. *Pediatrics, 122*, 1119–1126. doi:10.1542/peds.2008-2174

Gonzalez, A., & MacMillian, H. (2008). Preventing child maltreatment: An evidence-based update. *Journal of Postgraduate Medicine, 54*, 280–286.

Hoilette, L., Blumkin, A., Baldwin, C., Fiscella, K., & Szilagyi, P. (2013). Community health centers: Medical homes for children? *Academic Pediatrics, 13*, 436–442. doi:10.1016/j.acap.2013.06.006

Heermann, J.A., Wilson, M.E., Wilhelm, P.A. (2005). Mothers in the NICU: Outsider to partner. *Pediatric Nursing, 31*, 176–181.

Klitzner, T., Rabbitt, L., & Chang, R. (2010). Benefits of care coordination for children with complex disease: A pilot medical home project in a resident teaching clinic. *Journal of Pediatrics, 156*, 1006–1010.

Kuo, D., Melguizo-Castro, M., Goudie, A., Nick, T., Robbins, J., & Casey, P. (2014). Variation in child health care utilization by medical complexity. *Maternal and Child Health Journal, 19*, 40–48. doi:10.1007/s10995-014-1493-0

Martin, J., Hamilton, B., Osterman, M., Curtain, S., & Matthews, T. (2013). Division of vital statistics. Births: Final data for 2012. *National Vital Statistics Reports, 62*, 1–69.

Martricardi, S., Agostino, R., Fedeli, C., & Motorosso, R. (2013). Mothers are not fathers: Differences between parents in the reduction of stress levels after a parental intervention in a NICU. *Acta Paediatrica, 102*, 8–14.

McAnulty, G., Duffy, F., Bernstein, J., Butler, S., Zurakowski, D., Als, H. (2009). Effects of the newborn individualized developmental care and assessment program (NIDCAP) at age 8 years: Preliminary data. *Clinical Pediatrics, 49*, 258–270.

Miles, M.S., Holditch-Davis, D., Schwartz, T., Scher, M. (2007). Depressive symptoms in mothers of prematurely born infants. *Journal of Developmental and Behavioral Pediatris, 28*, 36–44.

Minkovitz, C.S., Strobino, D., Mistry, K.B., Scharfstein, D.O., Grason, H., Hou, W., Ialongo, N., Guyer, B. (2007). Healthy Steps for Young Children: Sustained results at 5.5 years. *Pediatrics, 120*, e658–e668.

Mouradian, L. E. (2013). An art-based occupation group reduces parent anxiety in the NICU: A mixed methods study. *Journal of Occupational Therapy, 67*, 692–700.

Moyer, V. (2013). Primary care interventions to prevent child maltreatment: U.S. Preventive Services Task Force recommendation statement. *Annals of Internal Medicine, 159*, 289–295. doi:10.7326/0003-4819-159-4-201308200-00667

Nandyal, R. (2014). Commentary on community violence and pregnancy health behaviors and outcomes. *Southern Medical Journal, 107*, 518–519. doi:10.14423/SMJ.0000000000000142

Nandyal, R., Owora, A., Risch, E., Bard, D., Bonner, B., & Chaffin, M. (2013). Special care needs and risk for child maltreatment reports among babies that graduated from the neonatal intensive care. *Child Abuse & Neglect, 37*, 1114–1121. doi:10.1016/j.chiabu.2013.04.003

Paradis, H., Sandler, M., Manly, J., & Valentine, L. (2013). Building healthy children: Evidence-based home visitation integrated with pediatric medical homes. *Pediatrics, 132*(Suppl 2), S174–S179. doi:10.1542/peds.2013-1021R

Parekh, A.K., Kronick, R., Tavenner, M. (2014). Optimizing health for persons with multiple chronic conditions. JAMA, 312, 1199–1200. doi:10.1001/jama.2014.10181

Powell, K.A., Wilson, K. (eds.) (2000). *Living miracles: Stories of hope from parents of premature babies*. New York, NY: St.Martins's Press.

Risch, E., Owora, A., Nandyal, R., Chaffin, M., & Bonner, B. (2014). Risk for child maltreatment among infants discharged from a neonatal intensive care unit: A sibling comparison. *Child Maltreatment, 19*, 92–100. doi:10.1177/1077559514539387

Robison, M., Pirak, C., & Morrell, C. (2000). Multidisciplinary discharge assessment of the medically and socially high-risk infant. *The Journal of Perinatal & Neonatal Nursing, 13*, 67–86.

Smith, V., SteelFisher, G., Salhi, C., & Shen, L. (2012). Coping with the neonatal intensive care experience: Parents' strategies and views of staff support. *Journal of Perinatal and Neonatal Nursing, 26*, 343–352.

Stoll, B., Hansen, N., Bell, E., Shankaran, S., Laptook, A., & Walsh, M. (2010). Neonatal outcomes of extremely preterm infants from the NICHD neonatal research network. *Pediatrics, 126*, 443–456. doi:10.1542/peds.2009-2959

Tyson, J., Parikh, N., Langer, J., Green, C., & Higgins, R. (2008). Intensive care for extreme prematurity: Moving beyond gestational age. *New England Journal of Medicine, 358*, 1672–1681. doi:10.1056/NEJMoa073059

Chapter 3
Enhancing Coping and Resilience Among Families of Individuals with Sickle Cell Disease

Sunnye Mayes and Ashley Baker

Sickle cell disease (SCD) is an inherited illness that is accompanied by lifelong medical complications. Management of illness-related symptoms has the potential to cause detrimental effects on the whole family system, thus adaptive coping with this disease is important to establish. SCD was first identified in 1910 by Dr. James Herrick, an internal medicine physician from Chicago, Illinois. He described his findings as "peculiar elongated and sickle-shaped red blood cell corpuscles in a case of severe anemia" (Herrick, 1910; p. 181). SCD is an inherited blood disorder due to homozygosity for the abnormal hemoglobin, Hb S. When deoxygenated, Hb S polymers elongate, causing distortion of the red blood cell into a sickle or crescent shape that impairs the blood cells' passage through narrow blood vessels, resulting in painful vasoocclusive episodes (Bunn, 1997).

Several genotypes exist in SCD: Hb SS, Hb Sβ° thalassemia, Hb Sβ+ thalassemia, and Hb SC (NIH, 2002). The clinical manifestations of SCD vary among the major genotypes. Hb SS and Hb Sβ° thalassemia are commonly referred to as sickle cell anemia (SCA) because they are similar (and most severe) in clinical manifestations. It is estimated that between 90,000 and 100,000 individuals in the United States have SCD. Most individuals with SCD are of African ancestry or self-identify as black, while fewer are of Hispanic, Middle Eastern, or Asian Indian descent, but SCD is not exclusive to these ethnicities.

People who inherit one sickle cell gene and one normal gene have sickle cell trait. It is estimated that 1 in 12 African Americans has sickle cell trait (US CDC, 2013). Individuals with trait have a 50% chance of passing the trait on to their children. Sickle cell trait is generally viewed as a benign condition without any of

---

S. Mayes, Ph.D. (✉) • A. Baker, M.D.
Department of Pediatrics, University of Oklahoma Health Sciences Center, Section of Pediatric Hematology/Oncology, 1200 Children's Avenue, Ste. 14500, Oklahoma City, OK 73104, USA
e-mail: sunnye-mayes@ouhsc.edu; ashley-baker@ouhsc.edu

the vasoocclusive symptoms of sickle cell disease; however, it has been associated with rare but fatal renal medullary cancer, exertional rhabdomyolysis, and exercise-related deaths (Tsaras et al., 2009).

3.1 Medical Complications and Treatments

Vasoocclusion and hemolysis are the clinical hallmarks of SCD. In addition to pain episodes, vasoocclusion may also result in a variety of organ system complications, which can lead to disabilities or death. The chronic hemolysis of SCD is associated with mild-to-moderate anemia, which is more severe in the Hb SS and Sβ° thalassemia genotypes (West, Weathers, Smith, & Steinberg, 1992).

Infection is the leading cause of SCD-associated death worldwide, particularly in less developed countries. Repeated episodes of sickling and ischemic damage cause the spleen to become scarred and atrophied, impairing or eliminating the ability of the spleen to remove bacteria from the blood (Booth, Inusa, & Obara, 2010). In 1985, Pearson and colleagues discovered that splenic dysfunction often occurs within the first 6–12 months of life among children with sickle cell anemia. Without normal splenic function, patients are at risk for overwhelming infection and are 30–600 times more likely to develop invasive pneumococcal disease than their healthy peers (Halasa et al, 2007).

The first major breakthrough in infection control with SCD occurred in 1986, when Gaston and colleagues demonstrated that prophylactic oral penicillin reduced the risk of invasive pneumococcal disease by 84% in children under 3 years of age. This discovery led to widespread implementation of newborn screening to detect SCD.

Another key strategy in the prevention of infection is vaccination. Introduction of the pneumococcal conjugate vaccine led to a significant reduction in the incidence of pneumococcal infection in children under the age of 5 (Halasa et al., 2007). All newborns identified with SCD are recommended to receive twice daily prophylactic penicillin until age 5, as well as pneumococcal vaccination and meningococcal vaccination (NIH, 2002). Annual influenza vaccination is also recommended to prevent infections from progressing into bacterial pneumonia.

Episodes of acute pain, or "crises," are the most common type of vasoocclusive event and the primary reason for individuals with SCD to seek medical care. Platt and colleagues (1991) reported that pain frequency peaks between the ages of 19 and 39 years. They also found that more frequent pain is associated with a higher mortality rate among adults with SCD. There is wide variability in the severity and frequency of acute painful episodes experienced by patients and most pain events are managed at home. SCD-related pain can affect any area of the body; the chest, extremities, and back are the most common sites. Sickle cell pain often becomes chronic and can result in decreases in quality of life (QOL; Smith et al., 2008). The treatment approach for individuals with pain should include timely administration of appropriate doses of parenteral opiates and other analgesics.

Acute Chest Syndrome (ACS) is the second most common cause of hospitalization in SCD and the leading cause of death (Platt et al., 1994). ACS typically presents as a sudden onset of a combination of fever, cough, chest pain, or shortness of breath accompanied by a new infiltrate on chest X-ray. The most common cause is infection from viruses, bacteria, or mycoplasma, but ACS may also result from bone marrow embolism, intrapulmonary aggregates of sickled cells, atelectasis, or pulmonary edema (Vichinsky et al., 2000). ACS can rapidly progress to respiratory failure or death. Treatment includes antibiotics, supplemental oxygen, and transfusion therapy. Long-term complications may include pulmonary hypertension and chronic lung disease.

Without primary prevention, it is estimated that 11% of children with Hb SS will experience a stroke by the age of 20 and this risk increases with age (Ohene-Frempong et al., 1998). An additional 22% will have silent cerebral infarcts by 14 years of age. Silent infarcts in children can present with nonfocal signs, such as developmental delay and poor or declining school performance. Patients who have sustained a previous stroke or silent infarct are at an elevated risk for recurrent strokes and are generally treated with regular transfusion therapy (Miller et al., 2001; Pegelow et al., 1995).

Stroke can be prevented by use of Transcranial Doppler (TCD) screening. This process detects increased blood flow in the Circle of Willis (a strong predictor of future strokes). All children and adolescents with SCA are recommended to receive annual TCD screening. Chronic transfusion therapy is indicated for all individuals with elevated TCD results for prevention of stroke (Adams et al., 1998).

In addition to the major complications listed earlier, vasoocclusion may affect many other parts of the body. Avascular necrosis (AVN or osteonecrosis) is caused by bone death due to compromised blood supply. It occurs in 10% of persons with SCD, and the hip joint is the most commonly affected site (followed by the humeral head; NIH, 2002). AVN leads to progressive joint destruction, causing chronic severe pain and disability. Therapy is usually conservative, with nonsurgical management including physical therapy and analgesics until joint replacement becomes necessary (Milner et al, 1991). Priapism (i.e., unwanted, often painful erections) affects as many as 35% of males with SCD. Self-limited, recurrent episodes may lead to chronic or persistent priapism, affecting quality of life or resulting in impotence (Olujohungbe et al., 2001).

Adult SCD patients are also at risk for other complications, such as cardiac dysfunction (a major cause of death in adult patients), chronic kidney disease (affecting an estimated that 4–18% of adult SCD populations; Ataga & Orringer, 2000), and other renal complications (e.g., proteinuria, hypertension, and focal segmental glomerulosclerosis). SCD may also affect the retina, manifesting as proliferative retinopathy, which can result in blindness (Nagpal, Goldberg, & Rabb, 1977). The risk of proliferative retinopathy is higher in Hb SC disease than in Hb SS disease.

3.1.1 Medical Management of SCD

Hydroxyurea is the only FDA-approved medication to treat SCD. Its primary effect is to increase the concentration of fetal hemoglobin, as well as lower the number of circulating leukocytes and reticulocytes and decrease their expression of adhesion molecules. It also increases red blood cell size and improves cellular deformability, increasing blood flow and reducing vasoocclusion. Hydroxyurea therapy greatly reduces the frequency of painful episodes and ACS events as well as the need for red blood cell transfusions and hospitalizations (Charache et al, 1995). Long-term hydroxyurea treatment has also been shown to reduce mortality (Voskaridou et al, 2010).

Transfusion of SCD patients with normal donor erythrocytes reduces the percentage of circulating erythrocytes that contain Hb S. Indications for blood transfusion in SCD include surgical procedures involving general anesthesia, primary or recurrent stroke prevention, and instances in which there is a high risk of mortality such as ACS, severe anemia, and splenic sequestration. Transfusions are associated with multiple risks or complications, including hyperviscosity, alloimmunization, and iron overload (Chou, 2013). Therefore, transfusions should be administered based on risk-benefit assessments.

The only proven curative therapy for patients with SCD is allogeneic stem cell transplantation from HLA-matched sibling donors. Novel transplant approaches such as reduced toxicity conditioning and the use of alternative allogeneic donors (such as matched unrelated donors, unrelated cord blood donors, and familial haploidentical donors) are currently under investigation (Talano & Cairo, 2015).

3.1.2 Prognosis Among Individuals with SCD

Survival of individuals with SCD is reduced compared to those without SCD, but the prognosis has improved with the institution of comprehensive care that includes newborn screening, immunizations, antibiotics, and hydroxyurea. The mortality rate for infants and children has improved in large part because of the decrease in sepsis from early use of prophylactic antibiotics and immunizations. Over half of affected individuals survive into their fifth decades. The median age of death for those with Hb SS is 42 years for men and 48 years for women. The median age of death for those with Hb SC disease is 60 years for men and 68 years for women (Platt et al., 1994). These rates are from the prehydroxyurea era and future statistics are expected to improve.

3.2 Neurocognitive Effects

Children and adolescents with SCD also demonstrate a number of neurocognitive difficulties associated with their illness. These difficulties range from subtle impairments to more significant cognitive deficiencies. Children and adolescents with SCD who have sustained silent cerebral vascular accidents (CVAs) have been documented to have lower IQ scores than their peers who have not experienced this complication (Armstrong et al., 1996). Furthermore, Steen and colleagues (1998) noted that children with histories of silent CVA earned lower full-scale IQ scores on the Wechsler Intelligence Scale for Children. Not surprisingly, the elevated risk for CVA among children and adolescents with SCD has significant potential to negatively affect their cognitive functioning and schoolwork.

Additional work has also identified elevated academic risks among children and adolescents with SCD who have not experienced known central nervous system (CNS) injury. Noll and colleagues (2001) found that children with SCD with no evidence of overt stroke, in comparison to age, gender, and race-matched peers without a chronic illness, evidenced significantly lower verbal, attention/memory, and overall scores. Kral and Brown (2004) also found significant differences in teacher ratings of executive functioning skills among children and adolescents with abnormal TCD findings. Teacher ratings indicated significant elevations in working memory, problem-solving, planning and organizational abilities, and their ability to self-monitor. Parents also reported elevations in inhibitory control, problem-solving, flexibility, and emotional modulation, but not at a clinically significant level.

In summary, the CNS findings among youth with SCD are often conflicting and difficult to predict. SCD genotype has not been consistently related to neuropsychological functioning (Grueneich et al., 2004). Children and adolescents with known CVAs are at greater risk for neurocognitive difficulties, but those with silent CVAs or abnormal imaging findings also demonstrate a slightly elevated risk. Previous studies have found significant variability in cognitive and neurocognitive functioning. Deficits in executive functioning skills have been noted among youth with abnormal imaging results, although some of these elevations may not cause significant academic impairment for all affected students.

3.2.1 Academic Risk Factors

Differential educational opportunities are another concern that affects children and adolescents with SCD. In a study conducted in a comprehensive sickle cell clinic population, 92% of parents reported experiencing at least one type of difficulty with their child's education (Mayes et al., 2011). The majority of these families (46%) reported experiencing both educational and health-related problems, while 34% reported only experiencing difficulty with health accommodations provided at school (or lack thereof), and 12% reported difficulties solely with educational work. Medical parameters associated with SCD were significantly related to these difficulties with educational accommodations. Lower average hemoglobin level (excluding the participants receiving chronic transfusion therapy), greater disease severity (based on genotype), and longer duration of hospitalizations were associated with greater educational concerns. These findings are consistent with other studies of academic functioning among children and adolescents with SCD; Ievers-Landis and colleagues (2001) also found that a majority of parents (70.3%) reported academic concerns among their students with SCD.

3.3 Resilience and Coping Among Individuals and Families Living with SCD

Manifestations of SCD have the potential to affect all family members. Numerous studies have examined resilience and coping among children and adolescents with SCD. Additionally, it is generally an illness that persists throughout the lifetime and complications are likely to continue, and potentially worsen, throughout child and adolescent development and into adulthood. Thus, resilience and coping strategies will also be examined among caregivers and families of children and adolescents with SCD, as well as adults coping with this chronic illness.

3.3.1 Family Coping with SCD

Stressors associated with SCD have the potential to extend beyond the patient to caregivers and other family members. Many siblings of children and adolescents with SCD may not be directly affected but may have SCD trait. They carry the knowledge that they have the potential to pass the trait along to their children, resulting in sickle cell disease, with potential for associated anxiety or guilt. Furthermore, parents may experience distress about their role in the inheritance of the illness by their affected children. In addition to heritability concerns, the disruption associated with having a child with SCD has the potential to cause elevated family stress associated with management of a chronic illness (e.g., school absenteeism, missed work for parents and/or adolescents, missed social opportunities, stress associated with pain, increased medical bills).

Karlson and colleagues (2012) examined risk and resiliency among families of children and adolescents with SCD. Overall, most caregivers reported low levels of distress and high resiliency. This study found that the risk for patient and sibling emotional problems, family problems, and parent stress tended to decrease over time as families continued to adapt to living with a child with the disease. Older children demonstrated increased risk for emotional difficulties. Children and adolescents of caregivers with lower education levels were at increased risk for emotional and behavioral problems. The authors found an increased risk for sibling and emotional behavior problems was associated with having more children in the home and greater financial difficulties. Increased risk for parenting stress was associated with less caregiver education, more children in the home, and greater financial difficulties. Clearly, risks for various family members have been identified that may be targeted for treatment interventions.

Gold and colleagues (2011) found that greater frequency of emergency room (ER) visits among children and adolescents with SCD was associated with poorer psychological adjustment among their siblings. This finding may indicate difficulties associated with prolonged separation among family members. These researchers also found that higher levels of family expressiveness and lower levels of conflict were associated with improved sibling adjustment, indicating potential for family interventions.

Overall family functioning also has the potential to affect coping outcomes among families of children and adolescents with SCD. Ievers and colleagues (1998) examined 67 caregivers of children and adolescents with SCD to assess effects of family functioning and social support on the relationship between child stressors and caregiver psychological adaptation. Family functioning moderated the effect of children's externalizing behavioral problems to caregiver hostility. Thus, greater familial cohesiveness and adaptive functioning decreased possible detrimental effects of the relationship between child externalizing behavior and caregiver hostility. Higher frequency of disruptive behavior was related to elevated caregiver distress, including elevations on ratings of depression, hostility, and anxiety. Clearly, overall family functioning has the potential to play a significant role, positively or negatively, on child and adolescent adaptation to management of their chronic illness.

Thompson and colleagues (1999) conducted a study evaluating neurocognitive skills, family functioning, and behavioral problems among children and adolescents with SCD. They evaluated a large sample of 289 children and adolescents and their families. Youth completed a neuropsychological battery and magnetic resonance imaging (MRI) of their brains. Twenty-two percent of participants demonstrated elevated ratings of internalizing problems and 18% demonstrated elevated ratings of externalizing problems. There were no changes in behavioral or emotional difficulties by gender, SCD genotype, or MRI status. Children and adolescents living with single parents demonstrated more behavioral problems. Significant relations were found between externalizing behavioral problems and maternal education and neurocognitive functioning. There was no significant relationship between MRI findings and frequency of behavioral problems. The authors found a significant relationship between behavior problems, lower levels of supportive family functioning, and higher levels of conflictual family functioning. Thus, conflictual family functioning, but not neurocognitive functioning, was related to parent-reported behavioral problems among children with SCD.

Kell and colleagues (1998) found that higher ratings of family competence were associated with lower levels of internalizing and externalizing behavior problems among adolescents with SCD. These findings were especially salient for the younger adolescents and females in the sample. Family competence was associated with lower ratings of externalizing problems. The authors also investigated individual risk factors. They found that boys reported more internalizing symptoms than girls and adolescents who had previously sustained strokes also had a higher prevalence of parent-reported internalizing problems.

Palermo, Riley, and Mitchell (2008) studied the relationship between socioeconomic (SES) distress, pain, and medical outcomes among families of children and adolescents with SCD. Understandably, they found that higher pain ratings were associated with greater child and adolescent disability and decreased health-related quality of life (HRQOL). They also found several outcomes regarding the associations between SES and neighborhood distress and QOL outcomes. Specifically, child- and adolescent-reported pain was not related to family or neighborhood SES distress, although higher income was associated with less child-reported disability and improved HRQOL. Their model examined individual characteristics of the child (age, disease severity, pain intensity, and depression), familial SES variables (income, parent education), and neighborhood SES characteristics as predictors of physical and psychosocial HRQOL. Individual child characteristics did not demonstrate any significant predictors, but did explain 20% of the variance in physical HRQOL. Higher parental education and lower neighborhood SES distress were significant predictors of improved physical HRQOL. Their model explained 48% of the variance in psychosocial HRQOL. Depression and disease severity were significant predictors of psychosocial functioning, with greater depression and disease severity associated with less optimal psychosocial functioning. Individual/family SES contributed an additional 26% of variance to the model and family income and parent education were significant predictors but not necessarily in the expected directions. Higher income was associated with lower psychosocial HRQOL and higher parental education was associated with better psychosocial HRQOL. Neighborhood distress did not provide a significant contribution to the psychosocial HRQOL model.

Sharpe, Brown, Thompson, and Eckman (1994) examined strategies used to cope with pain among families of children and adolescents with SCD. Specifically, they examined medical (disease severity), demographic (SES), child (adjustment and adaptive behaviors), maternal (reports of maternal psychopathology), and family variables to identify predictors of engagement or disengagement coping styles. Engagement coping strategies included problem-solving, solicitation of social supports, use of cognitive-behavioral skills, such as restructuring and open expression of emotions. Disengagement coping strategies included avoidance, criticism of oneself, wishful or magical thinking, and withdrawal. The authors found that SES was negatively correlated with disengagement coping styles. Maternal use of engagement coping strategies was associated with greater internalizing symptoms in children, increased family adaptability, and decreased maternal psychiatric symptoms. Higher disengagement coping by mothers was associated with greater family cohesiveness, more negative thinking/pessimistic attributional style among children, lower ratings of adaptive functioning in their children, and elevated reports of child externalizing behavioral symptoms. Medical coping (i.e., use of hydration, rest, massage, warm heat, and analgesic medication) was significantly related to use of engagement coping in mothers.

Sharpe and colleagues (1994) then analyzed predictors of maternal coping styles, examining child adjustment, child adaptive behavior, family functioning, maternal psychopathology, and SES as predictor variables. Family adaptability predicted a significant amount of variance in maternal engagement coping; SES did not add a significant contribution to the model. Ratings of child internalizing symptoms accounted for 11% of the variance in maternal disengagement coping, with an additional 6% explained by SES. They also found a significant negative relationship between family adaptability and use of disengagement coping strategies among the children and adolescents. Consequently, youth who reported more frequent use of disengagement coping were rated by their mothers as having higher levels of internalizing symptoms, negative thought patterns, and pessimistic thinking.

Findings from the literature regarding family functioning indicate that overall family functioning can have beneficial or detrimental effects on children and adolescents with SCD as well as other family members. These findings indicate that the functioning of the entire family unit is an important consideration in ensuring optimal psychosocial functioning–in other words, resilience–among children and adolescents with SCD.

3.3.2 Coping in Children

Consistent with the literature for other chronic illnesses, the consensus of the current psychosocial functioning of children and adolescents with SCD demonstrates that many youth are adjusting as well as their healthy peers, while a subset of youth demonstrate adjustment difficulties. Burlew and colleagues (2000) concluded that psychosocial variables have tended to be stronger predictors of adjustment than medical severity variables. Given the often-unpredictable nature of the disease courses that comprise SCD, this finding is not entirely surprising.

Anie and colleagues (2002) conducted a study measuring pain ratings, coping strategies, and health service use (e.g., days spent in the hospital and ER visits) among children and adolescents with SCD. The coping strategies they examined included (1) active coping (i.e., ignoring pain, use of calming self-statements, increasing activity, distraction, reinterpretation of pain, and prayer and hope), (2) affective coping (i.e., catastrophizing, anger self-statements, fear self-statements, isolation), and (3) passive adherence coping (i.e., obtaining sufficient hydration, resting, and use of heating pads or massage). None of the coping strategies predicted the number or duration of pain crises. Passive adherence did explain 15.5% of the variance in pain coping, indicating that use of these passive strategies was associated with more intense pain (or perhaps that these interventions were more likely to be implemented under more extreme perceptions of pain). Conversely, active coping accounted for 16.4% of the variance in health service use, indicating that individuals who respond to pain crises with active coping responses were more likely to seek hospitalization, regardless of perceived pain level.

Barakat, Schwartz, Salamon, and Radcliffe (2010) conducted a randomized controlled trial of a pain intervention for adolescents with SCD. Each family was randomly assigned to receive a brief pain intervention or a disease education intervention, delivered in their homes. Pain, psychosocial, and health-related variables were assessed at baseline, immediately following the intervention, and 1 year later. Although scores improved, the researchers did not find significant changes in outcome variables from pre- to postintervention or 1-year follow-up. Post hoc analyses did demonstrate statistically significant improvements in disease self-efficacy and transition knowledge, indicating that although the study's primary hypotheses were not supported, other positive outcomes were associated with the intervention.

Chen, Cole, and Kato (2004) conducted a review of empirically supported psychosocial interventions for pain and adherence in SCD and used the American Psychological Association Division 12 Task force (Chambless) criteria to evaluate the results. Cognitive-behavioral techniques were categorized as probably efficacious for SCD-related pain. Although many other interventions were included in the analyses, they did not meet criteria for empirical efficacy, indicating that SCD further research in SCD behavioral pain management intervention is clearly needed.

Gil and colleagues (1997) conducted a laboratory pain task among children and adolescents with SCD and examined their coping responses. Older children demonstrated more accurate discrimination between pain stimuli than younger participants, with their overall model explaining 19% of variance in sensory discrimination. Coping attempts was a significant predictor, indicating that children and adolescents who used more coping strategies demonstrated less accurate sensory discrimination than those who reported less frequent use of coping strategies. The authors hypothesized that this decreased accuracy allowed them to cope with their discomfort more effectively and noted that the response is similar to discrimination results following administration of analgesic pain medication. Children who used active cognitive and behavioral coping strategies reported lower levels of pain, suggesting that instruction in cognitive-behavioral skills could help them to achieve better overall pain management.

To further examine the potential benefits of cognitive-behavioral coping strategies, Gil and colleagues (2001) examined daily coping practice among children and adolescents with SCD. Participants were randomly assigned to receive coping skills training or a standard care condition. Participants in the coping group were assigned to practice coping skills daily using relaxation audio files. Participants in the coping intervention reported a significantly more active pain management approach, in comparison to their peers in the standard care condition. When children practiced coping strategies on days that they experienced pain, they demonstrated fewer health care visits and school absences, and less disruption from household activities than when they experienced pain on nonpractice days. There were no differences in reports of depression or anxiety based on group assignment. It may be that a more targeted intervention approach is warranted to adequately address these internalizing symptoms. Despite this finding, the overall study results indicated that, in addition to enhanced pain management, cognitive-behavioral coping skills have the potential to reduce numerous negative consequences of pain episodes, such as social and academic declines and increased medical utilization and costs.

Gil and colleagues (2001) did find several differences in coping practices among participants in their study. Younger children practiced coping skills more frequently than their older counterparts. Girls practiced coping skills more frequently than boys. Counterintuitively, children and adolescents with more chronic disease complications were less likely to practice coping skills. Several parent variables also predicted more frequent coping practice. Higher parental education achievement, divorced parent status, and parental employment were associated with more frequent coping skills practice for the children and adolescents in these categories. Children and adolescents were also more likely to practice coping skills when their reported pain levels were higher. Interestingly, higher pain and greater coping practice was not related to use of pain medications.

Gil and colleagues (2003) conducted a follow-up study examining pain and coping skills of adolescents. They tracked daily stress, mood, pain, health-care use, and activity among adolescents with SCD over a 6-month period. Elevated stress and negative mood were associated with increased same-day pain, health care utilization, and reduced social activity. Increased positive mood was associated with decreased pain, fewer health-care visits, and greater activity participation. Elevations in pain were associated with higher stress levels and less positive mood on subsequent days. Consistent with most adherence research, younger adolescents were more likely to complete their daily diaries. Similarly, Ievers-Landis et al. (2001) found that the number of caregiver-reported difficulties associated with their child's negative emotions regarding SCD were positively associated with frequency of hospitalizations and school absences in the past month.

Fisak and colleagues (2012) undertook a study to provide a comprehensive evaluation of variables contributing to HRQOL among children and adolescents with SCD. Disease severity and medical complication variables explained a significant 34% of variance in QOL ratings. Frequency of pain crises and disease genotype were the only significant predictors of QOL ratings. Barriers to health care accounted for a significant amount of variance (78%) in the relationship between adherence and QOL. Finally, frequency of pain crises, disease genotype, adherence and self-care behaviors, and barriers to adherence were entered into a regression model predicting total QOL ratings. This overall model was significant and predicted 49% of the variance in QOL. Disease type, pain crisis frequency, and adherence barriers emerged as significant predictor variables, with less severe disease type, lower pain crisis frequency, and fewer adherence barriers associated with higher QOL. These findings highlight the importance of assessing and comprehensively managing pain and adherence-related behaviors.

Thompson and colleagues (1994) examined stability of adjustment of children and adolescents with SCD over a 10-month period. They found that poor adjustment was constant over time, but there was little stability in meeting criteria for diagnoses from the Diagnostic and Statistical Manual. Mothers were more consistent in their ratings than child self-reports. Pain coping strategies accounted for a significant amount of change in child-reported symptoms and mother-reported internalizing concerns, indicating benefits to both emotional and physical functioning. They did not find any significant changes over time in illness severity, frequency of pain crises, number of child complications, maternal anxiety, or maternal-reported behavioral problems among children and adolescents. They did find a reduction in child symptoms from time one to time two. Child pain coping strategies demonstrated a significant contribution to adjustment at follow-up. Negative thinking at follow-up accounted for 19% of the variance in mother-reported internalizing difficulties. Maternal anxiety did not contribute to behavioral problems.

Promising results have also been found for electronically administered coping interventions. McClellan and colleagues (2009) conducted a home-based technology intervention for pain management among youth with SCD. This intervention collected information from daily pain diaries and coping skills practice sessions using the wireless handheld devices. This feasibility study provided information on the usefulness of home-based diary reporting. The authors had high rates of participation among participants.

Snyder's Hope Theory has also been examined as a possible mechanism for coping with SCD. Hope Theory posits that hope is comprised of two components (i.e., pathways and agency) that interact to encompass overall hope (Snyder et al., 1997). The pathways component is the belief in one's ability to find a means to achieve a goal. The agency component is the belief about one's ability to initiate and complete the necessary steps to achieving a stated goal. Snyder's contention is that an individual's perception of goals (e.g., illness-related goals) can affect overall management of their illness, including illness-related stressors. Thus, hopeful thinking patterns have the capacity to facilitate pathways thinking to achieve preferred health outcomes and agentic thinking to implement the necessary steps to do so.

Lewis and Kliewer (1996) examined mediator/moderator models of hope, coping, and adjustment among children and adolescents with SCD. They found that higher ratings of hope predicted physical symptoms of anxiety, but coping did not mediate the relationship between hope and physical manifestations of anxiety. They also found a strong negative relationship between hope and anxiety (i.e., higher levels of hope were related to lower levels of anxiety) when patients used distraction coping. Avoidance coping was associated with increased reports of anxiety. Thus, interventions aimed to increase hopeful thinking may be beneficial, particularly when combined with specific coping interventions.

Ziadini, Patterson, Pulgaron, Robinson, and Barakat (2011) examined resilience among adolescents with SCD and HRQOL and coping as predictors of adaptive behaviors. Higher ratings of QOL were significantly associated with higher ratings on interpersonal relationships and self-esteem. Adherence was positively correlated with personal adjustment, interpersonal relations, and self-esteem. Hope was associated with self-esteem. Hope and QOL were significant predictors of relations with parents and were associated with increased adaptive behavior. Adaptive behavior did not differ by QOL at lower levels of hope. Interaction between adherence and QOL was a significant predictor of interpersonal relations. At low levels of adherence, lower reported QOL was associated with less adaptive behavior. At higher levels of adherence, there was no relationship between adaptive behavior and QOL.

Although not much research is currently available regarding acceptance and commitment therapy (ACT) in pediatric SCD, Masuda and colleagues (2011) conducted a case study of an intervention conducted with a male adolescent with SCD. They found that following an ACT intervention, he demonstrated significant improvements in psychological flexibility and parental acceptance; however, further randomized clinical trials will be warranted to more definitively recommend this treatment.

Findings from these studies indicate that active coping strategies that are traditionally considered helpful in pediatric pain management are not consistently useful among children and adolescents experiencing pain from SCD-related crises. Cognitive-behavioral intervention techniques, including addressing pain-related thought patterns, implementation of relaxation activities, positive self-statements, and creative use of distraction, have been associated with the most statistically robust improvements in child and adolescent pain and adherence coping with SCD. Increased positive mood has shown beneficial effects on pain levels, medical visits, and social interactions. Children and adolescents with SCD should be encouraged to take active steps to help manage their chronic illness (Casey & Brown, 2003). Examples of strategies they may incorporate include participation in medication adherence regimens, maintaining regular fluid intake, engaging in appropriate physical activity, and maintaining adequate warmth. Coping often depends on the interaction between personal and environmental variables and may help to explain some of these inconsistent findings. Negative coping strategies, on the other hand, do have the anticipated negative effects on coping and can extend to increased medical utilization and greater school absenteeism.

3.3.3 Caregiver Coping

Assuming the role of primary caregiver for a child with a chronic illness, such as SCD, is a daunting task with many inherent stressors. Familial and demographic characteristics have the ability to support or hinder these efforts. Single parenting is one of these characteristics. Mullins and colleagues (2011) found that single mothers of children and adolescents with chronic illness demonstrated higher levels of perceived vulnerability and parenting stress than caregivers from two-parent families; however, income was a mediating variable and these effects disappeared with higher incomes. Thus, a significant amount of single-parenting stress is likely associated with financial limitations.

Cousino and Hazen (2013) examined a different component of parenting stress. They conducted a systematic review of parenting stress among parents of children and adolescents with chronic illness. They found a consistent relationship between greater parenting stress among caregivers of children with chronic illness, compared to parents of healthy children. They found that greater parenting stress was associated with greater responsibility for treatment management and was also significantly associated with poorer psychological adjustment in both caregivers and the children with chronic illness. They did not find relationships between parenting stress and illness duration or severity across illness populations.

Moskowitz and colleagues (2007) conducted a study where mothers of children with SCD were interviewed regarding amount of time spent providing care for the child, health care utilization, illness stigma, and caregiver mental health. They found that, compared to children with HIV, children with SCD had significantly lower functional status and more hospitalizations. Caregivers of children with HIV and SCD had significantly higher depressed mood scores than caregivers of healthy children; caregiving burden was comparable in both groups. The authors speculated that the perceived burden of care for SCD may pose particular challenges to caregivers due to the unpredictable nature of the disease. This finding provides support that specific features of SCD may make it a unique stressor that affects families differentially from other chronic illnesses.

Logan and colleagues (2002) examined parenting characteristics and health utilization variables among families of adolescents with SCD. Frequency of SCD-related stress explained the largest portion of variance in medical service utilization, followed by greater parental knowledge of SCD. Parent–adolescent relationship quality did not contribute significantly to the model. Disease severity was the strongest predictor of emergency medical service use.

Ievers-Landis and colleagues (2001) examined specific SCD-related parenting stressors. Caregivers primarily reported difficulties associated with nutrition, management of pain episodes, and management of disease-related emotions. Parents of boys reported more problems than parents of girls, including greater social concerns and negative affect associated with addressing these concerns. Caregiver emotional intensity of managing their child's disease-related emotions was significantly associated with frequency of hospitalizations and ER visits within the previous month. Thus, parents and caregivers of youth with SCD clearly have global chronic illness stressors as well as SCD-specific stressors to navigate.

Previous research has documented the effects of caregiver coping on overall family adjustment. Brown and colleagues (2000) found an indirect effect between caregiver coping on child adjustment through the caregivers' adjustment. They found that 35% of caregivers in their sample of caregivers of children and adolescents with SCD met criteria for poor adjustment. Use of disengagement coping by caregivers was associated with greater internalizing difficulties among the children and adolescents and overall poorer adjustment among caregivers. These findings suggest that how caregivers adjust to having a child with SCD has the potential to affect their children's coping as well.

Brown and colleagues (2006) conducted a study to assess caregiver adjustment and perception of their child's disease severity. They found that caregiver and child social adjustment accounted for a significant amount of variance, beyond what would be accounted for by subjective disease severity, demographics, and biological disease severity. Less optimal psychological adjustment of caregivers and communication patterns among children were associated with increased ER use, after controlling for objective disease severity levels and demographics. Child social adjustment, especially quality of peer relationships, accounted for a significant portion of variance in ER use, beyond what would be expected for socioeconomic status and disease-related characteristics. Thus, social functioning has the power to affect both family perceptions of the illness, as well as actual medical utilization rates.

Connelly and colleagues (2006) examined perceptions of disease severity, caregiver adjustment, and biological disease markers among 58 children and adolescents with SCD. They found that psychological adjustment of caregivers and biological disease markers were the most significant predictors of chronic disease severity. They found that caregivers perceived their child's disease as more severe (and displaying more severe symptoms) than the children and adolescents themselves. Ratings of functional limitations and pain were consistent between informants. Discrepancies between caregivers and other informants were significantly associated with more problematic psychological adjustment for caregivers. Thus, caregiver adjustment has the potential to play a significant role in the child's medical treatment and should be routinely assessed as a part of comprehensive care, when available.

> **Box 3.1. Focus on Practice**
> Before I worked in healthcare, I taught in a teacher-preparation program. One of the courses that I taught was Child Health, Safety, and Nutrition; I remember covering chapters on common childhood illnesses and diagnoses, and I always believed that I offered my students a very comprehensive and holistic view of the child as an integrated physical, social, and cognitive individual. Then I went to work as a behavioral health professional in a Sickle Cell Disease (SCD) clinic, and all that changed. Suddenly, I could recall only one single paragraph in our text book that was devoted to Sickle Cell, leaving my students and myself under the impression that Sickle Cell Disease was rare, mild, and not life threatening. I was guilty of perpetuating a "don't worry about it" attitude in the face of a disease that was very threatening to life, physical well-being, and even academic progress. Becoming "in the know" about the serious nature of Sickle Cell changed the course of my career, and I frequently reflect on the people who need to know about SCD, such as counselors and teachers, but for whom this information is rarely included in training programs. It's hard to limit the lessons I've learned to just three things because I had so much learning to do, but I suppose I would want to tell new clinicians or teachers this: (1) Respect pain and know that it is real; (2) Contact the SCD clinic in your city or state to learn about proper first aid, hydration, and restrictions on activity. Follow those guidelines; and (3) take early signs of learning problems very seriously in kids with SCD, and keep trying to get help until someone responds. Don't give up on kids with SCD.
> Ginger Welch, Ph.D.
> Former Pediatric Psychology Fellow, Hem/Onc Sickle Cell Clinic

3.3.4 Coping in Adults with SCD

Thompson and colleagues (1992) examined a transactional model of psychological adjustment among a sample of adults with SCD. They found that higher levels of adjustment were associated with fewer perceived daily stressors, lower stress regarding disease-related tasks, higher adherence-focused pain management strategies, and family functioning with high levels of support and low levels of conflict and control. The authors estimated that these variables explained 44–50% of the variance in their model.

McCrae and Lumley (1998) examined the relationship between coping, somatic awareness, and illness-related worrying among adults with SCD. Patterns of negative thinking or passive adherence were positively associated with increased frequency, severity, and duration of pain episodes and frequency of hospital admissions. They found that greater reports of negative affectivity were associated with negative thought patterns, somatic awareness, greater frequency and duration of pain episodes, and greater frequency of hospitalizations. Patients scoring higher on negative thinking/passive adherence reported more frequent pain crises, greater pain severity, and greater activity restrictions during pain episodes. Increased levels of somatic awareness were associated with increased duration of pain crises and frequency of hospital admissions, regardless of frequency, duration, or severity of pain. Although several behavioral associations were noted, coping attempts were unrelated to all SCD-related health measures.

Gil and colleagues (1992) conducted a 9-month follow-up of adults with SCD who participated in a study of a pain-coping intervention. They found that greater reports of negative thinking and passive adherence were associated with greater activity restriction and more frequent medical utilization during pain crises (i.e., more frequent and longer hospitalizations). Individuals who reported increases in negative thinking and passive adherence over time experienced further decreases in activity level during pain crises, indicating that these behaviors are associated with further deterioration of appropriate coping skills. Pain coping strategies were relatively stable over time for individuals who did not receive the intervention, indicating that participants tended to prefer certain patterns of coping behaviors. Men used more coping attempts than women, but also reported higher ratings on negative thinking and passive adherence. Younger patients experienced more frequent visits to the ER and hospital.

Gil and colleagues (1996) examined training in cognitive coping skills and pain coping and perception among adults with SCD. Participants were randomly assigned to receive either a cognitive coping skills intervention or education about SCD. Individuals who received the coping skills training reported increased coping attempts, decreased negative thinking, and lower reports of laboratory-induced pain. Overall, coping participation was associated with better discrimination of pain intensities, compared to controls. Use of coping skills was not associated with frequency, duration, or severity of pain episodes.

These effects were reexamined at 3 months posttreatment (Gil et al., 2000) and diary data regarding coping practice and medical utilization were also examined. Outcome measures included coping, pain perception, and clinical parameters. Participants who received the coping intervention reported significantly lower pain levels during laboratory pain tasks and used coping strategies more often than non-intervention participants at 3-month follow-up. Based on diary data, when patients practiced coping strategies on days they experienced pain, they experienced fewer medical contacts than on days when strategies were not implemented. At 3 month follow-up, there were significant group differences in use of coping strategies, but not for negative thinking. Participants in the coping condition were more stoic with their initial laboratory pain perceptions, but differences in sensory discrimination were not maintained at follow-up. Thus, while these findings are promising, further work is needed to determine how to maintain some of these positive treatment effects.

Gil and colleagues (2004) extended their examination of diary findings and asked adults with SCD to complete daily diaries of mood, stress, pain, medical utilization, and activity. They found that increased reports of stress and negative mood were associated with increases in pain (up to 2 days later), increased use of health care services, and missed work. Based on these findings, the authors estimated that pain may be a more powerful component in the pain-mood and pain-stress cycles. Greater positive mood was associated with lower pain on the same and subsequent days (up to 2 days later), less health care utilization, and less work absenteeism, indicating the capacity for positive mood to offset negative consequences of pain. Mean stress ratings among participants were significantly greater on pain than non-pain days. On pain days, participants reported less positive mood and higher ratings of negative mood. For 82% of pain days, no health care contact was initiated. Obviously, pain was a significant predictor of health care utilization. After controlling for pain, mood significantly predicted health care utilization and work absences. Examining medical adherence variables, the authors found that drinking sufficient fluids was significantly associated with less pain, overexertion was associated with increased pain ratings, and exposure to cold temperature was the strongest predictor of pain. These findings highlight the importance of following medical advice regarding activities to prevent or lessen pain crises.

3.4 Summary and Conclusions

Children and adolescents with SCD face many disease-related challenges. They may experience unexpected episodes of severe vasoocclusive pain, breathing difficulties, and neurocognitive complications, such as stroke. For the most part, children and adolescents handle these difficulties with remarkable resiliency; however, there is a small subpart of individuals who demonstrate clinically significant behavioral or emotional difficulties. Active coping strategies tend to be more effective in managing the negative consequences associated with this chronic illness. Furthermore, caregiver coping has been demonstrated to have a significant effect on child and adolescent functioning and is clearly an area that needs further attention in research and clinical efforts. Positive overall family functioning has been empirically shown to have the potential to counteract some of the negative effects associated with SCD. Thus, the entire family system is critical for achieving optimal coping with this illness.

Moving forward with coping research among youth with SCD, more multimethod multiinformant evaluations of family functioning are warranted (McClellan & Cohen, 2007). The extant research does demonstrate some reporter differences in parent and child/adolescent self-reports, with parents and caregivers often over-reporting child pain and distress. This finding is significant, given that it can negatively affect parental coping, which can translate into less adaptive child adjustment. Larger sample sizes and more multisite research collaborations will also help to provide more generalizable and robust results. Additional longitudinal results are also warranted to help identify developmental trends in coping and longer term effects of the investigated interventions.

SCD is a chronic and pervasive disease and the effects that children and adolescents experience can exert negative consequences on siblings. While some of these effects have been documented, further research is clearly warranted to further identify risk factors and treatment interventions for other family members who are likely to be impacted by this illness. Additionally, overall family functioning has been shown to have the power to exert positive or negative influences on child and adolescent functioning and stressors associated with unaffected siblings should not be ignored.

As children and adolescents with SCD mature and reach adulthood, they experience new challenges associated with transition to adult-care services. Many coping strategies that work for the pediatric populations (e.g., cognitive behavioral pain management interventions and following medical advice, such as maintaining adequate hydration and avoiding cold temperatures) have demonstrated efficacy among adult populations; however, further research is clearly needed to determine the best methods of maintaining use of these strategies over time and identifying newer and improved methods of management of this illness.

3.5 Implications for Understanding Family Resilience

The introduction of SCD into the family system has the potential to cause stress and disruption to all family members. This disruption may manifest in physical symptoms of the disease, emotional ramifications of having the illness (e.g., disappointment about athletic aspirations, mood disturbance associated with medical complications), financial hardships (e.g., medical bills, missed work), social impairment (e.g., difficulty maintaining relationships due to frequent hospitalizations or illnesses), and academic difficulties (e.g., cognitive complications, school absenteeism). This list is not inclusive of all of the potential difficulties faced by families of individuals with SCD but may help to highlight some of the specific issues that may be of concern.

Illness-related risks have the potential to affect the entire family system in multiple ways. For example, healthy siblings may be separated from their parents and siblings for the duration of prolonged hospitalizations. Parents may experience employment instability and elevated stress due to caregiving demands. Extended family members may be asked to take a greater role in childcare responsibilities. How family members feel about these situations has significant potential to determine their resilience, in other words, if they cope in an adaptive or maladaptive manner. The extant literature base has likely just begun to scratch the surface of uncovering the best management and intervention strategies for these concerns.

3.5.1 Implications for Practice and/or Policy

Children and adolescents with SCD face many disease-related obstacles. They can benefit from specific policy implementations to facilitate their optimal functioning. Newborn screening to detect SCD is an example of a medical policy that has been put into place nationwide in the United States but is not regularly occurring worldwide. In SCD treatment centers, treatment protocols for prophylactic penicillin, scheduled vaccinations, regular TCD screening, treatment with chronic transfusion therapy as needed, and greater use of hydroxyurea can also help to improve the health of individuals with SCD and to prevent or delay negative effects associated with the disease.

One example of a more potentially widespread policy in the medical environment is ensuring that individuals with SCD receive prompt medical attention when they seek emergency or outpatient services. Delaying of antibiotic administration may be life threatening and improper timing of analgesic medication has significant risks for decreased QOL. Medical facilities can address these concerns by implementing policies ensuring that patients with SCD receive prompt administration of antibiotic and analgesic medications. Many hospitals institute similar policies (Pokala et al., 2012) and this is a feasible and cost-efficient first step that can be taken by emergency departments to improve patient care.

In the academic environment, students with SCD are at risk for experiencing neurocognitive dysfunction. Additionally, frequent school absenteeism is associated with increased risk for social deficits. Ensuring that all students with SCD have appropriate medical plans and accommodations in the classroom (i.e., Section 504 Plans or Individualized Education Plans) is one step that can help improve academic and social outcomes. Parents may also be educated about formal education plans and peer victimization policies to become more effective advocates. Students may be taught specific problem-solving and social skills to help them navigate difficult peer encounters. Policies emphasizing the importance of establishing formal education plans are recommended for comprehensive SCD programs. Further research with these interventions can best inform the specific skills needed in these situations.

Comprehensive SCD programs are encouraged to implement regular screening for psychological functioning during routine sickle cell clinic appointments. Such screening can help to identify potential risk factors for psychological distress (e.g., peer victimization) and can help to identify early symptoms of depression, anxiety, and other psychiatric concerns (Mayes et al., 2011). Early intervention can help to prevent greater functional impairments from occurring and can serve to enhance overall family resilience.

3.6 Future Directions

Research on transition to adulthood consistently indicates that successful transition can have a significant protective effect on medical care, adherence, and mortality (Hamideh & Alvarez, 2013). Unfortunately, there are few well-controlled studies examining the critical ingredients for a successful adolescent-to-adult transition program. Clearly, interventions in this area have significant potential to affect resilience and adoption of appropriate health maintenance behaviors among individuals with SCD and additional investigations are definitely warranted in this area.

In sum, individuals with SCD, despite facing a significant amount of risk, adversity and uncertainty in their illness, demonstrate remarkable resilience. For the subset of individuals who do experience behavioral and/or emotional difficulties, cognitive-behavioral interventions have shown the most promise to address these concerns. Clearly, coping and resilience research encompassing medical management, as well as cognitive and social functioning, continues to be warranted in the SCD population and there are obvious benefits to including caregivers and other important family members in coping interventions, particularly those targeted to children and adolescents.

Discussion Questions

1. What is the best way to encourage regular physical activity and exercise and also allow necessary accommodations to prevent physical overexertion?
2. Families are encouraged to advocate for themselves and inform medical providers what medications and treatments work most effectively for them, yet when many patients attempt to do so they are perceived as drug seeking. What is the best way to manage this problem?
3. What supports can be put into place to facilitate the transition to adult services?
4. Sickle cell disease predominately affects families of African American descent. How does race or ethnicity affect stress and coping levels?

References

Adams, R. J., McKie, V. C., Hsu, L., Files, B., Vichinsky, E., Pegelow, C., et al. (1998). Prevention of a first stroke by transfusions in children with sickle cell anemia and abnormal results on transcranial Doppler ultrasonography. *New England Journal of Medicine, 339*, 5–11. doi:10.1056/NEJM199807023390102

Anie, K. A., Steptoe, A., Ball, S., Dick, M., & Smalling, B. M. (2002). Coping and health service utilization in a UK study of paediatric sickle cell pain. *Archives of Diseases of Childhood, 86*, 325–329. doi:10.1136/adc.86.5.385

Armstrong, F. D., Thompson, R. J., Wang, W., Zimmerman, R., Pegelow, C. H., Miller, S., et al. (1996). Cognitive functioning and brain magnetic resonance imaging in children with sickle cell disease. Neuropsychology Committee of the Cooperative Study of Sickle Cell Disease. *Pediatrics, 97*(6 Pt 1), 864–870.

Ataga, K. I., & Orringer, E. P. (2000). Renal abnormalities in sickle cell disease. *American Journal of Hematology, 63*, 205–211. doi:10.1002/(SICI)1096-8652(200004)63:4<205::AID-AJH8>3.0.CO;2-8

Barakat, L. P., Schwartz, L. A., Salamon, K. S., & Radcliffe, J. (2010). A family-based randomized controlled trial of pain intervention for adolescents with sickle cell disease. *Journal of Pediatric Hematology Oncology, 32*, 540–547.

Booth, C., Inusa, B., & Obaro, S. K. (2010). Infection in sickle cell disease: A review. *International Journal of Infectious Diseases, 14*, e2–e12. doi:10.1016/j.ijid.2009.03.010

Brown, R. T., Connelly, M., Rittle, C., & Clouse, B. (2006). A longitudinal examination predicting emergency room use in children with sickle cell disease and their caregivers. *Journal of Pediatric Psychology, 31*, 163–173. doi:10.1093/jpepsy/jsj002

Brown, R. T., Lambert, R., Devine, D., Baldwin, D., Baldwin, K., Casey, R., et al. (2000). Risk-resistance adaptation model for caregivers and their children with sickle cell syndromes. *Annals of Behavioral Medicine, 22,* 158–169. doi:10.1007/BF02895780

Bunn, H. F. (1997). Pathogenesis and treatment of sickle cell disease. *New England Journal of Medicine, 337,* 762–769. doi:10.1056/NEJM199709113371107

Burlew, K., Telfair, J., Colangelo, L., & Wright, E. C. (2000). Factors that influence adolescent adaptation to sickle cell disease. *Journal of Pediatric Psychology, 25,* 287–299.

Casey, R. L., & Brown, R. T. (2003). Psychological aspects of hematologic diseases. *Child and Adolescent Psychiatric Clinics of North America, 12,* 567–584.

Charache, S., Terrin, M. L., Moore, R. D., Dover, G. J., Barton, F. B., Eckert, S. V., et al. (1995). Effect of hydroxyurea on the frequency of painful crises in sickle cell anemia. *The New England Journal of Medicine, 332,* 1317–1322. doi:10.1056/NEJM199505183322001

Chen, E., Cole, S. W., & Kato, P. M. (2004). A review of empirically supported psychosocial interventions for pain and adherence outcomes in sickle cell disease. *Journal of Pediatric Psychology, 29,* 197–209. doi:10.1093/jpepsy/jsh021

Chou, S. T. (2013). Transfusion therapy for sickle cell disease: A balancing act. *Hematology American Society of Hematology Education Program, 439–446.* doi:10.1182/asheducation-2013.1.439

Connelly, M., Wagner, J. L., Brown, R. T., Rittle, C., Cloues, B., & Taylor, L. (2006). Informant discrepancy in perceptions of sickle cell disease severity. *Journal of Pediatric Psychology, 30,* 443–448. doi:10.1093/jpepsy/jsi068

Cousino, M. K., & Hazen, R. A. (2013). Parenting stress among caregivers of children with chronic illness: A systematic review. *Journal of Pediatric Psychology, 38,* 809–828. doi:10.1093/jpepsy/jsto49

Fisak, B., Belkin, M. H., von Lehe, A. C., & Bansal, M. M. (2012). The relation between health-related quality of life, treatment adherence and disease severity in a paediatric sickle cell disease sample. *Child: Care, Health and Development, 38,* 204–210. doi:10.1111/j.1365-2214.2011.01223.x

Gaston, M. H., Verter, J. I., Woods, G., Pegelow, C., Kelleher, J., Presbury, G., et al. (1986). Prophylaxis with oral penicillin in children with sickle cell anemia. *The New England Journal of Medicine, 314,* 1593–1599. doi:10.1056/NEJM198606193142501

Gil, K. M., Abrams, M. R., Phillips, G., & Williams, D. A. (1992). Sickle cell disease pain: 2. Predicting health care use and activity level at 9-month follow-up. *Journal of Consulting and Clinical Psychology, 60,* 267–273.

Gil, K. M., Anthony, K. K., Carson, J. W., Redding-Lallinger, R., Daeschner, C. W., & Ware, R. E. (2001). Daily coping practice predicts treatment effects in children with sickle cell disease. *Journal of Pediatric Psychology, 26,* 163–173.

Gil, K. M., Carson, J. W., Porter, L. S., Ready, J., Valrie, C., Redding-Lallinger, R., et al. (2003) Daily stress and mood and their association with pain, health-care use, and school activity in adolescents with sickle cell disease. *Journal of Pediatric Psychology, 28*(5), 363–373. doi:10.1093/jpepsy/jsgo26

Gil, K. M., Carson, J. W., Porter, L. S., Scipio, C., Bediako, S. M., & Orringer, E. (2004). Daily mood and stress predict pain, health care use, and work activity in African American adults with sickle-cell disease. *Health Psychology, 23,* 267–274.

Gil, K. M., Carson, J. W., Sedway, J. A., Porter, L. S., Schaeffer, J. J. W., & Orringer, E. (2000). Follow-up of coping skills training in adults with sickle cell disease: Analysis of daily pain and coping practice diaries. *Health Psychology, 19,* 85–90.

Gil, K. M., Edens, J. L., Wilson, J. J., Raezer, L. B., Kinney, T. R., Schultz, W. H., et al. (1997). Coping strategies and laboratory pain in children with sickle cell disease. *Annals of Behavioral Medicine, 19,* 22–29.

Gil, K. M., Wilson, J. J., Edens, J. L., Webster, D. A., Abrams, M. A., Orringer, E., et al. (1996). Effects of cognitive coping skills training on coping strategies and experimental pain sensitivity in African American adults with sickle cell disease. *Health Psychology, 15,* 3–10.

Gold, J. I., Treadwell, M., Weissman, L., & Vichinsky, E. (2011). The mediating effects of family functioning on psychosocial outcomes in healthy siblings of children with sickle cell disease. *Pediatric Blood and Cancer, 57*, 1055–1061.

Grueneich, R., Ris, M. D., Ball, W., Kalinyak, K. A., Noll, R., Vannatta, K., et al. (2004). Relationship of structural magnetic resonance imaging, magnetic resonance perfusion, and other disease factors to neuropsychological outcome in sickle cell disease. *Journal of Pediatric Psychology, 29*, 83–92. doi:10.1093/jpepsy/jsho12

Halasa, N. B., Shankar, S. M., Talbot, T. R., Arbogast, P. G., Mitchel, E. F., Wang, W. C., et al. (2007). Incidence of invasive pneumococcal disease among individuals with sickle cell disease before and after the introduction of the pneumococcal conjugate vaccine. *Clinical Infectious Diseases, 44*, 1428–1433. doi:10.1086/516781

Hamideh, D., & Alvarez, O. (2013). Sickle cell disease related mortality in the United States (1999-2009). *Pediatric Blood and Cancer, 60*, 1482–1486. doi:10.1002/pbc.24557

Herrick, J. B. (1910). Peculiar elongated and sickle-shaped red blood corpuscles in a case of severe anemia. *Archives of Internal Medicine, 6*, 517–521.

Ievers, C. E., Brown, R. T., Lambert, R. G., Hsu, L., & Eckman, J. R. (1998). Family functioning and social support in the adaptation of caregivers of children with sickle cell syndromes. *Journal of Pediatric Psychology, 23*, 377–388.

Ievers-Landis, C. E., Brown, R. T., Drotar, D., Bunke, V., Lambert, R. G., & Walker, A. A. (2001). Situational analysis of parenting problems for caregivers of children with sickle cell syndromes. *Developmental and Behavioral Pediatrics, 22*, 169–178.

Karlson, C. W., Leist-Haynes, S., Smith, M., Faith, M. A., Elkin, T. D., & Megason, G. (2012). Examination of risk and resiliency in a pediatric sickle cell disease population using the Psychosocial Assessment Tool 2.0. *Journal of Pediatric Psychology, 37*, 1031–1040. doi:10.1093/jpepsy/jss087

Kell, R. S., Kliewer, W., Erickson, M. T., & Ohene-Frempong, K. (1998). Psychological adjustment of adolescents with sickle cell disease: Relations with demographic, medical, and family competence variables. *Journal of Pediatric Psychology, 23*, 301–312.

Kral, M. C., & Brown, R. T. (2004). Transcranial Doppler ultrasonography and executive dysfunction in children with sickle cell disease. *Journal of Pediatric Psychology, 29*, 185–195. doi:10.1093/jpepsy/jsho20

Lewis, H. A., & Kliewer, W. (1996). Hope, coping, and adjustment among children with sickle cell disease: Tests of mediator and moderator models. *Journal of Pediatric Psychology, 21*, 25–41.

Logan, D. E., Radcliffe, J., & Smith-Whitley, K. (2002). Parent factors and adolescent sickle cell disease: Associations with patterns of health service use. *Journal of Pediatric Psychology, 27*, 475–484.

Masuda, A., Cohen, L. L., Wicksell, R. K., Kemani, M. K., & Johnson, A. (2011). A case study: Acceptance and commitment therapy for pediatric sickle cell disease. *Journal of Pediatric Psychology, 36*(4), 398–408. doi:10.1093/jpepsy/jsq118

Mayes, S., Wolfe-Christensen, C., Mullins, L. L., & Cain, J. P. (2011). Psychoeducational screening in pediatric sickle cell disease: An evaluation of academic and health concerns in the school environment. *Children's Health Care, 40*, 101–115. doi:10.1080/02739615.2011.566465

McClellan, C. B., & Cohen, L. L. (2007). Family functioning in children with chronic illness compared with healthy controls: A critical review. *Journal of Pediatrics, 150*, 221–223. doi:10.1016/jpeds.2006.11.063

McClellan, C. B., Schatz, J. C., Puffer, E., Sanchez, C. E., Stancil, M. T., & Roberts, C. W. (2009). Use of handheld wireless technology for a home-based sickle cell pain management protocol. *Journal of Pediatric Psychology, 34*, 564–573. doi:10.1093/jpepsy/jsn121

McCrae, J. D., & Lumley, M. A. (1998). Health status in sickle cell disease: Examining the roles of pain coping strategies, somatic awareness, and negative affectivity. *Journal of Behavioral Medicine, 21*, 35–55.

Miller, S. T., Macklin, E. A., Pegelow, C. H., Kinney, T. R., Sleeper, L. A., Bello, J. A., et al. (2001). Silent infarction as a risk factor for overt stroke in children with sickle cell anemia: A report from the Cooperative Study of Sickle Cell Disease. *Journal of Pediatrics, 139*, 385–390.

Milner, P. F., Kraus, A. P., Sebes, J. I., Sleeper, L. A., Dukes, K. A., Embury, S. H., et al. (1991). Sickle cell disease as a cause of osteonecrosis of the femoral head. *The New England Journal of Medicine, 325*, 1476–1481. doi:10.1056/NEJM199111213252104

Moskowitz, J. T., Butensky, E., Harmatz, P., Vichinsky, E., Heyman, M. B., Acree, M., et al. (2007). Caregiving time in sickle cell disease: Psychological effects in maternal caregivers. *Pediatric Blood and Cancer, 48*, 64–71. doi:10.1002/pbc.20792

Mullins, L. L., Wolfe-Christensen, C., Chaney, J. M., Elkin, T. D., Wiener, L., Hullmann, S. E., et al. (2011). The relationship between single-parent status and parenting capacities in mothers of youth with chronic health conditions: The mediating role of income. *Journal of Pediatric Psychology, 36*, 249–257. doi:10.1093/jpepsy/jsqo80

Nagpal, K. C., Goldberg, M. F., & Rabb, M. F. (1977). Ocular manifestations of sickle hemoglobinopathies. *Survey of Ophthalmology, 21*, 391–411.

National Institutes of Health. (2002). *The management of sickle cell disease.* Washington, DC: US. Department of Health and Human Services.

Noll, R. B., Stith, L., Gartstein, M. A., Ris, M. D., Grueneich, R., Vannatta, K., et al. (2001). Neuropsycholocial functioning of youths with sickle cell disease: Comparison with non-chronically ill peers. *Journal of Pediatric Psychology, 26*, 69–78.

Ohene-Frempong, K., Weiner, S. J., Sleeper, L. A., Miller, S. T., Embury, S., Moohr, J. W., et al. (1998). Cerebrovascular accidents in sickle cell disease: Rates and risk factors. *Blood, 91*, 288–294.

Olujohungbe, A. B., Adeyoju, A., Yardumian, A., Akinyanju, O., Morris, J., Westerdale, N., et al. (2011). A prospective diary study of stuttering priapism in adolescents and young men with sickle cell anemia: Report of an international randomized control trial—The Priapism in Sickle Cell Study. *Journal of Andrology, 32*, 375–382. doi:10.2164/jandrol.110.010934

Palermo, T. M., Riley, C. A., & Mitchell, B. A. (2008). Daily functioning and quality of life in children with sickle cell disease pain: Relationship with family and neighborhood socioeconomic distress. *The Journal of Pain, 9*, 833–840. doi:10.1016/j.pain.2008.04.002

Pearson, H. A., Gallagher, D., Chilcote, R., Sullivan, E., Williams, J., Espeland, M., et al. (1985). Developmental pattern of splenic dysfunction in sickle cell disorders. *Pediatrics, 76*, 392–397.

Pegelow, C. H., Adams, R. J., McKie, V., Abboud, M., Berman, B., Miller, S. T., et al. (1995). Risk of recurrent stroke in patients with sickle cell disease treated with erythrocyte transfusions. *Journal of Pediatrics, 126*, 896–899.

Platt, O. S., Brambilla, D. J., Rosse, W. F., Milner, P. F., Castro, O., Steinberg, M. H., et al. (1994). Mortality in sickle cell disease. Life expectancy and risk factors for early death. *New England Journal of Medicine, 330*, 1639–1644.

Platt, O. S., Thorington, B. D., Brambilla, D. J., Milner, P. F., Rosse, W. F., Vichinsky, E., et al. (1991). Pain in sickle cell disease—Rates and risk factors. *The New England Journal of Medicine, 325*, 11–16. doi:10.1056/NEJM199107043250103

Pokala, H., Harris, S., Steckel, T., Dow, G., Hagemann, T., & Chemotherapy staff nurses of the Jimmy Everest Center for Childhood Cancer and Blood Disorders. (2012). *Fever and antibiotic delivery time in immune-compromised patients.* Poster presented at University of Oklahoma Health Sciences Center Quality Improvement Symposium.

Sharpe, J. N., Brown, R. T., Thompson, N. J., & Eckman, J. (1994). Predictors of coping with pain in mothers and their children with sickle cell syndrome. *Journal of the American Academy of Child and Adolescent Psychiatry, 33*, 1246–1255. doi:10.1097/00004583-199411000-00005

Smith, W. R., Penberthy, L. T., Bovbjerg, V. E., McClish, D. K., Roberts, J. D., Dahman, B., et al. (2008). Daily assessment of pain in adults with sickle cell disease. *Annals of Internal Medicine, 148*, 94–101. doi:10.7326/0003-4819-148-2-200802250-00004

Snyder, C. R., Hoza, B., Pelham, W. E., Rapoff, M., Ware, L., Danovsky, M., et al. (1997). The development and validation of the Children's Hope Scale. *Journal of Pediatric Psychology, 22*, 399–421. doi:10.1093/jpepsy/22.3.399

Steen, R. G., Reddick, W. E., Mulhern, R. K., Langston, J. W., Ogg, R. J., Bieberich, A. A., et al. (1998). Quantitative MRI of the brain in children with sickle cell disease reveals abnormalities unseen by conventional MRI. *Journal of Magnetic Resonance Imaging, 8*, 535–543. doi:10.1002/jmri.1880080304

Talano, J. A., & Cairo, M. S. (2015). Hematopoietic stem cell transplantation for sickle cell disease: State of the science. *European Journal of Haematology, 94*, 391–399. doi:10.1111/ejh.12447

Thompson, R. J., Armstrong, F. D., Kronenberger, W. G., Scott, D., McCabe, M. A., Smith, B., et al. (1999). Family functioning, neurocognitive functioning and behavior problems in children with sickle cell disease. *Journal of Pediatric Psychology, 24*, 491–498.

Thompson, R. J., Gil, K. M., Abrams, M. R., & Phillips, G. (1992). Stress, coping, and psychological adjustment of adults with sickle cell disease. *Journal of Consulting and Clinical Psychology, 60*, 433–440.

Thompson, R. J., Gil, K. M., Keith, B. R., Gustafson, K. E., George, L. K., & Kinney, T. R. (1994). Psychological adjustment of children with sickle cell disease: Stability and change over a 10-month period. *Journal of Consulting and Clinical Psychology, 62*, 856–860.

Tsaras, G., Owusu-Ansah, A., Boateng, F. O., & Amoateng-Adjepong, Y. (2009). Complications associated with sickle cell trait: A brief narrative review. *The American Journal of Medicine, 122*, 507–512. doi:10.1016/j.amjed.2008.12.020

U.S. Centers for Disease Control and Prevention. (2013). *Sickle cell disease: Data and statistics*. Retrieved March 8, 2014, from http://www.cdc.gov/ncbddd/sicklecell/data.htm

Vichinsky, E. P., Neumayr, L. D., Earles, A. N., Williams, R., Lennette, E., Dean, D., et al. (2000). Causes and outcomes of the acute chest syndrome in sickle cell disease. *The New England Journal of Medicine, 342*, 1855–1865. doi:10.1056/NEJM200006223422502

Voskaridou, E., Christoulas, D., Bilalis, A., Plata, E., Varvagiannis, K., Stamatopoulos, G., et al. (2010). The effect of prolonged administration of hydroxyurea on morbidity and mortality in adult patients with sickle cell syndromes: Results of a 17-year, single-center trial (LaSHS). *Blood, 115*, 2354–2363.

West, M. S., Wethers, D., Smith, J., & Steinberg, M. (1992). Laboratory profile of sickle cell disease: A cross-sectional analysis. The Cooperative Study of Sickle Cell Disease. *Journal of Clinical Epidemiology, 45*, 893–909. doi:10.1016/0895-4356(92)90073-V

Ziadini, M. S., Patterson, C. A., Pulgaron, E. R., Robinson, M. R., & Barakat, L. P. (2011). Health-related quality of life and adaptive behaviors of adolescents with sickle cell disease: Stress processing moderators. *Journal of Clinical Psychology in Medical Settings, 18*, 335–344. doi:10.1007/s10880-011-0254-3

Chapter 4
Translational Research and Clinical Applications in the Management of Cystic Fibrosis

Alexandra L. Quittner, Christina J. Nicolais, Estefany Saez-Flores, and Ruth Bernstein

Advancements in the diagnosis and treatment of cystic fibrosis (CF) have led to significant increases in life span. Recent data from the Cystic Fibrosis Foundation Registry (CFF, 2016) indicates that the median projected survival for an infant born with CF today is 39 years. In 2014, 50.7% of the CF population in the United States was comprised of adults. These increases in survival have been attributed to universal newborn screening for CF, the development of new medications to prevent and treat pulmonary exacerbations (Cohen-Cymberknoh, Shoseyov, & Kerem, 2011; Wainwright et al., 2015), and in the case of certain genotypes, modification of the underlying protein defect (Ramsey et al., 2011). For many patients, the treatment regimen now takes 2-4 hours per day (Sawicki, Sellers, & Robinson, 2009). Although these improvements in prognosis and disease progression are welcome, they have also dramatically increased patient and family perceptions of treatment burden (Sawicki et al., 2009, 2013). In addition, a recent international study indicates that both patients with CF and parent caregivers are at increased risk for depression and anxiety in comparison to community samples (Quittner, Goldbeck, et al., 2014). Thus, this chronic illness poses a unique set of challenges for individuals living with CF and their families.

Cystic fibrosis is a life-shortening, recessive genetic disorder affecting approximately 1 in 2500 live births worldwide (Ratjen et al., 2015). It is the result of having two mutations of the CF gene, which disrupt the exchange of salt and water across cell membranes, affecting multiple organs including the lungs, pancreas, liver, and

---

A.L. Quittner, Ph.D. (✉)
Department of Psychology and Pediatrics, University of Miami,
Coral Gables, FL 33146, USA
e-mail: aquittner@miami.edu

C.J. Nicolais, M.S. • E. Saez-Flores, B.A. • R. Bernstein, M.S.
Department of Psychology, University of Miami, Coral Gables, FL, USA
e-mail: nicolaisc@miami.edu; rbernstein@miami.edu

© Springer International Publishing Switzerland 2017
G.L. Welch, A.W. Harrist (eds.), *Family Resilience and Chronic Illness*,
Emerging Issues in Family and Individual Resilience,
DOI 10.1007/978-3-319-26033-4_4

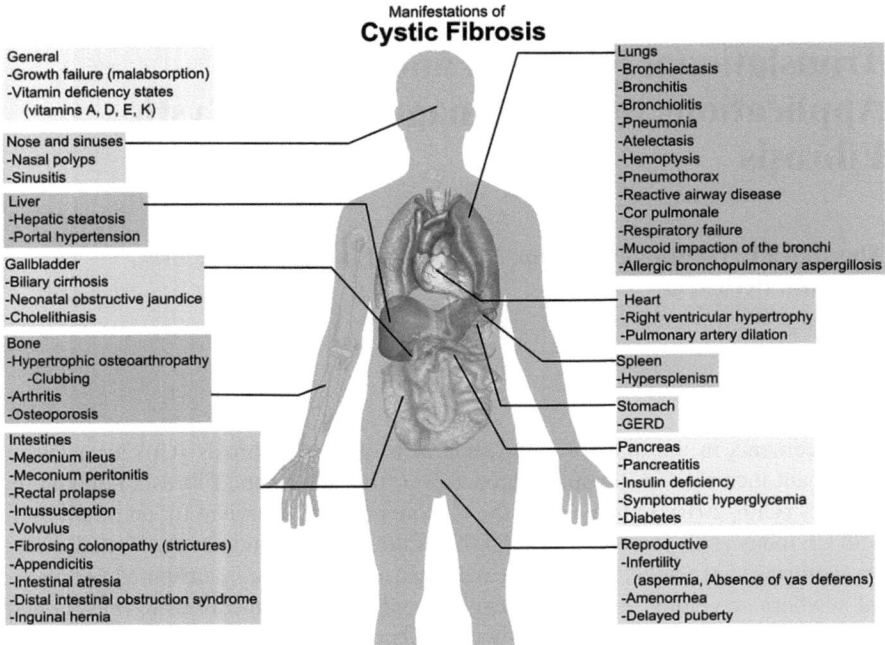

Fig. 4.1 Multisystemic effects of cystic fibrosis (Marcdante, Kliegman, Behrman, & Jenson, 2010). Reproduced with permissions from Wikimedia Commons

reproductive systems (Wallis, 2012; See Fig. 4.1). By 2010, all 50 US states and Washington, DC, implemented standardized newborn screening for CF (CFF, 2016) to increase early detection. Early diagnosis is critical to initiation of pancreatic enzymes for those who need them (>85%) to facilitate early weight gain and growth (Davis, 2006). In 2014, 64% of new diagnoses were identified as a result of an abnormal newborn screen (CFF, 2016). Early diagnosis and aggressive treatment have led to better health outcomes and longer survival (Accurso, Sontag, & Wagener, 2005; Farrell et al., 2005).

The majority of treatments are considered palliative and are aimed at slowing the secondary effects of the disease (e.g., pulmonary exacerbations, CF-related diabetes) and often include nebulized medications, inhaled antibiotics, airway clearance, pancreatic enzymes, and increased caloric intake (Ratjen et al., 2015). More recently in 2012, the first disease-modifying drug, Ivacaftor, received FDA approval for individuals ages 6 years and older who have the G551D mutation. Although a promising avenue for drug development, this represents only 4% of the CF population in the U.S. and Ivacaftor is extremely costly (approximately $373,000 per year), which is a potential barrier for adoption (O'Sullivan, Orenstein, & Milla, 2013).

Despite significant advances in the diagnosis and treatment of CF, it remains one of the most challenging chronic conditions to manage. Several key issues will be discussed in this chapter, including adherence to prescribed treatments, effects of

CF on family functioning and psychological distress, impact of infection control procedures on social functioning, and the difficulties of transitioning pediatric patients to adult care.

4.1 Literature Review and Implications

4.1.1 Adherence

4.1.1.1 Adherence to CF Treatments

Adherence to the prescribed treatment regimen for CF is one of the greatest challenges faced by individuals with CF and their families (Lomas, 2014; Quittner, Alpern, & Blackwell, 2012). The current regimen is primarily palliative, aimed at reducing respiratory and digestive symptoms, boosting calories, and improving growth. Recently, the first disease-modifying drug was approved for those with the G551D mutation, which represents approximately 4% of the US population (Ramsey et al., 2011). Despite major advances in the diagnosis and treatment of CF, management of this disease continues to be extremely time consuming and complex, requiring 2–4 h per day (Sawicki et al., 2009, 2013).

Routine, prescribed treatments for CF include airway clearance (twice a day for 20 min), enzymes with each meal and snack, boosting calories (up to 200% of the Recommended Daily Allowance), inhaled medications (i.e., Pulmozyme once a day; hypertonic saline twice a day for 20 min; cycling inhaled antibiotics twice a day for 20 min), fat soluble vitamins, and Azithromycin 3 days per week. Patients have reported substantial difficulties completing these treatments each day and perceive the regimen to be highly burdensome (Geller & Madge, 2011; Sawicki et al., 2013).

Rates of adherence to this regimen are quite low. A recent national study, using medication possession ratios from a national pharmacy database, indicated that adherence to pulmonary medications alone was 50% or less across the life span, from ages 6 to 70 years (Quittner, Zhang, et al., 2014; Fig. 4.2). In addition, a substantial decline in adherence was noted during adolescence. Poor adherence is related to a variety of negative health outcomes, including increased pulmonary exacerbations, more frequent hospitalizations, worse lung function, worse health-related quality of life, and increased symptoms of depression (Eakin, Bilderback, Boyle, Mogayzel, & Riekert, 2011; Hilliard, Eakin, Borrelli, Green, & Riekert, 2015; Quittner, Zhang, et al., 2014).

To date, few interventions have been tested to improve adherence (Goldbeck et al., 2014). Recently, a comprehensive intervention to improve knowledge of disease management, treatment skills, and adherence behaviors was conducted in adolescents at 18 CF Center in the US (iCARE; I Change Adherence and Raise Expectations). Preliminary evidence indicated that relative to standard care, the intervention group evidenced improvements in some areas of knowledge, in the

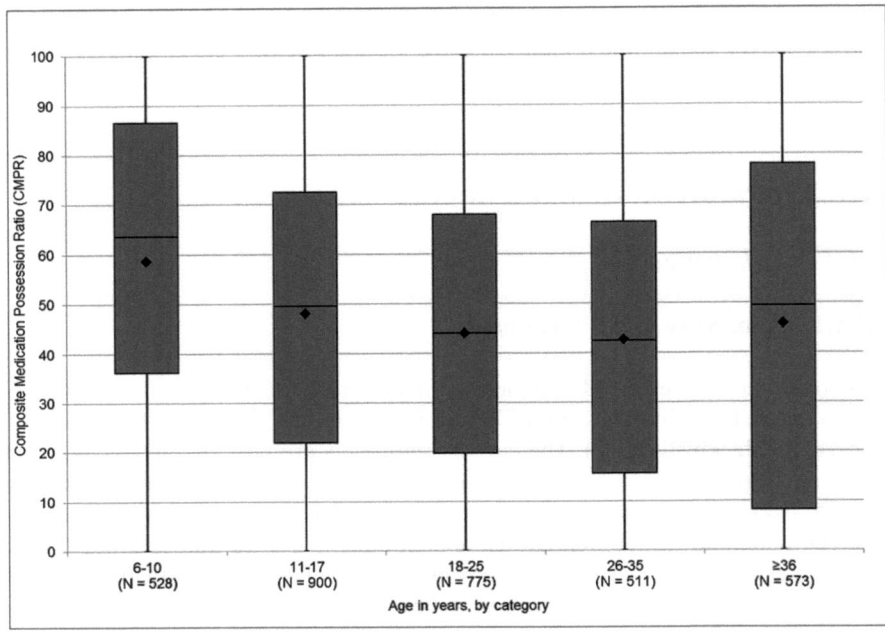

Fig. 4.2 Composite Medication Possession Ratio (CMPR) by age in years. The lower quartile, median, and upper quartile are represented by the bottom, midline, and top of each box, respectively. Minimum and maximum CMPR values are represented by the end points of the vertical lines. The CMPR is a composite measure of adherence to all prescribed pulmonary medication that evaluates medication possession based on prescription refill data (Quittner, Zhang, Marynchenko & Chopra, 2014). Reproduced with permissions from CHEST Publications

skills utilized to perform their treatments, and in health outcomes, such as BMI percentile and lung function. Brief, behavioral approaches have demonstrated the best efficacy in changing adherence behaviors and are more likely to be utilized in busy specialty clinics (Bernard & Cohen, 2004; Bradley, Madge, Morton, Quittner, & Elborn, 2012; Duff & Latchford, 2010; Marciel et al., 2010).

4.1.1.2 Impact of Adherence on Family Functioning

Family structure can affect the way in which families manage the treatment regimen (Gayer & Ganong, 2006). In a large study of 318 mothers at six CF centers, standardized questionnaires assessed adherence, family functioning, and child health over the past year. Mothers reported that they took primary responsibility for performing daily treatments and caring for their child with CF. Similar results were found for the mothers who were single, separated, divorced, or repartnered. Single mothers, however, took responsibility for a larger proportion of the daily treatments when the child was sick and reported a lack of support from others (e.g., family members, friends). Ratings of family coherence and regular routines were significantly associated with completing daily treatments among single mothers.

It is clear that family functioning is impacted by the burden of caring for a child with CF. Adherence is particularly associated with family functioning and some CF illness-management tasks are associated with more family dysfunction than others. Increasing calorie intake and enzyme use are two such requirements of illness management. Children with pancreatic-insufficient CF must adhere to a high calorie diet (120–150% of normal requirements; Matel & Milla, 2009) due to higher resting energy expenditure, typically low Body Mass Index (55% meeting BMI goals ages 2–19 years; CFF, 2016), and malfunction in pancreatic enzyme production. In addition to increased calorie intake, pancreatic enzyme replacement therapy is required for individuals with pancreatic-insufficient CF. These individuals must take oral pancreatic enzymes prior to meals to break down fats, proteins, and carbohydrates in the stomach. Enzyme therapy is a prescribed treatment for 87.3% of individuals with CF. Even when children take enzymes orally they may have inadequate energy intake (Morrison, Rawe, McCracken, Redmond, & Dodge, 1994). Children are often noncomplaint with enzyme use and increased calorie intake, which can be frustrating for parents who understand that poor nutritional status may be detrimental to recovery from infections and disease complications (Berlinski, Fan, Kozinetz, & Oermann, 2002).

Because of these disease management requirements, mealtimes can be contentious for families of children with pancreatic-insufficient CF. Thus, mealtimes provide an especially vivid snapshot of CF family functioning. Studies (e.g., Everhart, Fiese, Smyth, Borschuk, & Anbar, 2014) have used the Mealtime Observations Coding System (MICS) to observe the behaviors of families during video recorded typical mealtimes. The MICS coding system assesses family functions including task accomplishment, communication, interpersonal involvement, behavior control, role allocation, and affect regulation.

Results of mealtime observation studies using the MICS vary by the age of the family member with CF. In one study of 33 families with an infant or toddler with CF (ages 6–36 months) and 33 matched control families, video recordings of typical family mealtimes were coded using the MICS. Families also completed a measure assessing frequencies of problematic mealtime behaviors. Results demonstrated that families of children with CF have lower overall mealtime functioning, and lower communication, interpersonal involvement, behavioral control, affect management, and roles scores than non-CF families. In families with CF, better functioning was associated with fewer mealtime behavior problems though this difference was not related to weight status or calorie consumption (Mitchell, Powers, Byars, Dickstein, & Stark, 2004).

In another study with 28 families of children with CF (age 6–12.9 years) and 27 age-matched healthy peers, families with children with CF showed lower overall mealtime functioning (as measured by the MICS) compared to families without a child with CF (Janicke, Mitchell, & Stark, 2005). Families with a child with CF also had lower functioning in the specific domains of communication, affect management, interpersonal involvement, and behavioral control.

A third study observed 19 families of children and adolescents (ages 8–19) with CF (Everhart et al., 2014). Parents completed the Treatment Adherence Rating Scale (TARS), a measure assessing adherence to their prescribed treatment regimen in the previous 2 weeks, and videos of families during typical mealtimes were coded using the MICS. Family functioning fell in the "unhealthy" range in all subscales of the MICS aside from role allocation. Lower socioeconomic status in these families was also associated with lower family functioning. Better family functioning was associated with better adherence to antibiotics but worse adherence to enzymes.

Another study of children and adolescents examined how adherence is associated with family relationship quality (DeLambo, Ivers-Landis, Drotar, & Quittner, 2004). Ninety-six children and adolescents with CF, ages 9–16 years, and their parents participated. When parents were married, both parents were required to participate. Parent and child participants individually completed the TARS and together they completed a 20 min discussion about CF-related conflictual issues and non-CF conflictual issues. The Iowa Family Interaction Rating Scale assessed the quality of family relationships demonstrated during the 20 min discussion. Results showed that relationship quality, as observed in conflict discussions, was associated with both child and parent reports of adherence to airway clearance and aerosolized medication treatments.

4.1.1.3 Family Interventions to Improve Adherence

The treatment burden inherent in CF places strain on the child, on the parent, and on family interaction. Child resistance to treatment is common in CF and has led to awareness of need for behavioral management strategies to improve treatment adherence. To date, few examples of proposed interventions exist and most lack empirical validation. One single-subject design study provides an example of a time-out-based discipline intervention to improve adherence (McClellan, Cohen & Moffett, 2009). This intervention, as studied, requires parents to give clear and defined instruction and time-out when children do not comply. This preliminary study showed hopeful improvements in compliance and problem behaviors. Thus, behavioral interventions like time-out may increase adherence and parent–child communication across the lifespan, though further research will be required to validate this type of intervention.

4.1.2 Translations and Applications

Two key suggestions for clinical application can be drawn from the literature just reviewed:

1. Use brief behavioral approaches to improve adherence to CF treatments.
2. Target child and parent problem-solving skills so as to increase effective communication and functioning within the family (Quittner et al., 2010).

Families are also impacted by, and can impact issues other than, adherence as can be seen in the extant research about psychological distress and family functioning when a child has CF.

4.2 Family Functioning and Psychological Distress

4.2.1 Impact of Family Functioning on the Child

Parent functioning can play a significant role in how well functioning the family is as a whole. One study by Quittner and colleagues (Quittner, Espelage, Opipari, Carter, & Eid, 1998) examined 33 couples caring for a child with CF and 33 couples matched on patient age and gender, sibling age and gender, health history, parent age and education, years married or cohabitating, parent employment and health history, and family income. Couples were required to complete a demographic interview and daily phone diaries to assess their activity patterns and mood, as well as the frequency of positive interactions between the parents. Additionally, couples individually sorted cards with various household and childcare tasks written on them in two ways: "How do you and your spouse divide these tasks?" and "How would you like you and your spouse to divide these tasks?." Results showed significantly more marital role strain in couples parenting a child with CF compared to couples parenting matched controls. Specifically, on the diary and self-report measures, parents of children with CF reported more role frustration, conflict over child-rearing issues, and time spent caring for children, as well as fewer positive interactions with their partner. Mothers of children with CF reported more parenting stress, and more medical care responsibilities, than fathers of children with CF and parents of non-ill children. Couples parenting children with CF also engaged in fewer recreation activities and spent less time in recreation than parents of matched controls. Despite this, parents of children with CF spent more time playing with their children than matched controls. Notably, this study was published in 1998 when life expectancy for children with CF was much lower, but treatment burden was also lower. Thus, generalizations of these findings should be made with caution.

Many studies have found that better family functioning is associated with better child functioning. One Australian study sought to examine the relations between functioning of families with an adolescent (ages 12–18 years) with CF and adolescent functioning (Szyndler, Towns, van Asperen, & McKay, 2005). Questionnaires assessing disease-specific health-related quality of life, psychopathology, and family dynamics were completed by 52 adolescents with CF. Results indicated that family cohesion (family commitment and support), expressiveness (encouragement to express feelings directly), and organization (planning of family events and responsibilities) were associated with better adolescent mental health. Family conflict was associated with poorer clinically measured physical health. Family cohesion was associated with better physical functioning, energy, emotional functioning, and body image, as well as fewer eating problems as measured by a disease-specific quality of life questionnaire.

> **Box 4.1. Implications for Practice**
> For our family, cystic fibrosis is so much more than the name of a disease. From the moment our daughter was diagnosed at 2 weeks of age, it became our reality and our new way of life. We were thrust into a world as new parents where, instead of just worrying about sleepless nights, colic and dirty diapers, we were facing a harsh new reality that included expensive medications, hours of treatments, and the possibility of a shortened life span for our precious new bundle of joy. We were told our child's lungs would begin to fill with a thick, sticky mucus and that many repeated lung infections would lead to a loss of lung function. While holding our infant, we were told about the possibility of a lung transplant in her future. Then we were given a life expectancy that was completely unacceptable. We were crushed, but we knew we had to be strong for our daughter. In the beginning, it was incredibly hard for us. Trying to administer pills and breathing treatments to an infant takes some getting used to. While those areas have gotten easier as she has grown, there are aspects of this ugly disease that never become less difficult to swallow. Our hearts stop each time a throat swab comes back positive for bacteria, or any time the pulmonary function test percentages drop. It never becomes easier to hear the words hospitalization or surgery thrown around. The hopes and dreams we have for her future are coupled with fear and worry. The hardest part, however, is watching our child endure pill taking, breathing treatments, throat swabs, X-rays, blood draws, GI tubes, surgeries, and more while showing strength unparalleled by most adults. We ache for her, we wish we could take it from her, and we are in awe of her—her strength, courage, and determination—all at the same time. Cystic fibrosis can dictate a large portion of her life…but it cannot steal her spirit.
>
> —Alyssa Siler, Parent

4.2.2 Depression and Anxiety in Families with CF

Individuals living with chronic illnesses and their caregivers are at increased risk for elevated symptoms of depression and anxiety (Fauman, Pitch, Han, Niedner, Reske, & LeVine, 2011; Pinquart & Shen, 2011), and these psychological symptoms negatively affect disease management and health outcomes (Moussavi et al., 2007). In CF specifically, psychological distress has been associated with worse adherence, worse health outcomes and health care utilization, and worse health-related quality of life (Havermans, Colpaert, & Dupont, 2008; Riekert, Bartlett, Boyle, Krishnan, & Rand, 2007; Smith, Modi, Quittner, & Wood, 2010).

Recently, an international screening study in nine countries measured symptoms of depression and anxiety in 6088 patients with CF and 4102 parent caregivers (The International Depression Epidemiological Study [TIDES]; Quittner, Goldbeck,

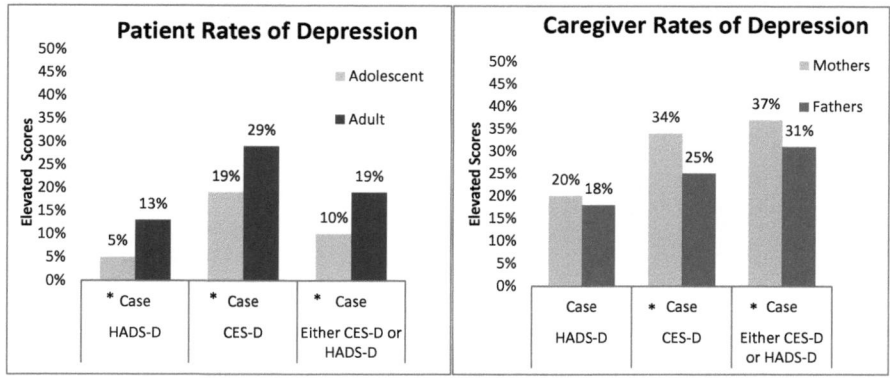

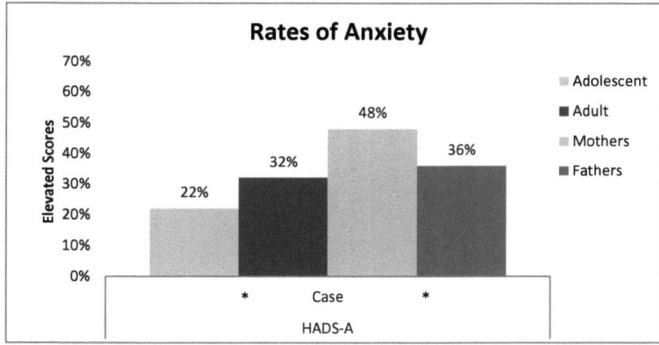

Fig. 4.3 Rates of depression and anxiety by respondent. *$p < 0.001$, HADS-D = Hospital anxiety and depression scale-depression, HADS-A = Hospital anxiety and depression scale-anxiety. CES-D = Center for epidemiologic studies depression scale (Quittner, Goldbeck, et al., 2014) Reproduced with permissions from BMJ Publishing Group, Ltd

et al., 2014). In the US alone, 1207 patients were screened, with 25% reporting elevations in depression and 35% reporting elevated symptoms of anxiety. Across all countries, 17% of patients with CF reported elevations in depression and 30% reported elevations in anxiety, which are two times the rates found in community samples (Dierker et al., 2001; Eisenberg, Gollust, Golberstein, & Hefner, 2007). We also found evidence of comorbid psychological distress. In 1122 dyads, adolescents with CF were 2.39 times more likely to be above the cut-off for depression if either parent was elevated and they were 2.22 times more likely to be anxious if a parent was elevated (see Fig. 4.3).

These results led to the formation of an international guidelines committee on mental health in CF. This committee has formally recommended annual screening of these symptoms in patients ages 12 and older and in parents of children with CF birth to age 17, using the PHQ-9 and GAD-7 (Quittner et al., 2016; see Fig. 4.4).

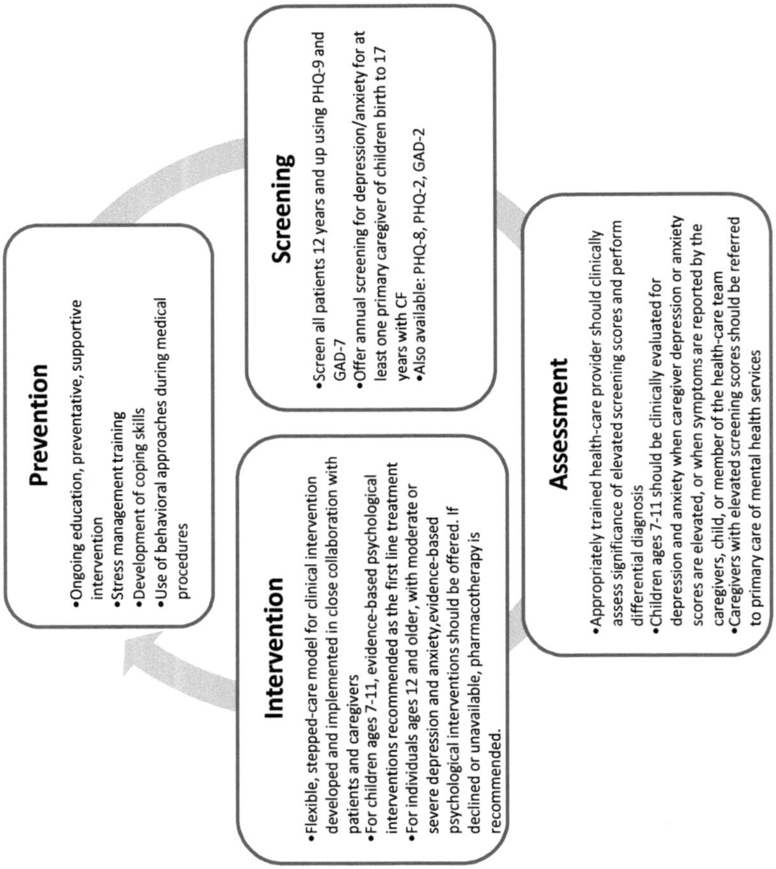

Prevention
- Ongoing education, preventative, supportive intervention
- Stress management training
- Development of coping skills
- Use of behavioral approaches during medical procedures

Screening
- Screen all patients 12 years and up using PHQ-9 and GAD-7
- Offer annual screening for depression/anxiety for at least one primary caregiver of children birth to 17 years with CF
- Also available: PHQ-8, PHQ-2, GAD-2

Assessment
- Appropriately trained health-care provider should clinically assess significance of elevated screening scores and perform differential diagnosis
- Children ages 7-11 should be clinically evaluated for depression and anxiety when caregiver depression or anxiety scores are elevated, or when symptoms are reported by the caregivers, child, or member of the health-care team
- Caregivers with elevated screening scores should be referred to primary care of mental health services

Intervention
- Flexible, stepped-care model for clinical intervention developed and implemented in close collaboration with patients and caregivers
- For children ages 7-11, evidence-based psychological interventions recommended as the first line treatment
- For individuals ages 12 and older, with moderate or severe depression and anxiety, evidence-based psychological interventions should be offered. If declined or unavailable, pharmacotherapy is recommended.

Fig. 4.4 Assessing and treating depression and anxiety in CF

In addition to annual screening, the committee recommended the use of preventative methods, including psychoeducation to normalize these symptoms and cognitive-behavioral interventions to improve coping skills.

4.2.3 Impact of CF on Siblings

Having a sibling with a serious chronic illness affects not only parents but healthy siblings (Williams, 1997). Given the time-consuming nature of the treatments for CF, parents often find it difficult to spend equal amounts of time with each sibling. Two studies have found evidence of parental differential treatment, with more time and attention dedicated to the child with CF compared to the healthy sibling, and harsher discipline strategies reported by the healthy child (Foster et al., 2001; Quittner & Opipari, 1994). Parents themselves are aware that they spend less time with other siblings, particularly when the child with CF is sick or hospitalized. Parents may also be less tolerant of the healthy siblings' misbehavior but in most cases, this is unintentional. In contrast, parents also identify the benefits of growing up with a sibling with CF, such as increased personal growth, maturation, and family closeness (Williams, Ridder, Setter, & Liebergen, 2009).

Benefits in quality of life have also been found among healthy siblings. In a Belgian study at two CF centers, quality of life (QoL) and impact of illness were measured in 39 healthy children who had a brother or sister with CF (Havermans et al., 2010). Surprisingly, siblings of patients with CF scored higher on all of the QoL scales compared to healthy controls, including feeing healthier, having less bodily pain, better physical functioning, fewer behavior problems, and feeling more positive about their role in family activities. These findings may be the result of observing a sibling dealing with treatments and illnesses on a daily basis, which changed their perspective on their own QoL. However, siblings of children who had recently been hospitalized reported more negative impacts than those whose siblings were not hospitalized. Evidence of long-term resilience was found in a longitudinal study among young adults who had grown up with a sibling with CF (Wennström, Isberg, Wirtberg, & Ryden, 2011). The authors found no differences in self-esteem between siblings of young adults with CF compared to a healthy reference group. Thus, healthy siblings are at-risk for parental differential treatment while they are growing up, particularly during medical crises, but also report benefits in terms of increased maturity. Parents could benefit from greater awareness of the healthy child's needs and encouragement to equalize their time and attention.

4.2.4 Protective Factors in Children with CF

Families and children with CF are relatively resilient and generally function well at home and at school, particularly when their health is stable. For example, themes extracted from exploratory qualitative interviews with young adults with CF, ages

20–26 years, in Minneapolis, Minnesota, suggested that they resemble their peers in important ways, such as having jobs and friends, participating in social activities, and setting long-term goals (Palmer & Boisen, 2002). Adolescents with CF reported that they found meaning in their daily treatments by considering it a positive time to devote to themselves. They also reported that having CF allowed them to view life events with more perspective and not worry about unimportant things. Furthermore, they reported that they live fuller lives and appreciate life events more because of their limited life expectancy. Participants also reported having strengths and skills as a result of having CF, including a better ability to maneuver the health care system and insurance than their peers, and being more compassionate, caring, and sensitive. Although adults with CF reported gaining independence later than their siblings without CF, they also perceived themselves as more mature earlier in their lives (Palmer & Boisen, 2002).

Adolescents with CF also use a number of coping skills and adaptive strategies to manage their feelings about having CF. One of these is optimism. Szyndler and colleagues (2005) found that most adolescents (ages 12–18 years) with CF were hopeful and positive about their futures. A second study of 25 adolescents used a questionnaire-based approach and found that better acceptance of the diagnosis was associated with less disability (defined as limitations in physical and psychological functioning), anxiety, and depression (Casier et al., 2008). Optimistic acceptance, a construct representing a combination of optimism and acceptance, is characterized by a positive, confident, determined, and perspective-driven way of coping with CF. In a study of adolescents and young adults, patients completed the CF Coping Questionnaire. Results indicated that most participants with CF used optimistic acceptance (a scale on the questionnaire) to manage their feelings about CF (Abbott et al., 2001). Importantly, optimistic acceptance has been associated with better adherence in adolescents and young adults with CF. Another study showed that optimism was associated with better social functioning, emotional responses, interpersonal relationships, future concerns, and physical functioning (as measured by the Cystic Fibrosis Quality of Life Questionnaire; Abbott, Hart, Morton, Gee, & Conway, 2008) in adults with CF. Thus, psychological interventions which increased optimism and acceptance might be effective for improving both adaptation to CF and adherence to the treatment regimen.

While children with CF engage in protective practices, there are also a number of behaviors and attitudes associated with negative outcomes in children with CF. For example, Abbot and colleagues previously discussed study identified distraction as a coping mechanism associated with only partial adherence to treatment regimens (Abbott et al., 2001). Also in this study, avoidant coping (i.e., avoiding thinking about CF to decrease distress) was associated with nonadherence to physiotherapy and enzymes, but more adherence to exercise therapy.

Finally, in a cross-sectional study, 46 individuals with CF, 128 individuals with Type 1 Diabetes (mean age of 14.7), and their caregivers completed questionnaires about the adolescent's spiritual coping, behavior, and attribution styles. Participants with CF had negative spiritual coping skills (defined as feelings of uncertainty, struggle, and rejection by a God figure) that were associated with more internalizing problems (Reynolds, Mrug, & Guion, 2013). These findings demonstrate the importance of optimistic coping and suggest a positive impact of positive spiritual coping on health outcomes.

4.3 Interventions to Improve CF Family Functioning

One behavioral intervention to improve family functioning targeted family mealtime and has demonstrated effectiveness with regard to its impact on affect management (Janicke, Mitchell, Quittner, Piazza-Waggoner, & Stark, 2008). The effectiveness of this behavioral intervention ("Be In Charge!") was compared to that of nutrition education alone. The "Be In Charge!" intervention targeted increasing caloric intake and weight gain in children age 4–12 years with CF. Parents and children met in separate, weekly, 90-min sessions. In sessions, parents received education about using a daily nutrition diary, meal-specific nutrition (i.e., snack, breakfast, lunch, dinner), and behavioral management strategies to motivate their children. The child group received nutritional education, behavioral practice eating a high-calorie meal in-session, and rewards for meeting daily energy goals. Each family also recorded three evening meals that occurred within the duration of the intervention and videos were coded using the MICS. This study yielded hopeful results with a number of families moving from unhealthy to healthy family interactions between baseline and a 1-year follow-up. In addition, more families in the intervention group significantly improved in affect management from pretreatment to 1-year follow-up compared to families in the nutrition education only group.

4.3.1 Translations and Applications

Three key suggestions for practice based on the research reviewed include:

1. Regularly screen children with CF and their parents for mental health problems including depression and anxiety. The International Depression Epidemiological Study suggests that patients and their parents complete the PHQ-9 and the GAD-7 annually (Quittner, Goldbeck, et al., 2014).
2. Make referrals for mental health interventions as necessary based on the results of annual screenings and their interactions with families affected by CF.
3. Introduce simple behavioral strategies in families of preschool-aged children with CF to improve family functioning and child behaviors at mealtimes (Janicke et al., 2008).

4.4 Impact of Infection Control Guidelines on Social Support

CF is currently the only chronic disease that requires complete patient segregation. This is due to the possible transmission of multiresistant bacteria between patients (e.g., *Pseudomonas aeruginosa, Burkholderia cepacia, MRSA, M. abscessus*), which can accelerate the severity of lung disease, leading to earlier mortality (Orchard & Bilton, 2014; Strausbaugh & Davis, 2007). To limit the risk of transmission of these pathogens among patients or between patients and providers, the Cystic Fibrosis Foundation (CFF) has published infection prevention and control (IP&C) guidelines, most recently in 2013 (Saiman et al., 2013). These strict guidelines advise healthcare providers to wear a fluid-resistant gown and latex gloves when caring for all individuals with CF. If a patient is suspected or confirmed to have a pathogen that is communicable through droplets (e.g., sneezing, coughing), masks and eye protection must also be worn.

Of the 77 guidelines in the 2013 update, one of the most impactful to CF patients is the recommendation for complete patient segregation. Patients are not allowed to be in the same waiting room, they must be separated by at least 6 ft, regardless of respiratory tract cultures, and they are advised not to meet outside the clinic for any social events (e.g., family education days, support groups, camps). Some CF centers have tried cohort segregation, scheduling patients who have the same pathogen on the same clinic day. The 2013 update to the IP&C guidelines recommends against cohort segregation because they could be harboring an unidentified pathogen, suggesting all patients with CF be separated regardless of their respiratory culture.

4.4.1 Clinical Implications and Interventions

Although it has been over 10 years since the release of the first IP&C guidelines (Saiman & Siegel, 2003), patients, providers, and families have found them challenging to implement. One of these challenges is educating the CF community about the importance of these guidelines. Zhou and colleagues (Zhou, Garber, & Saiman, 2008) found that, of 158 CF care centers, only 103 centers (65%) had written infection control policies, and many were not consistent with the IP&C recommendations. In a follow-up study by Garber and colleagues (2008), 49% of 528 healthcare providers at 25 randomly selected CF centers were either unaware or lacked access to guidelines. Thus, not having a copy of the guidelines was a significant barrier to both implementing and adhering to them (Garber et al., 2008). The authors concluded that additional education for providers was needed.

In terms of patient adherence to the infection control guidelines, Masterson and colleagues (Masterson, Wildman, Newberry, & Omlor, 2011) surveyed 74 individuals, ages 9 years through 43 years, at one CF center. They found that 27% of patients were not adherent to the guidelines and this was related to age, with older teens and young adults reporting more contact with friends and non-first-degree relatives with CF, than those who were 12 and younger. Those reporting poor adherence to the guidelines did not believe their risk of acquiring new pathogens was very high and they reported that having a close friend with CF was very helpful.

In a recent survey of 25 randomly selected CF Centers in the U.S., 532 patients, ages 16 years and up, and 867 family members of CF patients younger than 16 years, completed questions about their knowledge of and attitudes toward the infection control guidelines, as well as their own adherence to them (Miroballi et al., 2012). Surprisingly, only 65% of participants were aware of the CFF's infection control guidelines and 34% reported never discussing them with their healthcare team. Although 83% of the participants knew that CF pathogens could be transmitted between patients, only 64% understood that patients should avoid being in close contact with others with CF, even when not actively showing symptoms (e.g., coughing). Further, only 42% of respondents were confident in their ability to avoid close contact with other CF patients during clinic visits. A major predictor of better knowledge and a more adherent attitude was the number of discussions they had with their healthcare team about the guidelines. Just one discussion significantly increased the odds of higher knowledge scores (Miroballi et al., 2012). Thus, patient–provider communication appears to be a major barrier to adequate implementation.

One of the major consequences of implementing the IP&C guidelines is a decrease in social support, which is directly linked to higher self-esteem, better adherence, and improved health-related quality of life (Herzer, Umfress, Aljadeff, Ghai, & Zakowski, 2009). For example, peer support has been shown to positively affect treatment adherence, with friends reminding and encouraging teens to do their treatments, reducing social isolation, and increasing emotional support (Barker, Driscoll, Modi, Light, & Quittner, 2012).

Few studies have explored the psychosocial effects of the IP&C guidelines on CF patients and their families. An early study by Russo and colleagues (Russo, Donnelly, & Reid, 2006) surveyed 75 parents and 23 children at one CF center in Belfast, examining patient and parent attitudes toward the implementation of stricter infection control guidelines. Their infection control practices closely resembled the updated 2013 IP&C guidelines. Although most parents and pediatric patients agreed that segregation during hospital stays was important, participants anticipated that implementation would have negative effects on both patients and caregivers. Children mentioned issues such as boredom, limitations on movement, loneliness, anxiety, stigma, and social isolation.

In attempting to address potential decreases in peer-to-peer support, we developed a web-based peer support platform (i.e., CFfone) that allowed adolescents and adults with CF to communicate via phone or internet "chat" (Marciel, Saiman, Quittell, Dawkins, & Quittner, 2010). We sought to improve knowledge of disease management, social support, and adherence. The NIH mandated that we monitor the patients' "chat" to reduce misinformation and to identify those who were experiencing psychological distress. Although unexpected, we found that a significant percentage of adolescents on the CFfone website were posting information that reflected emotional distress (e.g., depressive thoughts, fears about upcoming medical procedures) and referrals to mental health professionals in their community were made on several occasions. Preliminary findings suggested that social support did improve in the study patients; however, there were few changes in knowledge or adherence (Quittner et al., 2013). Thus, peer-to-peer support for adolescents may have to be "moderated" by a trained health care provider to avoid these high-risk situations. Although electronic platforms may be one solution to patient segregation, a recent study (Helms, Dellon, & Prinstein, 2014) found that even with constant electronic interactions with other CF teens (over 7 hours per week via internet and phone), patients still reported in-person interactions, despite the risks of infection. Thus, improving peer support in CF is still a major challenge in need of intervention.

4.4.2 Translations and Applications

Two suggestions for clinical practice based on these findings include:

1. Assess infection control knowledge annually and remediate gaps in knowledge.
2. Inform patients of their culture results so that they can make informed decisions.

4.5 Transition from Pediatric to Adult Care

4.5.1 Transition of Responsibility

As children with CF grow older, there is a critical need to transition responsibility for the daily treatment regimen from parents to the young adolescent. The goal of transition of responsibility is that the parent shifts from a "complete director" of their child's medical care to near noninvolvement (Williams, Mukhopadhyay, Dowell, & Coyle, 2007). This process parallels the child's transition from an "overwhelming recipient" to an "independent administrator" of their medical care, with parental involvement returning only during periods of illness or hospitalization (Iles & Lowton, 2010).

Although most families transition the majority of responsibility to the teen by the age of 15, this transition is not always successful. In one study, participants ages 10–17 years at six pulmonary centers across three states completed a daily phone diary; additionally, electronic monitoring was used to track their use of nebulized medications (Modi, Marciel, Slater, Drotar, & Quittner, 2008). Older adolescents in this study spent less time with parents conducting medical activities compared to preadolescents, and preadolescents spent significantly less time completing treatments alone than adolescents. Data also suggested a pattern of decreasing parental supervision with age, though participants age 16 and 17 showed higher parental supervision than 15-year-old participants. Across all participants, those who spent more time supervised by their mother during treatments had better treatment adherence.

Other studies of young adults corroborate this research finding qualitatively with self-reports that they were generally responsible for their own care well before adulthood though they experienced difficulties taking the initiative to complete their care independently, without their parents' reminders and encouragement (Palmer & Boisen, 2002).

As adolescents become more responsible for their own care, they are also increasingly responsible for communicating their concerns directly to their care team. This open communication can be complicated by the long-standing personal relationship that most adolescents have with their pediatric care team (Iles & Lowton, 2008). By the time some patients with CF become adolescents, their care team is protective of them, exhibiting a familial relationship. Therefore, adolescents may avoid telling their care team about their medical issues for fear of worrying them, thereby further limiting open communication. In light of these problems, clinics have made recent efforts to improve communication with adolescent and young adult patients so that these patients are comfortable independently communicating with their CF care team. Many clinics now meet individually with adolescent patients before inviting parents into clinic rooms, or meet with the patient for the first part of the session and the parents and patient for the second part of the session. Other clinics have clinic days dedicated to treating adolescents and, on these days, format appointments so that they closely resemble adult clinic appointments.

As with their care team, adolescent and young adult CF patients often feel that they need to protect their parents from negative health information. One qualitative study of 50 individuals age 13–24 and 23 CF healthcare professionals in Southeast England concluded that patients may not effectively communicate health concerns to their parents (Iles & Lowton, 2010) in an attempt to protect them. Poor parent–child communication is problematic as young adults may not always be prepared for independence with regard to their care, and typically perceive some parental involvement as supportive.

According to semistructured interviews with 24 adolescents (ages 11–18) with CF from South Florida and Cincinnati, adolescents find specific parent behaviors especially supportive during the time of their increased medical independence. These behaviors include treatment reminders, assistance and monitoring, assistance with transportation to clinics, navigation of the medical system, and allowance of autonomy when making decisions (Barker et al., 2012).

The period of transition of disease management responsibility from the parent to the child parallels a transfer from a multidisciplinary care team in a pediatric clinic to a multidisciplinary care team in an adult clinic. This transfer is recommended at age 14 (Yankaskas, Marshall, Sufian, Simom, & Rodman, 2004) though the actual age of transfer may be highly varied (McLaughlin et al., 2008; CFF, 2016). According to interviews with young adults ages 12–24 years, a number of psychosocial issues can complicate this transfer to adult care (Iles & Lowton,

2008). These include the adolescents' concerns about leaving home; worries about how CF will impact the interpersonal relationships that they have and will have in the future; and anticipation of worsening health and the associated mental, physical, and financial difficulties. Many adolescents also worry about how they will manage their health without their pediatric multidisciplinary care team.

Although many families successfully complete the shift of responsibility from the parent to the patient without much consideration for the process, the transition is characterized by a number of events. First, with increasing child age, parental supervision of medical treatments decreases (Modi et al., 2008). The responsibility changes from being exclusively that of the parent to a collaboration of both the parent and the child. Collaboration happens when the adolescent shares information with the parent, when the adolescent requests the parent's opinion, and when both parties express their own points of view about health decisions (Miller, 2009). While parental supervision of medical responsibilities declines with age, parents typically remain involved in supervising the other aspects of their adolescents' lives (e.g., work, school; Modi et al., 2008) as expected of adolescent–parent relationships.

4.5.2 Interventions to Facilitate Transition to Adult Care

Clearly, the transition of responsibility and ownership is complicated and requires attention to ensure that it occurs successfully. One of the most effective ways of ensuring that children with CF become adults who are independently responsible for their health care is to include them early and often in their medical care. Table 4.1 provides recommendations for addressing typical challenges associated with the transition of responsibility from the parent to the adolescent. One of the primary recommendations is that children be included in the transition of responsibility in successive approximations, one responsibility at a time (Madan et al., 2014). For example, with regard to dornase alfa, an inhaled mucolytic, children with CF first become responsible around age 6 years for the small jobs of turning on the compressor, holding the t-bar, and turning off the compressor. As they proceed through childhood to adolescence they should gain responsibilities in treatment and ultimately take responsibility for the entire process from retrieving the medication from the refrigerator to replacing and cleaning the filter. This process can take place with all health care responsibilities associated with CF such that by late adolescence the child is fully responsible for all of his or her daily treatments in a gradual and structured manner.

Collaborative decision making is another way to structure the transition of responsibility from the parent to the child (Miller, 2009). As with the transition of treatment responsibility, health decision making should involve the child as early as possible. Including children with CF in medical decision making early in their lives helps them to gain knowledge about the management and symptoms of their disease. It similarly provides an opportunity for the parent to model effective health decision making. When developmentally appropriate, the parent should explain

Table 4.1 Challenges and recommendations for transition

Challenge	Recommendations
Clinic visit independence	Meet with the child independently beginning in early adolescence; meet jointly with parent(s) and adolescent (Madan et al., 2014)
Readiness for transfer	Measure disease management including knowledge and skills; use results to guide remediation and transition
Lack of disease knowledge and skills, poor adherence	Assess knowledge, skills, and adherence regularly, and remediate (Quittner, Alpern, & Blackwell, 2012; Sawicki et al., 2011)
	Include child early and often in the management of their disease to increase independence and competence (Flume, 2009)
	Discuss health insurance and system-related issues with family; include adolescents in discussions
Child communication with parents and providers	Train families in positive communication and shared decision making (Madan et al., 2014)
	Encourage children and adolescents to bring questions to clinic
"Letting go" of pediatric providers	Gradually transition from pediatric care to adult care. Begin discussion of transfer in late primary school years (Pai & Schwartz, 2011; Tuchman et al., 2010)
	Patient, pediatric provider, and adult provider meet before transfer to establish similarities and differences between pediatric and adult care and to "transfer trust" from the pediatric to the adult provider (Madan et al., 2014)
	Create a transfer plan so that the parent, child, and provider are adequately prepared for the transfer to adult care (Sawicki et al., 2011)
CF impedes normative transitions	Provide extra medical, mental health, and social support in periods of normative transition (e.g., college, marriage, living independently; Madan et al., 2014)
Lack of peer support	Encourage disclosure to peers who may assist with normalizing independence and behave in helpful and supportive ways (Modi, Quittner, & Boyle, 2010)
Anxiety and depression	Complete annual screening of anxiety and depression symptoms. Use these results to anticipate barriers to transfer and intervene with support from mental health providers as necessary (Quittner et al., 2016)

reasons for, and factors related to, treatment-related decisions. The parent should then begin asking the child's opinions. Children have described this behavior as helpful because, "there is value simply in being heard" (Miller, 2009, p. 258). The parent should gradually transition to a source of support and advice, with the child being the primary decision maker. Notably, this strategy is more effective when healthcare professionals also begin to speak directly to the adolescent, while still involving the parent in communication. This dialog reinforces the idea of collaborative communication. Similarly, by including children in the decision-making process, parents help them to understand the consequences and benefits of disease self-management, while also allowing the child to practice self-management in a scaffolded experience.

Systemic interventions with adolescents preparing to take on the responsibility for their own care are few though necessary with increasing projected life expectancies and more individuals with CF needing adult care. CF R.I.S.E. (Helmers, 2010) is a tool set developed to aid the transition of responsibility and transfer of care. This intervention includes assessments of CF knowledge, a responsibilities checklist to assess the adolescent's self-management, and a progress report to track movement toward transfer and achievement of intermediate transition goals. This system provides practitioners with assessments necessary to ensure that the transition of ownership progresses appropriately, to understand where gaps in knowledge and skills exist, and to prepare the adolescent for transfer to adult care. Programs like CF R.I.S.E. are necessary to ensure the smooth and successful transition of the child with CF into an adult with CF who is proficient in self-management.

Another multidimensional CF transfer model including a patient transition clinical pathway, collaboration with the adult clinic, and measurement of transfer readiness, has been evaluated and found feasible and acceptable (Gravelle, Paone, Davidson, & Chilvers, 2015). Using this model, participants complete age-appropriate clinical checklists and screening tools, education on knowledge and disease awareness, and disease and healthcare system skill-building. They also participate in a "CF Pre-graduation Workshop" approximately 1–2 years before their transfer to adult care that introduces them and their parents to local adult care teams and provides education about important issues for adolescents with cystic fibrosis like sexuality, self-advocacy, and medication adherence. Pilots of this intervention included pre- and post-surveys of patients and parents. Patients' disease knowledge improved pre- to postworkshop. Parents expressed gratitude for the opportunity to meet the adult CF teams. A final piece of this multidimensional intervention is a Cystic Fibrosis Readiness to Graduate Questionnaire which is currently awaiting validation. Initial use of these interventions in one clinic suggests that they are both feasible and acceptable to patients and care providers.

4.5.2.1 Fertility and Sexual Health

As adolescents transition to young adulthood and greater independence, they need current information about how CF affects sexual and reproductive health. A review of several studies indicates that systematic education about these issues is often not occurring in pediatric CF centers (Havermans, Abbott, Colpaert, & De Boeck, 2011), resulting in gaps in knowledge, misinformation, and risky sexual behaviors (Tsang, Moriarty, & Towns, 2010). For females with CF, there is often a delay in menarche of approximately 1–2 years, due to poor growth and nutrition (Tsang et al., 2010). This delay in puberty may be associated with negative psychosocial outcomes (e.g., low self-esteem, anxiety) and misunderstandings about the effects of CF on later family planning. For example, women with CF have greater challenges in becoming pregnant because of thick, sticky mucus in the cervix and fallopian tubes (Gage, 2012); however, they are able to conceive and have healthy children (Schechter et al., 2013). In a national sample of women ($N=1309$), ages

18–28, those who had experienced pregnancy and given birth were compared to those who had not. Comparisons indicated that women who had given birth had an increase in pulmonary exacerbations, respiratory symptoms, and illness-related outpatient clinic visits. However, there were no statistically significant differences between the groups in lung function, nutritional status, or mortality (Schechter et al., 2013). Note, however, there are concerns about these women's ability to perform daily treatments while caring for a young child and the possibility that the mother's health will decline while the child is still young (Gage, 2012; Schechter et al., 2013).

For males, fertility is the most significant problem. Approximately 98% of males exhibit azoospermia, defined as a lack of measurable sperm (Tsang et al., 2010). A semen analysis is required to determine if azoospermia is present in order to educate young men about their family planning options (Havermans, Abbott, Colpaert & De Boeck, 2011). Men with CF retrospectively reported that the appropriate age for semen analysis is 17–18 years and they also recommended that information about infertility treatments be provided to young men (Tsang et al., 2010), including sperm harvesting techniques (e.g., microsurgical epididymal sperm aspiration, percutaneous epididymal sperm aspiration, and testicular sperm aspiration; Ahmad, Ahmed, & Patrizio, 2013). They also noted that "they would have given a high priority to funding infertility treatments if they had been informed about this treatment option in adolescence" (Roberts & Green, 2005, p. 8).

Importantly, adolescents with CF are sexually active, have normal sexual libido, and engage in similar risk-taking behaviors as their non-CF age-matched peers (Havermans et al., 2011). In two recent surveys, individuals with CF demonstrated poor understanding of the need for and use of contraception, and few teens were aware that contraception use is necessary to protect against sexually transmitted infections (STIs). Approximately half of women with CF reported not using contraceptives, compared to 25% of women without CF; about one-third of men with CF indicated they did not need condoms (Havermans et al., 2011; Tsang et al., 2010).

Appropriate timing of these conversations is important to prevent STIs and consider family planning options. Women with CF reported that the appropriate age for this discussion is 12–14 years (Korzeniewska et al., 2009) and similarly, healthcare providers have indicated that the appropriate age for both males and females is between 13 and 14 years (Havermans et al., 2011). This often does not happen in practice because providers feel inadequate or uncomfortable when discussing fertility and sexual health issues with their patients. Potential barriers include lack of time, lack of privacy, and uncertainty about the timing of the conversation (Tsang et al., 2010).

Parents of children with CF have also reported dissatisfaction with their level of knowledge about their child's fertility and sexual health, making it difficult for them to discuss these issues with their adolescent. Looking back, parents suggested that the CF team institute a practice of reeducating parents about sexual health issues when their children are about 10 years of age. They also requested that up-to-date information on sexuality and fertility be provided in written form to parents and teens (Havermans et al., 2011).

4.5.3 Translations and Applications (See also Table 4.1)

Four suggestions for practice can be derived from this research:

1. Regularly measure disease management knowledge and skills and use results to target intervention and remediation.
2. Discuss CF specific and non-CF specific sexual health and fertility when developmentally appropriate (typically 12–14 years; Havermans et al., 2011).
3. Include children in decision making and management of their disease early and often.
4. Gradually transition adolescents into adult care using a patient-specific transition plan.

4.6 Conclusion and Future Directions

A number of important conclusions can be drawn from this chapter. First, the needs of individuals with cystic fibrosis are constantly changing alongside systemic changes in medicine and policy. For example, recently updated infection control guidelines (Saiman et al., 2013), the frequent release of new treatments such as Ivacaftor (CFF, 2016), and the increased projected life expectancy, all suggest an imperative need for interventions that address the increased burden and decreased social support associated with these changes. While those with cystic fibrosis would benefit from supportive interventions, their families would similarly benefit. This chapter highlights literature examining the impact of cystic fibrosis on affected families and clearly shows that family functioning plays a role in adherence to treatment and health outcomes (DeLambo et al., 2004). Positive family functioning is particularly predictive of positive mental and physical health outcomes. Thus, interventions targeting family communication and problem solving are necessary for this population. Additionally, while many adolescents and children with CF find benefits from having this disease (Palmer & Boisen, 2002), the TIDES study clearly shows that children with CF and their parents are at high risk for depression and anxiety, and demonstrates the necessity of yearly mental health screening. Finally, this chapter makes clear the significance of the transition to independence and self-management and demonstrates the need for systemic intervention to adequately prepare families for this transition.

Discussion Questions

1. What Family Adaptive Systems (FAS), as described in Henry, Morris, and Harrist (2015), might be most relevant to the issue of treatment adherence in families with a child with CF? Give hypothetical examples to support your choice.

2. *For Human Science students*: What normative developmental issues of adolescence are likely involved in the transition of disease management from parents to self for CF patients?
3. *For Health Science students*: The authors state that "...patient-provider communication appears to be a major barrier to adequate implementation" of infection control. Given limited time available during patient visits, how might communication about this topic be improved?
4. The authors report that recent studies found that "Approximately half of women with CF reported not using contraceptives, compared to 25% of women without CF." Why might that be the case?
5. Summarize what you learned in this chapter using "resilience" terminology as described in Luthar, Cicchetti, and Becker (2000; e.g., risk status, protective factors, protective-stabilizing factors, protective-enhancing factors, protective-reactive factors, vulnerable-stable factors, vulnerable-reactive factors).

References for Discussion Questions

Henry, C. S., Morris, A. S., & Harrist, A. W. (2015). Family resilience: Moving into the third wave. *Family Relations, 64*, 22–43. doi:10.1111/fare.12106

Luthar, S. S., Cicchetti, D., & Becker, B. (2000). The construct of resilience: A critical evaluation and guidelines for future work. *Child Development, 71*, 543–562. doi:10.1111/1467-8624.00164

References

Abbott, J., Dodd, M., Gee, L., & Webb, K. (2001). Ways of coping with cystic fibrosis: Implications for treatment adherence. *Disability and Rehabilitation: An International, Multidisciplinary Journal, 23*, 315–324. doi:10.1080/09638280010004171

Abbott, J., Hart, A., Morton, A., Gee, L., & Conway, S. (2008). Health-related quality of life in adults with cystic fibrosis: The role of coping. *Journal of Psychosomatic Research, 64*, 149–157. doi:10.1016/j.jpsychores.2007.08.017

Accurso, F. J., Sontag, M. K., & Wagener, J. S. (2005). Complications associated with symptomatic diagnosis in infants with cystic fibrosis. *The Journal of Pediatrics, 147*, S37–S41 doi:10.1016/j.jpeds.2005.08.034

Ahmad, A., Ahmed, A., & Patrizio, P. (2013). Cystic fibrosis and fertility. *Current Opinion in Obstetrics and Gynecology, 25*, 167–172. doi:10.1097/GCO.0b013e32835f1745

Barker, D. H., Driscoll, K. A., Modi, A. C., Light, M. J., & Quittner, A. L. (2012). Supporting cystic fibrosis disease management during adolescence: The role of family and friends. *Child: Care, Health and Development, 38*, 497–504. doi:10.1111/j.1365-2214.2011.01286.x

Berlinski, A., Fan, L. L., Kozinetz, C. A., & Oermann, C. M. (2002). Invasive mechanical ventilation for acute respiratory failure in children with cystic fibrosis: Outcome analysis and case-control study. *Pediatric Pulmonology, 34*, 297–303. doi:10.1002/ppul.10159

Bernard, R. S., & Cohen, L. L. (2004). Increasing adherence to cystic fibrosis treatment: A systematic review of behavioral techniques. *Pediatric Pulmonology, 37*, 8–16. doi:10.1002/ppul.10397

Bradley, J. M., Madge, S., Morton, A. M., Quittner, A. L., & Elborn, J. S. (2012). Cystic fibrosis research in allied health and nursing professions. *Journal of Cystic Fibrosis, 11*, 387–392. doi:10.1016/j.jcf.2012.03.004

Casier, A., Goubert, L., Huse, D., Theunis, M., Franckx, H., Robberecht, E., et al. (2008). The role of acceptance in psychological functioning in adolescents with cystic fibrosis: A preliminary study. *Psychology & Health, 23*, 629–638. doi:10.1080/08870440802040269

Cohen-Cymberknoh, M., Shoseyov, D., & Kerem, E. (2011). Managing cystic fibrosis: Strategies that increase life expectancy and improve quality of life. *American Journal of Respiratory and Critical Care Medicine, 183*, 1463–1471. doi:10.1164/rccm.201009-1478CI

Cystic Fibrosis Foundation. (2016). *Highlights of the 2014 patient registry data.*. Bethesda, MD: Cystic Fibrosis Foundation.

Davis, P. B. (2006). Cystic fibrosis since 1938. *American Journal of Respiratory and Critical Care Medicine, 173*, 475–482. doi:10.1164/rccm.200505-840OE

DeLambo, K. E., Ievers-Landis, C. E., Drotar, D., & Quittner, A. L. (2004). Association of observed family relationship quality and problem-solving skills with treatment adherence in older children and adolescents with cystic fibrosis. *Journal of Pediatric Psychology, 29*, 343–353. doi:10.1093/jpepsy/jsh038

Dierker, L. C., Albano, A., Clarke, G. N., Heimberg, R. G., Kendall, P. C., Merikangas, K. R., et al. (2001). Screening for anxiety and depression in early adolescence. *Journal of the American Academy of Child & Adolescent Psychiatry, 40*, 929–936. doi:10.1097/00004583-200108000-00015

Duff, A. J., & Latchford, G. J. (2010). Motivational interviewing for adherence problems in cystic fibrosis. *Pediatric Pulmonology, 45*, 211–220. doi:10.1002/ppul.21103

Eakin, M. N., Bilderback, A., Boyle, M. P., Mogayzel, P. J., & Riekert, K. A. (2011). Longitudinal association between medication adherence and lung health in people with cystic fibrosis. *Journal of Cystic Fibrosis, 10*, 258–264. doi:10.1016/j.jcf.2011.03.005

Eisenberg, D., Gollust, S. E., Golberstein, E., & Hefner, J. L. (2007). Prevalence and correlates of depression, anxiety, and suicidality among university students. *American Journal of Orthopsychiatry*. doi:10.1037/0278-6133.23.2.207

Everhart, R. S., Fiese, B. H., Smyth, J. M., Borschuk, A., & Anbar, R. D. (2014). Family functioning and treatment adherence in children and adolescents with cystic fibrosis. *Pediatric Allergy, Immunology, and Pulmonology., 27*, 82–86. doi:10.1089/ped.2014.0327

Farrell, P. M., Lai, H. J., Li, Z., Kosorok, M. R., Laxova, A., Green, C. G., et al. (2005). Evidence on improved outcomes with early diagnosis of cystic fibrosis through neonatal screening: Enough is enough! *The Journal of Pediatrics, 147*, S30–S36. doi:10.1016/j.jpeds.2005.08.012

Fauman, K. R., Pituch, K. J., Han, Y. Y., Niedner, M. F., Reske, J., & LeVine, A. M. (2011). Predictors of depressive symptoms in parents of chronically ill children admitted to the pediatric intensive care unit. *American Journal of Hospice and Palliative Medicine, 28*, 556–563. doi:10.1177/1049909111403465

Flume, P. A. (2009). Smoothing the transition from pediatric to adult care: Lessons learned. *Current Opinion in Pulmonary Medicine, 15*, 611–614. doi:10.1097/MCP.0b013e3283314dec

Foster, C., Eiser, C., Oades, P., Sheldon, C., Tripp, J., Goldman, P., et al. (2001). Treatment demands and differential treatment of patients with cystic fibrosis and their siblings: Patient, parent and sibling accounts. *Child: Care, Health and Development, 27*, 349–364. doi:10.1046/j.1365-2214.2001.00196.x

Gage, L. A. (2012). What deficits in sexual and reproductive health knowledge exist among women with cystic fibrosis? A systematic review. *Health & Social Work, 37*, 29–36. doi:10.1093/hsw/hls003

Garber, E., Desai, M., Zhou, J., Alba, L., Angst, D., Cabana, M., et al. (2008). Barriers to adherence to cystic fibrosis infection control guidelines. *Pediatric Pulmonology, 43*, 900–907. doi:10.1002/ppul.20876

Gayer, D., & Ganong, L. (2006). Family structure and mothers' caregiving of children with cystic fibrosis. *Journal of Family Nursing, 12*, 390–412. doi:10.1177/1074840706294510

Geller, D. E., & Madge, S. (2011). Technological and behavioral strategies to reduce treatment burden and improve adherence to inhaled antibiotics in cystic fibrosis. *Respiratory Medicine, 105*, S24–S31. doi:10.1016/S0954-6111(11)70024-5

Goldbeck, L., Fidika, A., Herle, M., & Quittner, A. L. (2014). Psychological interventions for individuals with cystic fibrosis and their families (Review). *The Cochrane Library, 6*, 1–152. doi:10.1002/14651858.CD003148.pub3

Gravelle, A. M., Paone, M., Davidson, A. G. F., & Chilvers, M. A. (2015). Evaluation of a multidimensional cystic fibrosis transition program: A quality improvement initiative. *Journal of Pediatric Nursing, 30*, 236–243. doi:10.1016/j.pedn.2014.06.011

Havermans, T., Abbott, J., Colpaert, K., & De Boeck, K. (2011). Communication of information about reproductive and sexual health in cystic fibrosis. Patients, parents and caregivers' experience. *Journal of Cystic Fibrosis, 10*, 221–227. doi:10.1016/j.jcf.2011.04.001

Havermans, T., Colpaert, K., & Dupont, L. J. (2008). Quality of life in patients with cystic fibrosis: Association with anxiety and depression. *Journal of Cystic Fibrosis, 7*, 581–584. doi:10.1016/j.jcf.2008.05.010

Havermans, T., Wuytack, L., Deboel, J., Tijtgat, A., Malfroot, A., De Boeck, A., et al. (2010). Siblings of children with cystic fibrosis: Quality of life and the impact of illness. *Child: Care, Health and Development, 37*, 252–260. doi:10.1111/j.1365-2214.2010.01165.x

Helmers, M. (2010). *Pediatric CF updates* [PDF document]. Retrieved from Presentation slides online web site. http://cfcenter.stanford.edu/education/ed_day/EdDay2010.html

Helms, S. W., Dellon, E. P., & Prinstein, M. J. (2014). Friendship quality and health-related outcomes among adolescents with cystic fibrosis. *Journal of Pediatric Psychology, 40*, 349–358. doi:10.1093/jpepsy/jsu063

Herzer, M., Umfress, K., Aljadeff, G., Ghai, K., & Zakowski, S. G. (2009). Interactions with parents and friends among chronically ill children: Examining social networks. *Journal of Developmental & Behavioral Pediatrics, 30*, 499–508. doi:10.1097/DBP.0b013e3181c21c82

Hilliard, M. E., Eakin, M. N., Borrelli, B., Green, A., & Riekert, K. A. (2015). Medication beliefs mediate between depressive symptoms and medication adherence in cystic fibrosis. *Health Psychology, 34*, 496–504. doi:10.1037/hea0000136

Iles, N., & Lowton, K. (2008). Young people with cystic fibrosis' concerns for their future: When and how should concerns be addressed, and by whom? *Journal of Interprofessional Care, 22*, 436–438. doi:10.1080/1356182080195032

Iles, N., & Lowton, K. (2010). What is the perceived nature of parental care and support for young people with cystic fibrosis as they enter adult health services? *Health & Social Care in the Community, 18*, 21–29. doi:10.1111/j.1365-2524.2009.00871.x

Jain, M., & Goss, C. (2014). Pulmonary, sleep, and critical care update: Update in cystic fibrosis 2013. *American Journal of Respiratory and Critical Care Medicine, 189*, 1181–1186. doi:10.1164/rccm.201402-0203UP

Janicke, D. M., Mitchell, M. J., Quittner, A. L., Piazza-Waggoner, C., & Stark, L. J. (2008). The impact of behavioral intervention on family interactions at mealtime in pediatric cystic fibrosis *Children's Health Care, 37*, 49–66. doi:10.1080/02739610701766891

Janicke, D. M., Mitchell, M. J., & Stark, L. J. (2005). Family functioning in school-age children with cystic fibrosis: An observational assessment of family interactions in the mealtime environment. *Journal of Pediatric Psychology, 30*, 179–186. doi:10.1093/jpepsy/jsi005

Korzeniewska, A., Grzelewski, T., Jerzyńska, J., Majak, P., Sołoniewicz, A., Stelmach, W., et al. (2009). Sexual and reproductive health knowledge in cystic fibrosis female patients and their parents. *The Journal of Sexual Medicine, 6*, 770–776. doi:10.1111/j.1743-6109.2008.01049.x

Lomas, P. (2014). Enhancing adherence to inhaled therapies in cystic fibrosis. *Therapeutic Advances in Respiratory Disease, 8*, 39–47. doi:10.1177/1753465814524471

Madan, A. S., Alpern, A. N., & Quittner, A. L. (2014). Transition from paediatric to adult cystic fibrosis care: A developmental framework. *Cystic Fibrosis, 64*, 272. doi:10.1016/S1521-6918(02)00150-6

Marcdante, K., Kliegman, R. M., Behrman, R. E., & Jenson, H. B. (2010). *Nelson essentials of pediatrics*. Philadephia, PA: Elsevier Health Sciences.

Marciel, K. K., Saiman, L., Quittell, L. M., Dawkins, K., & Quittner, A. L. (2010). Cell phone intervention to improve adherence: Cystic fibrosis care team, patient, and parent perspectives. *Pediatric Pulmonology, 45*, 157–164. doi:10.1002/ppul.21164

Masterson, T. L., Wildman, B. G., Newberry, B. H., & Omlor, G. J. (2011). Impact of age and gender on adherence to infection control guidelines and medical regimens in cystic fibrosis. *Pediatric Pulmonology, 46*, 295–301. doi:10.1002/ppul.21366

Matel, J. L., & Milla, C. E. (2009). Nutrition in cystic fibrosis. *Seminars in Respiratory and Critical Care Medicine, 30*(5), 579. doi:10.1055/s-0029-1238916

McClellan, C., Cohen, L., & Moffett, K. (2009). Time out based discipline strategy for children's non-compliance with cystic fibrosis treatment. *Disability and Rehabilitation, 31*, 327–336. doi:10.1080/09638280802051713

McLaughlin, S. E., Diener-West, M., Indurkhya, A., Rubin, H., Heckmann, R., & Boyle, M. P. (2008). Improving transition from pediatric to adult cystic fibrosis care: Lessons from a national survey of current practices. *Pediatrics, 121*, e1160–e1166. doi:10.1542/peds.2007-2217

Miller, V. A. (2009). Parent–child collaborative decision making for the management of chronic illness: A qualitative analysis. *Families, Systems & Health, 27*, 249–266. doi:10.1037/a0017308

Miroballi, Y., Garber, E., Jia, H., Zhou, J. J., Alba, L., Quittell, L. M., et al. (2012). Infection control knowledge, attitudes, and practices among cystic fibrosis patients and their families. *Pediatric Pulmonology, 47*, 144–152. doi:10.1002/ppul.21528

Mitchell, M. J., Powers, S. W., Byars, K. C., Dickstein, S., & Stark, L. J. (2004). Family functioning in young children with cystic fibrosis: Observations of interactions at mealtime. *Journal of Developmental & Behavioral Pediatrics, 25*, 335–346. doi:10.1097/00004703-200410000-00005

Modi, A. C., Marciel, K. K., Slater, S. K., Drotar, D., & Quittner, A. L. (2008). The influence of parental supervision on medical adherence in adolescents with cystic fibrosis: Developmental shifts from pre to late adolescence. *Children's Health Care, 37*, 78–92. doi:10.1080/02739610701766925

Modi, A. C., Quittner, A. L., & Boyle, M. P. (2010). Assessing disease disclosure in adults with cystic fibrosis: The adult data for understanding lifestyle and transitions (ADULT) survey disclosure of disease in adults with cystic fibrosis. *BMC Pulmonary Medicine, 10*, 46. doi:10.1186/1471-2466-10-46

Morrison, J. M., O'Rawe, A., McCracken, K. J., Redmond, A. O. B., & Dodge, J. A. (1994). Energy intakes and losses in cystic fibrosis. *Journal of Human Nutrition and Dietetics, 7*, 39–46. doi:10.1111/j.1365-277X.1994.tb00405.x

Moussavi, S., Chatterji, S., Verdes, E., Tandon, A., Patel, V., & Ustun, B. (2007). Depression, chronic diseases, and decrements in health: Results from the World Health Surveys. *The Lancet, 370*, 851–858. doi:10.1016/S0140-6736(07)61415-9

O'Sullivan, B. P., Orenstein, D. M., & Milla, C. E. (2013). Pricing for orphan drugs: Will the market bear what society cannot? *The Journal of the American Medical Association, 310*, 1343–1344. doi:10.1001/jama.2013.278129

Orchard, C., & Bilton, D. (2014). Antibiotic treatment of cystic fibrosis lung disease. *Cystic Fibrosis, 64*, 188.

Pai, A. L., & Schwartz, L. A. (2011). Introduction to the special section: Health care transitions of adolescents and young adults with pediatric chronic conditions. *Journal of Pediatric Psychology, 36*, 129–133. doi:10.1093/jpepsy/jsq100

Palmer, M. L., & Boisen, L. S. (2002). Cystic fibrosis and the transition to adulthood. *Social Work in Health Care, 36*, 45–58. doi:10.1300/J010v36n01_04

Pinquart, M., & Shen, Y. (2011). Depressive symptoms in children and adolescents with chronic physical illness: An updated meta-analysis. *Journal of Pediatric Psychology, 36*, 375–384. doi:10.1093/jpepsy/jsq104

Quittner, A. L., Abbott, J., Georgiopoulos, A. M., Goldbeck, L., Smith, B., Hempstead, S. E., ... & Crossan, A. (2016). International Committee on Mental Health in Cystic Fibrosis: Cystic Fibrosis Foundation and European Cystic Fibrosis Society consensus statements for screening and treating depression and anxiety. *Thorax, 71*, 26–34.

Quittner, A. L., Alpern, A. N., & Blackwell, L. S. (2012). Treatment adherence in adolescents with cystic fibrosis. In C. Castellani, S. Elborn, & H. Heijerman (Eds.), *Health care issues and challenges in the adolescent with cystic fibrosis* (pp. 77–91). Oxford, UK: Elsevier Inc.

Quittner, A. L., Espelage, D. L., Opipari, L. C., Carter, B., Eid, N., & Eigen, H. (1998). Role strain in couples with and without a child with a chronic illness: Associations with marital satisfaction, intimacy, and daily mood. *Health Psychology, 17,* 112. doi:10.1037/0278-6133.17.2.112

Quittner, A. L., Goldbeck, L., Abbott, J., Duff, A., Lambrecht, P., Solè, A., et al. (2014). Prevalence of depression and anxiety in patients with cystic fibrosis and parent caregivers: Results of the international depression epidemiological study across nine countries. *Thorax, 69,* 1090–1097. doi:10.1136/thoraxjnl-2014-205983

Quittner, A. L., & Opipari, L. C. (1994). Differential treatment of siblings: Interview and diary analyses comparing two family contexts. *Child Development, 65,* 800–814. doi:10.1111/j.1467-8624.1994.tb00784.x

Quittner, A. L., Riekert, K. A., Marciel, K. K., Kimberg, C. I., Eakin, M. N., & Zhang, J. (2010). Adolescent management of CF: Gaps in knowledge and treatment skills in the iCARE study. *Pediatric Pulmonology, 45*(S33), 199–200.

Quittner, A. L., Romero, S. L., Blackwell, L. S., McLean, K. A., Monzon, A. D., & Dawkins, K. (2013). Efficacy of an online social networking site: CFFone results. *Pediatric Pulmonology, 48*(S36), 135.

Quittner, A. L., Zhang, J., Marynchenko, M., Chopra, P. A., Signorovitch, J., Yushkina, Y., et al. (2014). Pulmonary medication adherence and health-care use in cystic fibrosis. *Chest, 146,* 142–151. doi:10.1378/chest.13-1926

Ramsey, B. W., Davies, J., McElvaney, N. G., Tullis, E., Bell, S. C., Dřevínek, P., et al. (2011). A CFTR potentiator in patients with cystic fibrosis and the G551D mutation. *New England Journal of Medicine, 365,* 1663–1672. doi:10.1056/NEJMoa1105185

Ratjen, F., Bell. S.C., Rowe, S.M., Goss, C.H., Quittner, A.L., Bush, A. Cystic fibrosis. *Nature Reviews Disease Primers.* Published online: 14 May 2015

Reynolds, N., Mrug, S., & Guion, K. (2013). Spiritual coping and psychosocial adjustment of adolescents with chronic illness: The role of cognitive attributions, age, and disease group. *Journal of Adolescent Health, 52,* 559–565. doi:10.1016/j.jadohealth.2012.09.007

Riekert, K. A., Bartlett, S. J., Boyle, M. P., Krishnan, J. A., & Rand, C. S. (2007). The association between depression, lung function, and health-related quality of life among adults with cystic fibrosis. *Chest Journal, 132,* 231–237. doi:10.1378/chest.06-2474

Roberts, S., & Green, P. (2005). The sexual health of adolescents with cystic fibrosis. *Journal of the Royal Society of Medicine, 98*(Suppl 45), 7.

Russo, K., Donnelly, M., & Reid, A. J. (2006). Segregation—The perspectives of young patients and their parents. *Journal of Cystic Fibrosis, 5,* 93–99. doi:10.1016/j.jcf.2005.12.002

Saiman, L., & Siegel, J. (2003). Infection control recommendations for patients with cystic fibrosis: Microbiology, important pathogens, and infection control practices to prevent patient-to-patient transmission. *Infection Control and Hospital Epidemiology, 24*(S5), S6–S52. doi:10.1086/503485

Saiman, L., Siegel, J. D., LiPuma, J. J., Brown, R. F., Bryson, E. A., Chambers, M. J., et al. (2013). Infection prevention and control guideline for cystic fibrosis: 2013 update. *Infection Control and Hospital Epidemiology, 35*(S1), S1–S67. doi:10.1086/676882

Sawicki, G. S., Ren, C. L., Konstan, M. W., Millar, S. J., Pasta, D. J., & Quittner, A. L. (2013). Treatment complexity in cystic fibrosis: Trends over time and associations with site-specific outcomes. *Journal of Cystic Fibrosis, 12,* 461–467. doi:10.1016/j.jcf.2012.12.009

Sawicki, G. S., Sellers, D. E., & Robinson, W. M. (2009). High treatment burden in adults with cystic fibrosis: Challenges to disease self-management. *Journal of Cystic Fibrosis, 8,* 91–96. doi:10.1016/j.jcf.2008.09.007

Sawicki, G. S., Whitworth, R., Gunn, L., Butterfield, R., Lukens-Bull, K., & Wood, D. (2011). Receipt of health care transition counseling in the national survey of adult transition and health. *Pediatrics, 128,* e521–e529. doi:10.1542/peds.2010-3017

Schechter, M. S., Quittner, A. L., Konstan, M. W., Millar, S. J., Pasta, D. J., & McMullen, A. (2013). Long-term effects of pregnancy and motherhood on disease outcomes of women with cystic fibrosis. *Annals of the American Thoracic Society, 10,* 213–219. doi:10.1513/AnnalsATS.201211-108OC

Smith, B. A., Modi, A. C., Quittner, A. L., & Wood, B. L. (2010). Depressive symptoms in children with cystic fibrosis and parents and its effects on adherence to airway clearance. *Pediatric Pulmonology, 45*, 756–763. doi:10.1002/ppul.21238

Strausbaugh, S. D., & Davis, P. B. (2007). Cystic fibrosis: A review of epidemiology and pathobiology. *Clinics in Chest Medicine, 28*, 279–288. doi:10.1016/j.ccm.2007.02.011

Szyndler, J. E., Towns, S. J., van Asperen, P. P., & McKay, K. O. (2005). Psychological and family functioning and quality of life in adolescents with cystic fibrosis. *Journal of Cystic Fibrosis, 4*, 135–144. doi:10.1016/j.jcf.2005.02.004

Tsang, A., Moriarty, C., & Towns, S. (2010). Contraception, communication and counseling for sexuality and reproductive health in adolescents and young adults with CF. *Paediatric Respiratory Reviews, 11*, 84–89. doi:10.1016/j.prrv.2010.01.002

Tuchman, L. K., Schwartz, L. A., Sawicki, G. S., & Britto, M. T. (2010). Cystic fibrosis and transition to adult medical care. *Pediatrics, 125*, 566–573. doi:10.1542/peds.2009-2791

Wainwright, C. E., Elborn, J. S., Ramsey, B. W., Marigowda, G., Huang, X., Cipolli, M., ... & Konstan, M. W. (2015). Lumacaftor–ivacaftor in patients with cystic fibrosis homozygous for Phe508del CFTR. *New England Journal of Medicine, 373*, 220–231.

Wallis, C. (2012). Diagnosis and presentation of cystic fibrosis. In R. W. Wilmott, T. F. Boat, A. Bush, V. Chernick, R. R. Deterding, & F. Ratjen (Eds.), *Kendig and Chernick's disorders of the respiratory tract in children*. Philadelphia, PA: Elsevier Saunders.

Wennström, I. L., Isberg, P. E., Wirtberg, I. I., & Rydén, O. O. (2011). From children to young adults: Cystic fibrosis and siblingship a longitudinal study. *Acta Paediatrica, 100*, 1048–1053. doi:10.1111/j.1651-2227.2011.02182.x

Williams, P. D. (1997). Siblings and pediatric chronic illness: A review of the literature. *International Journal of Nursing Studies, 34*, 312–323.

Williams, B., Mukhopadhyay, S., Dowell, J., & Coyle, J. (2007). From child to adult: An exploration of shifting family roles and responsibilities in managing physiotherapy for cystic fibrosis. *Social Science & Medicine, 65*, 2135–2146. doi:10.1016/j.socscimed.2007.07.020

Williams, P. D., Ridder, E. L., Setter, R. K., & Liebergen, A. (2009). Pediatric chronic illness (cancer, cystic fibrosis) effects on well siblings: Parents' voices. *Issues in Comprehensive Pediatric Nursing, 32*, 94–113. doi:10.1080/01460860902740990

Yankaskas, J. R., Marshall, B. C., Sufian, B., Simom, R. H., & Rodman, D. (2004). Cystic fibrosis adult care. *Chest, 125*, 1S–39S.

Zhou, J., Garber, E., & Saiman, L. (2008). Survey of infection control policies for patients with cystic fibrosis in the United States. *American Journal of Infection Control, 36*, 220–222. doi:10.1016/j.ajic.2007.05.009

Chapter 5
Improving Physician Self-Efficacy and Reducing Provider Bias: A Family Science Approach to Pediatric Obesity Treatment

Sally Eagleton, Colony S. Fugate, and Michael J. Merten

Human Sciences is an interdisciplinary and interdepartmental degree program that aims to provide a framework for students whose interests may span both the sciences and humanities. It provides a general scheme within which to arrange scientific knowledge about our lives. To achieve such a general view, one must have some knowledge of the various disciplines that study humankind in their own particular ways. Human scientists must have a detailed knowledge of some special parts of the field. Thus, human scientists provide both wide, scientific knowledge of the life of humans and a detailed understanding of the evidence in some areas.

Human scientists study the biological, social, and cultural aspects of human life in recognition of the need for interdisciplinary understanding of fundamental issues and problems confronting contemporary societies. Central topics include the evolution of humans, their behavior, molecular and population genetics, population growth and aging, ethnic and cultural diversity, and the human interaction with the environment, including conservation, disease, and nutrition. The study of both biological and social disciplines, integrated within a framework of human diversity and sustainability, should enable the human scientist to develop professional

---

S. Eagleton
Department of Human Development and Family Science, Oklahoma State University, 233 Human Sciences, Stillwater, OK 74078, USA
e-mail: sally.eagleton@okstate.edu

C.S. Fugate, D.O.
Center for Health Sciences, Oklahoma State University, Stillwater, OK 74074, USA
e-mail: colony.fugate@okstate.edu

M.J. Merten, Ph.D. (✉)
Department of Human Development and Family Science, Oklahoma State University, 233 Human Sciences, Stillwater, OK 74078, USA

Center for Family Resilience, Oklahoma State University, Stillwater, OK 74074, USA
e-mail: michael.merten@okstate.edu

© Springer International Publishing Switzerland 2017
G.L. Welch, A.W. Harrist (eds.), *Family Resilience and Chronic Illness*, Emerging Issues in Family and Individual Resilience, DOI 10.1007/978-3-319-26033-4_5

competencies suited to address such multidimensional human problems, particularly childhood obesity.

Through discovery and delivery of research-based knowledge, human scientists help individuals and families develop essential skills to successfully live and work in a complex world. These professionals are uniquely qualified to address many critical issues affecting individuals and families, such as maintaining a healthy lifestyle, managing finances, and creating supportive relationships with family members, friends, and coworkers. Interdisciplinary research that includes human scientists is needed to understand and treat complex problems like childhood obesity (Albrecht, Freeman, & Higginbotham, 2004). To date, research into the causes of childhood obesity has come primarily from biologically based disciplines, not from developmental science (Harrist et al., 2012). However, environmental factors, such as the patterns of obesogenic eating and/or low activity, and the factors that contribute to those patterns, appear to be the largest contributors of childhood obesity.

Family science, an academic discipline that combines aspects of social and natural science, deals with the relationship among individuals, families, and communities, and the environment in which they live. Family science offers an inclusive multidisciplinary approach to studying families. Individuals with a family science background understand the importance of family dynamics and relationships that can act either as protective or risk factors in childhood obesity. The purpose of this chapter is to contribute to the national dialogue surrounding pediatric obesity treatment by showing the increasing importance of providing primary care physicians with education and training in major concepts from family science.

We argue that this training will improve physician self-efficacy and reduce provider weight bias and stigma, which in turn, will lead to greater physician adherence to clinical practice guidelines, more effective treatment programs, and improved patient outcomes. We will first provide an overview of the prevalence and problem of childhood obesity in the United States. Second, because the health care setting (i.e., primary care physician) and the family are two overlapping contexts in the treatment of childhood obesity, we will discuss familial correlates of childhood obesity and describe the current clinical practice guidelines for the assessment, prevention, and treatment of childhood obesity. Next we will provide an overview of the literature surrounding provider adherence to the clinical practice guidelines and we will identify major barriers to their consistent and effective implementation. Finally, we will address the need for incorporating family science education into medical school curriculum and physician training to effectively treat childhood obesity within the health care setting and discuss how the unique family-physician interface can further our understanding of family resilience.

The dramatic rise in childhood obesity over the past 40 years has been declared a public health crisis (Lobstein, Baur, & Uauy, 2004) and a global epidemic (Theodore, Bray, & Kehle, 2009). Body mass index (BMI) is the most commonly used indicator of child overweight and obesity (Centers for Disease Control and Prevention [CDC], 2012). Childhood overweight and obesity are defined by gender- and age-specific percentile curves such that a $BMI \geq 85$th percentile and < 95th percentile is considered overweight, a BMI ≥ 95th percentile and < 99th percentile is considered obese, and a BMI ≥ 99th percentile is considered severely obese (Barlow, 2007). Although obesity rates among children aged 2–19 years of age in the United States remained relatively consistent from 2003–2004 to 2011–2012, childhood obesity prevalence remains remarkably high and in certain age groups obesity prevalence continues to rise. The most recent data from the National Health and Nutrition Examination Survey (NHANES) showed that 16.9% of all U.S. children and adolescents aged 2–19 years are obese and an additional 14.9% are overweight. Since 2003–2004, obesity rates have decreased among children aged 2–5 years (i.e., 13.9–8.4%), whereas obesity rates have increased among children aged 12–19 years (i.e., 17.4–20.5%) (Fryar, Carroll, & Ogden, 2014). National surveys have consistently shown that ethnic minority youth are disproportionately affected by obesity. Compared to 14% of non-Hispanic white children and adolescents, 22% of Hispanic and 21% of non-Hispanic black youth are obese (Ogden, Carroll, Kit, & Flegal, 2014). Data from Wave I (1994–1995) and Wave II (1996) of the National Longitudinal Study of Adolescent Health showed that compared to an obesity rate of 14% (male) and 10% (female) among non-Hispanic white adolescents, 39% of Native American boys were obese and 14% of Native American girls were obese (Harris, Gordon-Larsen, Chantala, & Udry, 2006). In addition to higher rates of childhood obesity among ethnic minorities, obesity risks are typically greater among low income, less educated, and rural populations (Institute of Medicine [IOM], 2012). It is often a greater challenge for at-risk populations to achieve and maintain a healthy weight due to inherent barriers of the built environment such as inadequate access to affordable healthy food and safe places to engage in physical activity (O'Dea, 2005). Further, access to quality obesity prevention, assessment, and treatment may be more difficult for these vulnerable youth.

Childhood obesity is associated with both immediate and long-term physical and psychosocial problems (CDC, 2012) and is both a direct and indirect burden to the economy (Lobstein et al., 2004). A recent study estimated that the total lifetime direct medical cost of an obese child compared to a normal weight child who remains normal weight into adulthood is $19,000 (Finkelstein, Graham, & Malhotra, 2014). A literature review conducted by Trogdon, Finkelstein, Hylands, Dellea, and Kamal-Bahl (2008) reported that the estimated costs for obesity-related absenteeism ranged from $79 per obese person to $3,995 per obese person, and this does not include indirect costs due to disability, premature mortality, or workers compensations claims. Although these estimates are based on adult employees, obese children typically have obese parents who may be experiencing these indirect costs. These issues may either contribute to or be a result of weight bias and stigma in the workplace, which is an understudied area of research. Increasingly, children and adolescents are diagnosed with health conditions that were previously considered exclusive to adults (Whitlock, Williams, Gold, Smith, & Shipman, 2005). Obese children are at an increased risk for cardiovascular problems (e.g., high blood pressure, high cholesterol), type II diabetes, gastrointestinal disorders, bone and joint problems, pulmonary related disorders such as asthma and sleep apnea, and some types of cancer (Arens & Muzumbar, 2010; Daniels, 2006; Hannon, Rao, & Arslanian, 2005;

Sutherland, 2008; Taylor et al., 2006; Thompson et al., 2007). Because obese children are likely to be obese in adulthood (Freedman, Khan, Dietz, Srinivasan, & Berenson, 2001; Freedman et al., 2005), obese children are at an even greater risk of serious health complications and chronic disease later in life (Daniels, 2006; Office of the Surgeon General, 2010).

Research examining the psychosocial correlates of childhood obesity has primarily focused on self-esteem, depression, body dissatisfaction, interpersonal relationships, suicidal behaviors, and academic achievement. Although this area of research has produced inconsistent results, it appears that obesity does increase the risk of adverse psychosocial problems in some children, especially in clinical samples (Wardle & Cooke, 2005). A literature review conducted by Puhl and Latner (2007) that examined sources of weight stigma in children's lives not only described how overweight youth experience bias from peers, educators, and parents, but also provided evidence that weight stigma may mediate the relationship between obesity and negative psychosocial outcomes, which may explain some of the mixed findings. Research has shown that a culmination of psychosocial stressors that obese youth often face results in reduced overall quality of life (Theodore et al., 2009). For example, Schwimmer, Burwinkle, and Varni (2003) found that compared to normal weight children severely obese children scored lower on a multidimensional health related quality of life measure and had scores that were comparable to children with a cancer diagnosis. For all of these reasons, it is clear that childhood obesity prevention and intervention must remain a public health priority. It remains unclear why current interventions have been relatively ineffective to date. Scholars have argued that some well-intentioned childhood obesity preventive efforts may actually do more harm than good (e.g., cause overweight youth to feel worse about themselves) (Neumark-Sztainer, 2005; O'Dea, 2005). Further, current evidence-based intervention strategies to reduce childhood obesity fail to address weight stigma and bias (Puhl & Latner, 2007). Increasing sensitivity to the psychosocial causes and consequences of obesity in childhood is a necessary target for improving current intervention programs.

Childhood obesity has proven to be frustrating and difficult to treat (Barlow, 2007). At a very basic level, obesity is caused by energy imbalance such that energy intake is not matched with energy expenditure (Sharma & Padwal, 2010). However, the etiology of obesity is complex and involves a combination of multiple biological and environmental influences. Ecological models (Bronfenbrenner, 1986; Bronfenbrenner & Morris, 1988) of childhood obesity propose that the development of childhood obesity is a function of influences from several interrelated contexts in which the child is imbedded, including the child's family and school as well as the local community and broader society (Davison & Birch, 2001; Harrison et al., 2011). These contexts are highly influential on the development of obesity and go beyond a child's ability to successfully balance energy. Due to the complexity of childhood obesity and the fact that effective interventions to date consists of multidisciplinary intensive programming (US Preventive Services Task Force (USPSTF), 2010), scholars have argued that efforts to reverse the obesity epidemic need to be primarily focused on prevention (Barlow, 2007; Lobstein et al., 2004). Although prevention is crucial to the long-term health of the nation's children, the current high and rising rates of child and adolescent obesity and increasing comorbid health complications speak to the equal importance of intervention.

According to Lobstein et al. (2004), "the greatest health problems will be seen in the next generation of adults as the present childhood obesity epidemic passes through to adulthood" (p. 4). Effective obesity prevention, assessment, and intervention that extends to all children and adolescents is imperative to ensure that existing weight-related comorbidities in obese children are subsided and that children with a healthy weight maintain a healthy weight and continue to practice healthy lifestyle behaviors. The health care setting is an important context for childhood obesity prevention and intervention because of the potential to reach the majority of U.S. children. The first contact that a child generally has with the health care system is a primary care physician, thus they are the first line of defense in the battle against childhood obesity (Han, Lawlor, & Kimm, 2010). However, health care provider offices, particularly primary care physicians, are an overlooked and seldom universally discussed avenue for obesity prevention and intervention.

Currently, there are evidence-based recommended clinical practice guidelines in place for the prevention, assessment, and treatment of childhood obesity; however, there is little evidence that these guidelines have made progress in reversing obesity trends. The current recommendations emphasize the importance of interactions between the provider and the child's family when discussing obesity treatment, yet little research has examined the influence of how interactions between the family and the physician (e.g., quality of interaction) influence child weight and/or comorbid conditions. Previous research has identified several barriers that may limit consistent and effective implementation of the clinical practice guidelines, and we believe that a lack of training in human sciences, particularly concepts related to family science, is a possible mechanism underlying these barriers.

5.1 Family Context of Childhood Obesity

Childhood obesity is a chronic health condition that is uniquely situated within the family. Both shared genes and environment contribute to child weight, with parental overweight being the strongest predictor of child weight (Whitaker, Wright, Pepe, Seidel, & Dietz, 1997). The inclusion of parents and families in obesity treatment increases its complexity (Skelton, Buehler, Irby, & Grzywacz, 2012), thus highlighting the need to understand home/family environment factors that are related to child overweight and obesity. Previous research has identified various familial correlates of pediatric overweight that include but are not limited to parenting behaviors, family functioning, and family food and lifestyle patterns (See Berge, 2009, for a review).

Parenting and familial factors that are consistently related to child weight are typically behaviors that encompass child health behaviors (e.g., dietary habits and physical activity). In general, parental modeling of healthy dietary behaviors, an authoritative feeding style marked by a balance of high demandingness and responsiveness, frequent family meals, and parental support of physical activity are inversely associated with child BMI, increased healthy dietary habits, and greater physical activity (Berge, Wall, Bauer, & Neumark-Sztainer, 2010; Larson, Neumark-Sztainer, Hannan, & Story, 2007; Mitchell et al., 2011; Sen, 2006; Tibbs et al., 2001). In contrast, lower home availability of healthy food, greater parental restriction of high-calorie foods, and overly controlling feeding practices are associated with higher child BMI and poor dietary intake (Cardel et al., 2012; Larson, Wall, Story, & Neumark-Sztainer, 2013; Sandvik, Gjestad, Samdal, Brug, & Klepp, 2010). Although moderators of these associations have been identified (e.g., child age, parental BMI, parental perception of child weight), for clinical purposes, these are issues that physicians need to be generally aware of when discussing treatment options with families.

There is evidence suggesting that broader parenting and family characteristics that are typically studied in relation to children's social and emotional development also predict child weight outcomes. According to Harrist et al. (2012) the link between broader family variables and child weight is likely due to underlying mechanisms such as poor child self-regulation; however, little research has examined potential mediating pathways. Although the findings are somewhat mixed, studies have shown that greater family cohesion is associated with lower BMI (Mellin, Neumark-Sztainer, Story, Ireland, & Resnick, 2002), whereas obese youth are more likely to experience greater family conflict compared to nonobese youth (e.g., Zeller et al., 2007). Research has also shown that negative family variables such as low support (e.g., Snoek, Engels, Janssens, & van Strien, 2007) and high parental control and rejection (e.g., Schuetzmann, Richter-Appelt, Schulte-Markwort, & Schimmelmann, 2008) are related to deviant eating behaviors such as emotional eating (eating to cope with negative emotions) or external eating (eating in response to external cues such as portion size). Characteristics of the child, such as eating behaviors related to excess energy intake, may help explain how negative family dynamics translate to child obesity. Although research has yet to determine how broader family functioning contributes to child weight, it is clear that poor parenting and dysfunctional family interactions put a child at risk for high BMI and may act as a barrier in a weight management program.

To our knowledge there are few studies focusing on how the health care setting interacts with the family context to predict child weight or treatment outcomes, and it is our belief that intervention efforts within the health care setting will have limited success if the appropriate family factors are not adequately considered in treatment plans. Thus, physician education and training surrounding familial correlates of child obesity will allow physicians to recognize aspects of the family environment that may hinder or support patient adherence to a treatment plan and/or positive outcomes.

5.2 Current Clinical Practice Guidelines for Childhood Obesity Treatment

In 1998 an expert committee established recommendations (Barlow & Dietz, 1998) for the evaluation and treatment of childhood obesity. Since then, there has been a substantial increase in the scientific evidence surrounding childhood obesity, and there has been considerable variability in how physicians approach childhood obesity treatment (Rausch, Rothbaum, & Hametz, 2011). Consequently, the American Medical Association, the Health Resources and Services Administration, and the Centers for Disease Control and Prevention appointed an expert committee representing 15 national health care organizations from various disciplines to provide updated recommendations for the prevention, assessment, and treatment of childhood overweight and obesity (Barlow, 2007). The remainder of this section will provide a brief description of the recommended guidelines (see Barlow, 2007, for a full description).

First, for *prevention*, the expert committee recommends that pediatric providers target all children starting at birth by advising parents and their families to implement and maintain a variety of healthy habits related to eating, physical activity, and sedentary behaviors. The goal of prevention is to encourage healthy lifestyle behaviors in all children to reduce the need for later intervention. Several office practices are also endorsed as a part of prevention. These practices include consistent and accurate documentation of BMI, procedures to ensure all children receive obesity prevention messages, and established practices for follow-up when a child is flagged as overweight or obese, to name a few.

Second, if a child is identified as overweight or obese (BMI-for-age at or above 85th %ile) the expert committee recommends *assessment* of medical and behavioral risks associated with excess weight before intervention is initiated. Primary care providers are responsible for evaluating a variety of weight-related health issues and risk factors that will determine the course of treatment if treatment is to follow. The medical screening that goes into the assessment of risks is based on the BMI percentile of the child. In general, as BMI increases the amount of screening increases. In addition, providers must take into account parental obesity, family medical history, the child's previous BMI pattern, and current medical conditions and health behaviors. The behavioral assessment of risks involves identifying obesity-promoting dietary and physical activity behaviors and assessing the family's ability and readiness to change modifiable behaviors. With an eye toward intervention, behavioral changes that the provider and family discuss must be realistic for the family to accomplish. Thus, it is very important for the physician to be familiar with the family's cultural values and beliefs that may influence diet and physical activity, and to assess potential resources and barriers to implement these changes.

Finally, the recommended *treatment* is a four-staged approach that increases in intensity. The initial stage and advancement to a subsequent stage depends on the child's age, degree of obesity, health risks, motivation, and previous responses to treatment. The first stage, "prevention plus," generally takes place in the provider setting and lasts approximately 3–6 months. This stage focuses on healthy lifestyle behaviors consistent with prevention except that the targeted outcome is generally weight maintenance or slowed weight gain that results in improved BMI percentile. Successful stage one treatment typically involves more frequent follow-up visits with the physician as well as goal setting. Stage two, "structured weight management," focuses on similar targeted behaviors introduced in stage one, but increases in both structure and support. With additional training, the provider's office can provide much of stage two treatments; however, referral to a dietician is often required and there are situations where a physician may need to refer a family to a counselor. The success of stage one and stage two largely depends on the ability of physicians, nurse practitioners, physician assistants, and nurses to provide appropriate treatment and external referrals when needed. Stage three is comprehensive multidisciplinary treatment that requires professionals from a variety of expertise and is beyond the capabilities of the health provider's office. Lastly, stage four is tertiary care intervention that may involve medication, a very low-calorie diet, or bariatric surgery and is typically only offered to severely obese patients with significant health risks that have previously attempted multidisciplinary treatment.

Stage three multidisciplinary treatment programs are the most successful in terms of long-term weight outcomes (Association of American Medical Colleges (AAMC), 2007). According to an online survey conducted by the Children's Hospital Association, there are currently only 85 existing stage three childhood obesity programs in the United States (Cook, Harris, Biddingers, & Hill, 2014). Due to the scarcity of these programs, treatment success depends on stage one and stage two treatment in which the primary care provider is primarily responsible for providing treatment. For providers to successfully implement the recommended stage one and two obesity treatment, physicians must have a well-rounded medical education that includes perspectives from the behavioral and social sciences in addition to physical and biological science (AAMC, 2011). Thus, education and training must incorporate all aspects of the evidence-based recommendations, including behavioral management and family interactions and dynamics. Further, physician education and training must be careful to avoid contributing to bias and stigma of obese patients and their families (AAMC, 2007). To avoid this, when developing obesity-related curricula, careful consideration must be given to the underlying causes of obesity as well as health care providers as a source of weight bias. We will now discuss existing barriers to successful implementation of the expert committee recommendations with an emphasis on how a lack of education and training in the behavioral and social sciences, as well as existing weight bias, contribute to these flaws.

5.2.1 *Barriers to Guideline Implementation*

Although the expert committee recommendations for the prevention, assessment, and treatment of childhood obesity are based on the most recent scientific evidence, there are several limitations that need to be addressed. In general, physician nonadherence to clinical guidelines is problematic across disciplines and determining the rationale behind nonadherence in childhood obesity treatment is necessary for recommendations to have a positive impact on patient outcomes. Further, evidence points to high rates of attrition in pediatric weight management (Skelton, Irby, Beech, & Rhodes, 2012) suggesting a gap between physician recommendations (e.g., increased physical activity) and behavior change. It is well established that parental involvement in pediatric weight management is extremely important (Epstein, Paluch, Roemmich, & Beecher, 2007) and the best practice recommendation for treatment is multicomponent family-based programs that include diet, physical activity, and behavioral and family counseling (American Dietetic Association [ADA], 2006). However, according to Skelton, Irby, Beech, and Rhodes (2012), there is not a clear definition of family-based treatment and a greater understanding of family function and dynamics is needed to guide effective treatment programs. As a result, physician training that goes beyond traditional medical school education and emphasizes a multidisciplinary approach that will promote positive family adaptation to weight management and behavioral interventions that likely influence the entire family may play an important role in successful treatment outcomes. It is apparent that a lack of knowledge surrounding general family function and processes may contribute to barriers to consistent guideline implementation.

A comprehensive review article that examined barriers to physician adherence to clinical practice guidelines stressed the diversity of barriers to guideline adherence including lack of awareness, familiarity, self-efficacy, and outcome expectancy, to name a few (Cabana et al., 1999). In relation to the clinical practice guidelines for childhood obesity prevention and intervention, research has shown that most physicians are aware of the updated guidelines and, on average, adhere to about 60 % of the recommendations (Harkins, Lundgren, Spresser, & Hampl, 2012). One study conducted 4 years after the release of the updated guidelines found that provider practices still vary widely and do not always follow the committee recommendations (Rausch et al., 2011). The study found low use of accurate BMI percentile cutoffs for childhood overweight and obesity, major discrepancies in sending recommended laboratory tests and patient referrals to specialists, and it was common practice for some providers to give health behavior messages not endorsed by the committee. In general, previous research points to three primary issues that contribute to a lack of physician adherence to the committee guidelines: (1) low physician self-efficacy, (2) a lack of training in behavioral counseling and family dynamics, and (3) a lack of awareness of the complexity of obesity and provider weight bias and stigma. Importantly, we maintain that physician training in family science is an essential first step in tackling these issues and improving physician adherence to the recommended guidelines.

5.2.2 Low Physician Self-Efficacy

Different from studies that have found physician discomfort providing obesity counseling (Jelalian, Boergers, Alday, & Frank, 2003; Kolagotla & Adams, 2004) most providers in the Rausch et al. (2011) study felt comfortable with obesity prevention counseling. However, they did not feel that their counseling was effective. The study did not examine why physicians felt that their counseling messages were not being received; however, other research suggests that low physician self-efficacy in certain areas and a lack of patient motivation and adherence may contribute to these types of sentiments. For example, Harkins et al. (2012) surveyed 194 pediatricians and family physicians practicing in the Midwest and found that the majority reported self-efficacy for the assessment of weight, dietary habits, and physical activity, but only about half reported self-efficacy in counseling and behavioral weight management strategies. Similarly, Story et al. (2002) found low self-perceived proficiency in the use of behavioral management strategies in the treatment of childhood obesity among registered dieticians, pediatric nurse practitioners, and pediatricians, with pediatricians being the most likely to report low proficiency in this area. This study also found low self-perceived proficiency in guidance of parenting techniques as well as addressing family conflicts. In the Harkins et al. (2012) study, physicians were asked whether certain strategies would facilitate pediatric weight management in their practice and the solutions with the highest number of physician endorsements were effective methods to increase patient motivation, effective methods to increase patient compliance, and effective methods to increase family support.

Research has shown that self-efficacy in treating pediatric obesity is positively associated with adherence to the expert committee recommendations (Harkins et al., 2012). Thus, it is likely that physicians are only implementing the recommendations in areas that they feel competent in, which in most cases is guidance in dietary intake and physical activity, but are not implementing the recommendations in areas related to behavior change and family dynamics. This is problematic because behavior change is a necessary component of obesity treatment, and behavioral changes in children are not likely to occur unless the entire family is committed to making healthy lifestyle changes.

5.2.3 *Lack of Training in Behavioral Counseling and Family Dynamics*

One method that can be used to increase patient motivation and adherence to treatment as well as to involve the entire family is the use of interviewing techniques such as motivational interviewing (MI). As opposed to a more traditional approach to behavior change that is physician centered and prescriptive, MI is a client-centered directive method for enhancing intrinsic motivation to change (Miller & Rollnick, 2002). Motivational interviewing also takes into account a family's readiness to change and attempts to reveal the values and concerns of the family through nonjudgmental questions and reflective listening. The expert committee recommendations emphasize the importance of the role of the family as well as the patient and family's willingness to acknowledge and address a potential problem (Barlow, 2007). Thus, the use of MI is recommended as a bridge between assessment and treatment such that the intervention is a collaboration between the provider and the family and allows the family and child to determine the highest priority behaviors to target for change. Although the committee endorses counseling techniques such as MI, these techniques and other behavioral management techniques for pediatric obesity treatment are not generally a part of physician education, and postgraduate training is limited (World Health Organization [WHO], 1997). In addition to counseling techniques, it is clear that there is a need for more targeted physician training in behavioral management strategies as well as family interactions and dynamics (Story et al., 2002). This additional education and training will provide physicians with the necessary skills to feel equipped in all aspects of childhood obesity treatment and may increase patient motivation and decrease attrition rates.

5.2.4 Weight Bias, Stigma, and Lack of Awareness of the Complex Causes of Obesity

Although behavior change is critical to working toward an improved BMI, Sharma and colleagues (Sharma, 2009, 2010; Sharma & Padwal, 2010) argue that effective obesity management requires more than targeting problematic behaviors (e.g., eating too much, not moving enough) that contribute to positive energy imbalance, and that health care providers must acknowledge all possible underlying determinants of obesity including mental, physical, and socioeconomic health, to develop a rich understanding of "why" a child is overweight or obese (Sharma, 2010). There are two important reasons for physicians to address the "why" of childhood obesity rather than simply examining the behaviors that contribute to obesity. First, understanding the primary factors that explain positive energy imbalance in a given child can help physicians develop a treatment plan that targets the root cause of health habits and behaviors that result in obesity (Sharma & Padwal, 2010). Second, treating the root cause of obesity is more likely to translate into long-term lifestyle changes and improvement in BMI rather than frustration and failures due to weight cycling (i.e., weight loss and regain; see Sharma, 2009).

Importantly, attention to the underlying causes of obesity will serve to challenge weight bias and stigmatization, which has increased in the United States over the past decade (Andreyeva, Puhl, & Brownell, 2008), and is particularly prevalent among health care professionals (Puhl & Brownell, 2001; Puhl & Heuer, 2009; Schwartz, Chambliss, Brownell, Blair, & Billington, 2003). Importantly, weight bias has several negative consequences for children, including increased risk of physical activity avoidance, maladaptive eating behaviors, depression, low self-esteem, and poor body image (Puhl & Heuer, 2009). These outcomes may impair efforts to make healthy lifestyle changes, especially if the source of perceived bias is from the child's physician. Research has shown that physicians and other health care providers exhibit both implicit and explicit weight bias. For example, studies show that discriminatory attitudes and beliefs are prevalent among health care providers, such as stereotypes that obese patients are lazy, dishonest, unintelligent, lack self-control, and are noncompliant to treatment (Puhl & Brownell, 2001; Puhl & Heuer, 2009). As a result, weight bias can compromise effective medical care and intervention efforts for obese patients (Puhl & Heuer, 2010). Unique to childhood obesity treatment, weight bias and stigma from a physician extends to children's parents. Often times parents report feeling blamed by the provider for their child's weight (Edmunds, 2005) and that when discussing their child's weight physician use of the terms "fat" and "obese" as opposed to "weight" and "unhealthy weight" are perceived as stigmatizing and not likely to motivate their child to lose weight (Puhl, Peterson, & Luedicke, 2011).

Research has shown that reductions in weight bias occur when training addresses the complex causes of obesity as well as the concepts of weight bias and stigma (Poustchi, Saks, Piasecki, Hahn, & Ferrante, 2013). A study conducted by Wiese, Wilson, Jones, and Neises (1992) found that an intervention targeted to reduce weight stigma among first year medical students was effective in reducing negative stereotypes (e.g., obese individuals are lazy and lack self-control). Compared to controls, students that received the intervention were less likely to blame the individual for their obesity. A more recent study sought to reduce antifat prejudice among health promotion/public health bachelor degree program students by randomly assigning students to one of three tutorial conditions (O'Brien, Puhl, Latner, Mir, & Hunter, 2010). Results showed reductions in implicit and explicit antifat prejudice among students in the tutorial condition that focused on the uncontrollable reasons for obesity (i.e., genes and environment), whereas students in the tutorial condition that emphasized controllable reasons for obesity (i.e., diet and exercise) showed increases in implicit antifat prejudice. It is crucial that when developing obesity medicine education and training that we are mindful of the fact that depending on how the etiology of obesity is presented can either reduce or exacerbate weight bias. Reducing weight bias among health care providers will not only aid physicians in developing more effective treatment plans that target the root cause of overweight and obesity, but can also increase patient motivation and adherence.

> **Box 5.1. Implications for Practice**
> I have developed education programs that address weight management, nutrition, and physical activity, plus information about the family's role in child obesity: how important they are for building self-esteem and for helping the child maintain or grow into a healthy weight. Health rather than weight is the focus. In addition to genetic differences, I think the family is such an important factor in obesity because there are usually underlying causes that impact unhealthy eating, and for children those often lie in the family. I agree physicians need training in family correlates of child obesity. When I worked as a dietician, a physician would just give me an order—for example, this patient needs 1200 cal a day—and that was all the input I got. I believe a team

> approach to treatment would be most successful. Sometimes a child cannot "hear" advice from the parent but might listen to someone outside the family. In my own family, we ate together at the table, went on family walks, and so on, but my son did not develop his own good habits until he took a nutrition class in college! Another benefit of taking a team approach is it could minimize bias. I have not observed physicians to be insensitive, but rather biased in terms of how they view the causes of obesity. They are trained in a science; they see the causes as physiological—calories in and calories out—so when developing a treatment plan, they look at the science angle, and just try to change that balance of calories. Unfortunately, just saying "eat less and exercise more" does not translate to action, particularly if there are family conflicts or stress. Physicians need to help families with the *how*: to work within the family, to impact motivation, to encourage. There is a difference between having knowledge and knowing how it works within the family. If medical providers were trained in a more interdisciplinary way, they would better understand the complexity of the situation and then could make better referrals to the proper programs. It would be great if the physician could be involved with the follow up. Not only would this demonstrate to the family that the doctor is aware of their progress, but it would also inform the doctor about programs for future referrals.
>
> —Janice Hermann, Ph.D., Professor and Cooperative Extension Service Nutrition Specialist. Dr. Hermann has been developing and providing nutrition education for Cooperative Extension Service Family and Consumer Science County Educators for 30 years.

5.3 Implications

A concerted effort to address the described barriers to consistent and effective implementation of the clinical practice guidelines for the prevention and treatment of childhood obesity is needed. Addressing these barriers by incorporating human and family sciences into physician training will likely increase physician self-efficacy in behavior change and family dynamics and reduce weight bias and stigma. In turn, it is our belief that improved physician self-efficacy and reduced weight bias and stigma will translate into more consistent and effective adherence to the clinical practice guidelines and better patient outcomes. Based on our review of the literature, it is clear that there are significant gaps in physician education and training, and a lack of training in behavioral and family sciences may be one reason for the limited improvements in childhood obesity prevalence since the dissemination of the guidelines in 2007. We will now discuss how filling these gaps and addressing these barriers can influence clinical practice and policy in childhood obesity treatment and how these ideas can be more broadly applied to a greater understanding of family resilience.

5.3.1 Implications for Practice and Policy

Due to the scarcity of stage three multidisciplinary treatment programs in the United States, a greater focus on improving stage one and stage two obesity treatment is imperative. One possible effective strategy to increase the success of stage one and two treatment is to develop obesity medicine curriculum that specifically addresses the described barriers through training and education in medical schools and residency programs. Current obesity medical curriculum lacks education and training in the behavioral and social sciences and as the national conversation regarding core curriculum in obesity medicine moves forward, our experience informs us that experts working to develop this curriculum should consider incorporating concepts from human and family science. Based on the executive summary from a multidisciplinary committee formed by Oklahoma State University that developed an interdisciplinary training program and clinical clerkship for the prevention, assessment, and treatment of childhood obesity (Fugate, Morgan, Bourdeau, Beier, & Huber, 2014), we propose four primary educational and training objectives to be implemented into future physician education and training. The four objectives are intended to be an initial foundation of training to address the described barriers; it is certainly not inclusive and should be built upon as research continues to develop.

The first objective outlined by the executive summary is to develop and apply skills necessary to assess, treat, and monitor overweight and obese children. This training involves becoming familiar with the expert committee recommendations for the assessment, prevention, and treatment of child and adolescent overweight and obesity and developing the skills to properly apply these guidelines when working with overweight or obese children and their families. The expert committee speaks to the importance of involving the patient's family in the treatment process. Thus, additional training under this objective will teach physicians how to interact with families to promote behavior change at the family level that goes beyond prescribing diet and physical activity to the patient. Physicians will learn the importance of asking questions and learning about a family's day-to-day life such that physicians are able to assess family risk factors (e.g., economic vulnerability) that may inhibit or make adherence to treatment more difficult as well as protective processes (e.g., strong family cohesion) that may facilitate positive adaptation to treatment recommendations.

The second objective is to establish a baseline understanding of the basic concepts in obesity medicine including causes, physiology, pathophysiology, and epidemiology. To meet this objective, training will teach physicians the tenets of each basic concept in obesity. This objective covers the complex causes of obesity, including genetic, environmental, socioeconomic status, and variations in family structure, thus emphasizing that the sum of uncontrollable factors (e.g., genes, environment) in the development of obesity is far greater than the sum of controllable factors (e.g., self-control). This is an important concept for providers to internalize in order to reduce any implicit or explicit weight bias that may contribute to ineffective treatment plans and/or attrition. In addition to understanding basic concepts in obesity research, this training will teach physicians basic concepts from family science (e.g., family processes, family resilience) emphasizing the complexities of families and their functioning. As a result, this training will provide physicians with the ability to connect concepts from obesity medicine and family science when considering childhood obesity treatment efforts.

Objective three is to acquire awareness of disease prevention models (e.g., transtheoretical model, social–ecological model) and how they apply to childhood obesity intervention efforts. Training under this objective allows physicians to realize the components of each model that can be targeted by their efforts alone and which components require family, school, and/or community support. This objective also contributes to physicians understanding that childhood obesity is a chronic condition that will likely require long-term maintenance. Incorporating an obesity treatment plan into a child's life is a significant adjustment that often requires family support, and understanding where the family fits into disease prevention models requires the integration of family science into this training. As a result, physicians will also be introduced to family theories that can provide guidance to physicians when developing a pediatric obesity treatment plan (See Skelton, Buehler, Irby, & Grzywacz, 2012, for a review of relevant theories).

Finally, the fourth outlined objective is to increase awareness of how intrapersonal factors such as knowledge, attitudes and beliefs, and environmental influences including family, culture, policy, and advocacy impact obesity rates. Individual and cultural differences surrounding the perception of overweight and obesity exist, such that some families may not view a child's excess weight as problematic. In these cases, suggestions from a physician to make certain lifestyle changes may not be effective and the physician will need skills to help a child or parent understand the implications of excess weight without placing blame on the parent or making the child feel ashamed. Such skills can be taught through training in counseling techniques such as motivational interviewing in which the physician engages in nonjudgmental questioning and reflective listening to gain an understanding of the family's readiness to change. The dialogue evoked by motivational interviewing may reveal that a large part of the family's identity stems from traditional foods that are culturally important and incorporated into the family's routine meals. Changing this aspect of the family meaning system, just one of four primary family adaptive systems (described below), may be met with resistance and a family may be more motivated to adhere to a treatment plan that focuses on increasing physical activity and possibly decreasing portion sizes as opposed to cutting out traditional foods that are important to the family's identity.

Similarly, developing a weight management plan may be more difficult to implement when environmental factors such as poverty, food insecurity, and an obesogenic built environment are barriers to a healthy lifestyle. A family adaptive system that physicians may need to address (especially in families with limited resources) is the family maintenance system, which is defined as family processes that contribute to basic needs in families (e.g., food, shelter, clothing; Henry, Morris, & Harrist, 2015). This objective also provides physicians with training on how to address psychosocial determinants of obesity, such as depression, low self-esteem, or bullying at school. Human and family science training under this objective will allow physicians to recognize that a psychosocial problem may be present, confidently refer patients to professionals in other related disciplines, and to create community contacts that will contribute to the successful implementation of an obesity treatment plan that effectively serves overweight children and their families.

Childhood obesity is a complex chronic condition and its treatment is challenging and likely to affect the entire family system, making the inclusion of provider training in family science of utmost importance. Although we do not underestimate that future research will identify additional avenues for effective family-based obesity prevention and intervention, primary care physicians are in a unique position to have a significant impact on obesity rates due to the volume of children and families they come into contact with. The literature surrounding the clinical practice guidelines suggests that the barriers to the consistent and effective implementation of stage one and stage two treatment are related to a lack of training in issues of family science (e.g., family interactions, behavioral counseling). Further, our advocacy for incorporating family science into medical school curriculum and physician training also provides a unique insight into a greater understanding of family resilience.

5.3.2 *Implications for Understanding Family Resilience*

The study of family resilience has focused primarily on family adaptation associated with risk at a family systems level. Henry et al. (2015) described two waves of research on family resilience as well as the beginning of a third wave. Wave one of family resilience was an extension of family stress theory that identified resilience as a family characteristic and wave two focused on the process of family resilience (i.e., pathways to adaptation) through ongoing reciprocal interactions at multiple ecological levels (i.e., individuals, subsystems, family systems, and ecosystems). According to Henry et al., the emerging third wave is a multidisciplinary framework in which positive family adaptation is possible via multiple family levels, family adaptive systems, and interactions with ecosystems. Importantly, the third wave of resiliency research has the opportunity to contribute to the development of multidisciplinary prevention and intervention programs, especially those that impact the entire family system.

Not only can the proposed physician education and training contribute to positive family adaptation in the face of child obesity treatment, but can also further our understanding of the third wave of family resilience by showing how the health care setting (i.e., primary care physicians) can foster family resilience when families are faced with a complex chronic condition such as childhood obesity. To help drive family resilience research into the third wave, Henry et al. (2015) developed the Family Resilience Model (FRM) with family adaptive systems (FAS) at the forefront of the model. Family adaptive systems, which regulate day-to-day family interactions and contribute to positive family functioning, can be targeted by physicians when creating a treatment plan for weight management. Patients and families will have greater adherence to treatment and children are likely to have better outcomes if the plan involves the entire family in behavioral and lifestyle changes that draw upon existing strengths and capabilities within the family system. Physicians can collaborate with families during a visit to determine which family adaptive system (i.e., emotion systems, control systems, meaning systems, or maintenance systems) may contribute to positive adaptation throughout treatment. For example, one way to encourage healthier dietary intake is to increase the frequency of family meals. Family meals require organization, planning, and some level of family cohesion to have a positive mealtime experience. As a result, more frequent family meals would be a better recommendation for a family with an emotion system marked by family connectedness, supportive communication, and emotion regulation as opposed to a family with an emotion system marked by defensive communication and emotional reactivity. Instead of resulting in increased intake of healthy foods, recommending frequent family meals to a family with a poor emotion system may actually contribute to stress, dysfunction, and increased family conflict resulting in little or no behavior change in terms of diet.

Behavior and lifestyle changes related to diet and exercise are the major tenets of child obesity treatment plans. Successful behavior change typically requires participation from the entire family and an approach that draws upon existing family strengths and capabilities. Using a family adaptive system that already contributes to positive family functioning may be the best opportunity for families to incorporate new patterns and routines into day-to-day life. Primary care physicians have the opportunity to promote family resilience in the face of child obesity treatment by helping families recognize how existing adaptive systems can be drawn upon to meet treatment goals and behavior change that will contribute to a healthier life for both patient and family. However, it appears that without adequate education and training in concepts related to family science (e.g., family interactions, family conflict) and behavioral counseling, physicians do not feel competent in addressing family issues which may in fact be the key to adherence to all aspects of the clinical practice guidelines, successful treatment plans, and improved child weight outcomes.

5.4 Conclusion and Future Directions

Due to frequent contact with children and their families, primary care physicians have the unique opportunity to provide all children with obesity prevention and intervention. It is well established that childhood obesity is complex and difficult to treat, and it is clear that primary care physicians are not adequately equipped to treat all aspects of childhood obesity, especially as it relates to behavioral counseling and family dynamics. The proposed family science education to be incorporated into obesity medicine curriculum nationwide will provide the necessary training to improve the effectiveness of stage one and stage two obesity treatment in which the physician is the primary catalyst to behavior change, improved BMI, and family resilience in the face of weight management. Barriers to effective implementation of the recommended guidelines will be challenged with training that works to reduce weight bias and stigma among physicians and to improve physician self-efficacy in behavioral counseling and family dynamics.

The interface between the family and the health care setting is a fertile ground for future research. Research is needed that examines how interactions between the health care provider and the family influence adherence to treatment and treatment outcomes and a better understanding of both provider and patient/family perceptions of these interactions are warranted. Studies that compare differences in family-provider interactions based on whether or not physicians have received education and training in behavioral counseling and family dynamics can help promote the training objectives outlined by the Oklahoma State University multidisciplinary committee described earlier. Although it is clear that stage three multidisciplinary treatment is the gold standard, multicomponent family-based approaches have rarely been studied outside of randomized clinical trials with motivated families (American Dietetic Association, 2006). Physicians have the opportunity to incorporate parents and families in child obesity treatment. Incorporating family science into medical school curricula will give future physicians an interdisciplinary education in obesity medicine that is central to human sciences that will provide physicians with the tools necessary to address a complex chronic condition such as childhood obesity. Training that emphasizes the physician's role in empowering and supporting families in the process of behavior change is one example of moving family resilience research into its third wave. Physicians trained in family science can learn to target specific family adaptive systems when designing a treatment plan that will ensure the family has strengths and capabilities to draw upon in the face of difficult behavior and lifestyle changes. Finally, research connecting disease prevention models with family theories may provide physicians with a greater understanding of risk and protective factors in pediatric obesity and more effective intervention designs.

To reverse the obesity epidemic it is necessary that changes take place within all contexts of children's environments, including schools, communities, and broader society. The proposed training program does not directly address these necessary changes, but it does provide physicians with a greater understanding of the various barriers to successful obesity treatment and encourages physicians to be advocates for structural changes in their communities that will support healthy lifestyles among families. With a lack of evidence-based stage three multidisciplinary obesity treatment programs in the United States, effective stage one and stage two obesity treatment are imperative. Training physicians to approach stage one and stage two treatment by addressing family interactions will allow physicians to collaborate with children and families to manage and hopefully overcome obesity and its adverse consequences.

Discussion Questions

1. How does the first two authors' discipline (family science) impact the working definition of "resilience" used in this chapter? How might you imagine a Pediatrician or Family Practice physician would define "resilience" before reading the chapter's argument? Compare and contrast the two.
2. Develop a research question based on one of the assertions made in this chapter (e.g., that increasing health providers' knowledge of family dynamics will decrease prevalence of child obesity) and design a quantitative study that could be used to examine it.
3. *For Human Science students*: The authors propose that physicians in training should learn "… basic concepts in obesity research, this training will teach physicians basic concepts from family science (e.g., family processes, family resilience) emphasizing the complexities of families and their functioning." Chose 5 key "family process" concepts that you think would be most important to include in a training curriculum, and explain why you chose those 5.
4. *For Health Science students*: Write a 1–2 paragraph script that you could use with a parent who has brought in an obese child for an annual check up. The script should introduce the issue of obesity being a "family issue." Make sure you are sensitive to the feelings of the parent and child while also guiding them toward a family-level treatment approach.

References

Albrecht, G., Freeman, S., & Higginbotham, N. (2004). Complexity and human health: The case for a transdisciplinary paradigm. *Culture, Medicine and Psychiatry, 22*, 55–92. doi:10.1521/jscp

American Dietetic Association (ADA). (2006). Position of the American Dietetic Association: Individual-, family-, school-, and community-based interventions for pediatric overweight. *Journal of the American Dietetic Association, 106*, 925–945. doi:10.1016/j.jada.2006.03.001

Andreyeva, T., Puhl, R. M., & Brownell, K. D. (2008). Changes in perceived weight discrimination among Americans, 1995–1996 through 2004–2006. *Obesity, 16*, 1129–1134. doi:10.1023/A:1005328821675

Arens, R., & Muzumbar, H. (2010). Childhood obesity and obstructive sleep apnea. *Journal of Applied Physiology, 108*, 436–444. doi:10.1152/japplphysiol.00689.2009

Association of American Medical Colleges (AAMC). (2007, August). *Contemporary issues in medicine: The prevention and Treatment of overweight and obesity. Medical school objectives report (Report VIII)*. Washington, DC: Association of American Medical Colleges.

Association of American Medical Colleges (AAMC). (2011, November). *Behavioral and social science foundations for future physicians. Report of the behavioral and social science expert panel*. Washington, DC: Association of American Medical Colleges.

Barlow, S. E. (2007). Expert committee recommendations regarding the prevention, assessment, and treatment of child and adolescent overweight and obesity: Summary report. *Pediatrics, 120*, S164–S192. doi:10.1542/peds.2007-2329C

Barlow, S. E., & Dietz, W. H. (1998). Obesity evaluation and treatment: Expert committee recommendations. *Pediatrics, 102*, e29. doi:10.1542/peds.102.3.e29

Berge, J. M. (2009). A review of familial correlates of child and adolescent obesity: What has the 21st century taught us so far? *International Journal of Adolescent Medicine and Health, 21*, 457–483. doi:10.1515/IJAMH.2009.21.4.457

Berge, J. M., Wall, M., Bauer, K. W., & Neumark-Sztainer, D. (2010). Parenting characteristics in the home environment and adolescent overweight: A latent class analysis. *Obesity, 18*, 818–825. doi:10.1038/oby.2009.324

Bronfenbrenner, U. (1986). Ecology of the family as a context for human development: Research perspectives. *Developmental Psychology, 22*, 723–742. doi:10.1037/0012-1649.22.6.723

Bronfenbrenner, U., & Morris, P. A. (1988). The ecology of human developmental processes. In W. Damon & N. Eisenberg (Eds.), *The handbook of child psychology* (pp. 993–1027). New York, NY: John Wiley & Sons.

Cabana, M. D., Rand, C. S., Powe, N. R., Wu, A. W., Wilson, M. H., Abboud, P. C., et al. (1999). Why don't physicians follow clinical practice guidelines? A framework for improvement. *The Journal of the American Medical Association, 282*, 1458–1464. doi:10.1001/jama.282.15.1458

Cardel, M., Willig, A. L., Dulin-Keita, A., Casazza, K., Beasley, T. M., & Fernandez, J. R. (2012). Parental feeding practices and socioeconomic status are associated with child adiposity in a multiethnic sample of children. *Appetite, 58*, 347–353. doi:10.1016/j.appet.2011.11.005

Centers for Disease Control and Prevention. (2012, April). *Overweight and obesity, basics about childhood obesity*. Retrieved from http://www.cdc.gov/obesity/childhood/basics.html.

Cook, S., Harris, J., Biddingers, S., & Hill, K. (2014, October). *Description of comprehensive, multidisciplinary weight management services at children's hospitals: A national survey*. Presented at the AAP National Conference and Exhibition, San Diego, CA.

Daniels, S. R. (2006). The consequences of childhood overweight and obesity. *The Future of Children, 16*, 47–67. doi:10.1353/foc.2006.0004

Davison, K. K., & Birch, L. L. (2001). Childhood overweight: A contextual model and recommendations for future research. *Obesity Reviews, 2*, 159–171. doi:10.1046/j.1467789x.2001.00036.x

Edmunds, L. P. (2005). Parents' perceptions of health professionals' responses when seeking help for their overweight children. *Family Practice, 22*, 287–292. doi:10.1093/fampra/cmh729

Epstein, L. H., Paluch, R. A., Roemmich, J. N., & Beecher, M. D. (2007). Family-based obesity treatment, then and now: Twenty five years of pediatric obesity treatment. *Health Psychology, 26*, 381–391. doi:10.1037/0278-6133.26.4.381

Finkelstein, E. A., Graham, W. C. K., & Malhotra, R. (2014). Lifetime direct medical costs of childhood obesity. *Pediatrics, 133*, 854–862. doi:10.1542/peds.2014-0063

Freedman, D. S., Kettel, L., Serdula, M. K., Dietz, W. H., Srinivasan, S. R., & Berenson, G. S. (2005). The relation of childhood BMI to adult adiposity: The Bogalusa Heart Study. *Pediatrics, 115*, 22–27. doi:10.1542/peds.2004-0220

Freedman, D. S., Khan, L. K., Dietz, W. H., Srinivasan, S. A., & Berenson, G. S. (2001). Relationship of childhood obesity to coronary heart disease risk factors in adulthood: The Bogalusa Heart Study. *Pediatrics, 108*, 712–718. doi:10.1542/peds.108.3.712

Fryar, C. D., Carroll, M. D., & Ogden, C. L. (2014, September). Prevalence of overweight and obesity among children and adolescents: United states, 1963–1965 through 2011–2012. Atlanta, GA: Centers for Disease Control and Prevention. Retrieved from http://www.cdc.gov/nchs/data/hestat/ obesity_child_11_12/obesity_child_11_12.pdf.

Fugate, C. S., Morgan, K., Bourdeau, T., Beier, C., & Huber, J. (2014). *Interdisciplinary training program for the prevention, assessment, and treatment of childhood obesity, OSU Planning Grant for Establishing an Interdisciplinary Program Executive Summary, 2012– 2013*. Unpublished executive summary, Oklahoma State University, Tulsa, Oklahoma.

Han, J. C., Lawlor, D. A., & Kimm, S. (2010). Childhood obesity. *The Lancet, 375*, 1737–1748. doi:10.1016/S0140-6736(10)60171-7

Hannon, T. S., Rao, G., & Arslanian, S. A. (2005). Childhood obesity and type 2 diabetes mellitus. *Pediatrics, 116*, 473–480. doi:10.1542/peds.2004-2536

Harkins, P. J., Lundgren, J. D., Spresser, C. D., & Hampl, S. E. (2012). Childhood obesity: Survey of physician assessment and treatment practices. *Childhood Obesity, 8*, 155–161. doi:10.1089/chi.2011.0062

Harris, K. M., Gordon-Larsen, P., Chantala, K., & Udry, J. R. (2006). Longitudinal trends in race/ethnic disparities in leading health indicators from adolescence to young adulthood. *Archives of Pediatrics and Adolescent Medicine, 160*, 74–81. doi:10.1001/archpedi.160.1.74

Harrison, K., Bost, K. K., McBride, B. A., Donovan, S. M., Grigsby-Toussain, D. S., Kim, J., et al. (2011). Toward a developmental conceptualization of contributors to overweight and obesity in childhood: The six-cs model. *Child Development Perspectives, 5*, 50–58. doi:10.1111/j.1750-8606.2010.00150.x

Harrist, A. W., Topham, G. L., Hubbs-Tait, L., Page, M. C., Kennedy, T. S., & Shriver, L. H. (2012). What developmental science can contribute to a transdisciplinary understanding of childhood obesity: An interpersonal and intrapersonal risk model. *Child Development Perspectives, 6*, 445–455. doi:10.1111/cdep.12004

Henry, C. S., Morris, A. S., & Harrist, A. W. (2015). Family resilience: Moving into the third wave. *Family Relations, 64*, 22–43. doi:10.1111/fare.12106

Institute of Medicine (IOM). (2012, May). *Accelerating progress in obesity prevention: Solving the weight of the nation (Report Brief)*. Washington, DC: The National Academy of Sciences. Retrieved from http://www.iom.edu/~/media/Files/Report%20Files/2012/APOP/APOP_rb.pdf.

Jelalian, E., Boergers, J., Alday, C. S., & Frank, R. (2003). Survey of physician attitudes and practices related to pediatric obesity. *Clinical Pediatrics, 42*, 235–245. doi:10.1177/000992280304200307

Kolagotla, L., & Adams, W. (2004). Ambulatory management of childhood obesity. *Obesity Research, 12*, 275–283. doi:10.1038/oby.2004.35

Larson, N., Neumark-Sztainer, D., Hannan, P. J., & Story, M. (2007). Family meals during adolescence are associated with higher diet quality and healthful meal patterns during young adulthood. *Journal of the American Dietetic Association, 107*, 1502–1510. doi:10.1016/j.jada.2007.06.012

Larson, N. I., Wall, M. M., Story, M. T., & Neumark-Sztainer, D. R. (2013). Home/family, peer, school, and neighborhood correlates of obesity in adolescents. *Pediatric Obesity, 21*, 1858–1869. doi:10.1002/oby.20360

Lobstein, T., Baur, L., & Uauy, R. (2004). Obesity in children and young people: A crisis in public health. *Obesity Review, 5*, 4–85. doi:10.1111/j.1467-789X.2004.00133.x

Mellin, A. E., Neumark-Sztainer, D., Story, M., Ireland, J., & Resnick, M. D. (2002). Unhealthy behaviors and psychosocial difficulties among overweight adolescents: The potential impact of familial factors. *Journal of Adolescent Health, 31*, 145–153. doi:10.1016/S1054-139X(01)003962

Miller, W. R., & Rollnick, S. (2002). *Motivational interviewing: Preparing people for change* (2nd ed.). New York, NY: Guilford.

Mitchell, J., Skouteris, H., McCabe, M., Ricciardelli, L., Milgromb, A. J., Baurc, X., et al. (2011) Physical activity in young children: A systematic review of parental influences. *Early Child Development and Care, 182*, 1411–1437. doi:10.1080/03004430.2011.619658

Neumark-Sztainer, D. (2005). Can we simultaneously work toward the prevention of obesity and eating disorders in children and adolescents? *International Journal of Eating Disorders, 38*. 220–227. doi:10.1002/eat.20181

O'Brien, K. S., Puhl, R. M., Latner, J. D., Mir, A. S., & Hunter, J. A. (2010). Reducing anti-fat prejudice in preservice health students: A randomized trial. *Obesity, 18*, 2138–2144. doi:10.1038/oby.2010.79

O'Dea, J. A. (2005). Prevention of child obesity: First, do no harm. *Health Education Research, 20*, 259–265. doi:10.1093/her/cyg116

Office of the Surgeon General. (2010). *The surgeon general's vision for a healthy and fit nation*. Rockville, MD: U.S. Department of Health and Human Services. Retrieved from http://www.surgeongeneral.gov/initiatives/healthy-fit-nation/obesityvision2010.pdf

Ogden, C. L., Carroll, M. D., Kit, B. K., & Flegal, K. M. (2014). Prevalence of childhood and adult obesity, 2011–2012. *The Journal of the American Medical Association, 311*, 806–814. doi:10.1001/jama.2014.732

Poustchi, Y., Saks, N. S., Piasecki, A. K., Hahn, K. A., & Ferrante, J. M. (2013). Brief intervention effective in reducing weight bias among medical students. *Family Medicine, 45*, 345–348.

Puhl, R. M., & Brownell, K. D. (2001). Bias, discrimination, and obesity. *Obesity Research, 9*, 788–805. doi:10.1038/oby.2001.108

Puhl, R. M., & Heuer, C. A. (2009). The stigma of obesity: A review and update. *Obesity, 17*, 941–964. doi:10.1038/oby.2008.636

Puhl, R. M., & Heuer, C. A. (2010). Obesity stigma: Important considerations for public health. *American Journal of Public Health, 100*, 1019–1028.

Puhl, R. M., & Latner, J. D. (2007). Stigma, obesity, and the health of the nation's children. *Psychological Bulletin, 133*, 557–580. doi:10.1037/0033-2909.133.4.557

Puhl, R. M., Peterson, J. L., & Luedicke, J. (2011). Parental perceptions of weight terminology that providers use with youth. *Pediatrics, 128*, e786–e793. doi:10.1542/peds.20103841

Rausch, J. C., Rothbaum, P., & Hametz, P. (2011). Obesity prevention, screening, and treatment: Practices of pediatric providers since the 2007 expert committee recommendations. *Clinical Pediatrics, 50*, 434–441. doi:10.1177/0009922810394833

Sandvik, C., Gjestad, R., Samdal, O., Brug, J., & Klepp, K. I. (2010). Does socio-economic status moderate the associations between psychosocial predictors and fruit intake in schoolchildren? The pro children study. *Health Education Research, 25*(25), 121–134. doi:10.1093/her/cyp055

Schuetzmann, M., Richter-Appelt, H., Schulte-Markwort, M., & Schimmelmann, B. G. (2008). Associations among the perceived parent–child relationships, eating behavior, and body weight in preadolescents. Results from a community-based sample. *Journal of Pediatric Psychology, 33*, 772–782. doi:10.1093/jpepsy/jsn002

Schwartz, M. B., Chambliss, H. O., Brownell, K. D., Blair, S. N., & Billington, C. (2003). Weight bias among health professionals specializing in obesity. *Obesity Research, 11*, 1033–1039. doi:10.1038/oby.2003.142

Schwimmer, J. B., Burwinkle, T. M., & Varni, J. W. (2003). Health-related quality of life of severely obese children and adolescents. *The Journal of the American Medical Association, 289*, 1813–1819. doi:10.1001/jama.289.14.1813

Sen, B. (2006). Frequency of family dinner and adolescent body weight status: Evidence from the national longitudinal survey of youth, 1997. *Obesity, 14*, 2266–2276. doi:10.1038/oby.2006.266

Sharma, A. M. (2009). Obesity is not a choice (editorial). *Obesity Reviews, 10*, 371–372. doi:10.1111/j.1467-789X.2009.00619.x

Sharma, A. M. (2010). M, M, M, & M: a mnemonic for assessing obesity. *Obesity Reviews, 11*, 808–809. doi:10.1111/j.1467-789X.2010.00766.x

Sharma, A. M., & Padwal, R. (2010). Obesity is a sign—over-eating is a symptom: an aetiological framework for the assessment and management of obesity. *Obesity Reviews, 11*, 362–370. doi:10.1111/j.1467-789X.2009.00689.x

Skelton, J. A., Buehler, C., Irby, M. B., & Grzywacz, J. G. (2012). Where are family theories in family- based obesity treatment?: conceptualizing the study of families in pediatric weight management. *International Journal of Obesity, 36*, 891–900. doi:10.1038/ijo.2012.56

Skelton, J. A., Irby, M. B., Beech, B. M., & Rhodes, S. (2012). Attrition and family participation in obesity treatment programs: Clinicians' perceptions. *Academic Pediatrics, 12*, 420–428. doi:10.1016/j.acap.2012.05.001

Snoek, H. M., Engels, R. C. M. E., Janssens, J. M. A. M., & van Strien, T. (2007). Parental behavior and adolescents' emotional eating. *Appetite, 49*, 223–230. doi:10.1016/j.appet.2007.02.004

Story, M. T., Neumark-Stzainer, D. R., Sherwood, N. E., Holt, K., Sofka, D., Trowbridge, F. L., et al. (2002). Management of child and adolescent obesity: Attitudes, barriers, skills, and training needs among health care professionals. *Pediatrics, 110*, 210–214.

Sutherland, E. R. (2008). Obesity and asthma. *Immunology and Allergy Clinics of North America, 28*, 589–602. doi:10.1016/j.iac.2008.03.003

Taylor, E. D., Theim, K. R., Mirch, M., Ghorbani, S., Tanofsky-Kraft, M., Adler-Wailes, D., et al. (2006). Orthopedic complications of overweight in children and adolescents. *Pediatrics, 117*, 2167–2174. doi:10.1542/peds.2005-1832

Theodore, L. A., Bray, M. A., & Kehle, T. J. (2009). Introduction to the special issue: Childhood obesity. *Psychology in the Schools, 46*, 693–694. doi:10.1002/pits.20408

Thompson, P. R., Obarzanek, E., Franko, D. L., Barton, B. A., Morrison, J., Biro, F. M., et al. (2007). Childhood overweight and cardiovascular disease risk factors: The national heart, lung, and blood institute growth and health study. *The Journal of Pediatrics, 150,* 18–25. doi:10.1016/j.jpeds.2006.09.039

Tibbs, T., Haire-Joshu, D., Schechtman, K. B., Brownson, R. C., Nanney, M. S., Houston, C., et al. (2001). The relationship between parental modeling, eating patterns, and dietary intake among African American parents. *Journal of the Academy of Nutrition and Dietetics, 101,* 535–541. doi:10.1016/S0002-8223(01)00134-1

Trogdon, J. G., Finkelstein, E. A., Hylands, T., Dellea, P. S., & Kamal-Bahl, S. J. (2008). Indirect costs of obesity: a review of the current literature. *Obesity Reviews, 9,* 489-500. doi: 10.1111/j.1467-789X.2008.00472.x

US Preventive Services Task Force (USPSTF). (2010). Screening for obesity in children and adolescents: US preventive services task force recommendation statement. *Pediatrics, 125,* 361–367. doi:10.1542/peds.2009-2037

Wardle, J., & Cooke, L. (2005). The impact of obesity on psychological well-being. *Best Practice & Research Clinical Endocrinology & Metabolism, 19,* 421–440. doi:10.1016/j.beem.2005.04.006

Whitaker, R. C., Wright, J. A., Pepe, M. S., Seidel, K. D., & Dietz, W. H. (1997). Predicting obesity in young adulthood from childhood and parental obesity. *The New England Journal of Medicine, 337,* 869–873.

Whitlock, E. P., Williams, S. B., Gold, R., Smith, P. R., & Shipman, S. A. (2005). Screening and interventions for childhood overweight: A summary of evidence for the US preventive services task force. *Pediatrics, 116,* e125–e144. doi:10.1542/peds.2005-0242

Wiese, H. J., Wilson, J. F., Jones, R. A., & Neises, M. (1992). Obesity stigma reduction in medical students. *International Journal of Obesity and Related Metabolic Disorders, 16,* 859–868.

World Health Organization (WHO). (1997, June). *Obesity: Preventing and managing the global epidemic. Report of a WHO consultation on obesity.* Geneva, Switzerland: World Health Organization.

Zeller, M. H., Reiter-Purtill, J., Modi, A. C., Gutzwiller, J., Vannatta, K., & Davies, W. H. (2007). Controlled study of critical parent and family factors in the obesigenic environment. *Obesity, 15,* 126–136. doi:10.1038/oby.2007.517

Chapter 6
Facing Changes Together: Teamwork and Family Resilience During Transition of Pediatric Solid Organ Transplant Patients to Adult Care

Noel Jacobs, Marilyn Sampilo, Dianne Samad, and Judith O'Connor

6.1 Introduction

Biliary atresia, congenital kidney disease, and congenital heart defects are just a few examples of previously fatal conditions in children and adolescents. Advancements in medical technology, procedures, and medications now allow chronically medicalized patients the chance to lead meaningful lives late into adulthood. Pediatric patients with acute and chronic liver, kidney, and heart diseases can be managed with surgical procedures, immunosuppressive medications, and specific organ support, such as dialysis. Solid organ transplantation (SOT) offers both sustained longevity and quality of life in patients where medical and surgical interventions fail.

Advancements in the field of SOT and immunosuppressive medications have transformed SOT from an experimental option to standard of care. Because SOT requires lifelong immunosuppression and medical management, these children and their families have exchanged a previously life terminating disorder for a chronic medical condition. At the heart of this change in care, however, is the fact that patients and their families are then left to cope with the added stressors of living with a lifelong medical condition. Given the importance of facilitating positive outcomes for youth as they transition to adult care, the medical team's role in fostering resilience for both the patient and family should be a point of emphasis in transition preparation.

The first critical step is to identify specific patient, family, and medical system characteristics, which could contribute to stress associated with adjustment and adaptation to chronic illness. Previous research has documented various positive health factors that may be related to increased resilience and positive outcomes in

---

N. Jacobs, Ph.D. (✉) • M. Sampilo, Ph.D. • D. Samad • J. O'Connor, M.D.
University of Oklahoma Health Sciences Center,
1200 Children's Avenue, Oklahoma City, OK 73104, USA
e-mail: noel-jacobs@ouhsc.edu

youth with chronic illness, including improved quality of life and sustained capabilities (Rolland & Walsh, 2006; Shapiro, 2002). These same characteristics can be targets of interventions for patients and families in transition programs, and a family resilience framework can provide the context for these types of interventions. Pediatric solid organ transplant centers could benefit from asking themselves questions that include: "How do our transition components strengthen, or challenge, the resilience we need to see in our patients' families?" and "How do we evaluate the interaction of family resilience and medical care to promote safe and successful transition?" These answers will help to guide and adapt transition education and support for benefit of the patient and family. This chapter will identify the components of transition readiness needed for safe movement of pediatric patients into adult care, identify successes by medical teams in this work, and consider the ways medical team collaboration may fit within a framework of family resilience.

6.2 Background

Since the mid-1900s, the world of organ transplantation has progressed in almost unimaginable ways. The very first successful solid organ transplant was a kidney transplant performed by Dr. Joseph Murray and Dr. David Hume in 1954 at Brigham Hospital in Boston, for which they were awarded a Nobel Prize. The first attempt at a human liver transplant was performed on March 1, 1963 at the University of Colorado by Dr. Thomas Starzl (Starzl, Marchioro, Rowlands, et al., 1964; Starzl, Marchioro, Vonkaulla, et al., 1963). Four years later, on July 23, 1967, the first successful human liver transplant was performed at the University of Colorado and 5 months later Dr. Christian Barnard successfully transplanted the first human heart (Moore et al., 2006; Starzl et al., 2010; Starzl et al., 1968). Due to the discovery of immunosuppression therapies to avoid graft loss, the number of SOT surgeries increased rapidly. This resulted in the need for a national regulatory organization and the United Network of Organ Sharing (UNOS) was established in 1984. Its purpose is to provide and govern ethical organ allocation and monitor transplant outcomes. In 2013 alone, according to UNOS statistics, a total of 28,953 solid organ transplants were performed with 1-year organ graft success rates averaging between 80% and 90%.

Indications for pediatric SOT vary with the organ affected, but in general, include both congenital and acquired conditions. Although the majority are congenital or acquired in infancy or childhood, most are not associated with a specific racial, ethnic, or socioeconomic status. Thus, these diseases and disorders are not limited in their reach or scope, affecting all types of families. Although the success rate for graft survival is excellent, the situation that confronts pediatric patients and providers after SOT is more challenging. In order to have sustained success, SOT recipients require lifelong immunosuppression to prevent rejection, a situation where the recipient's natural immune system attacks the donor organ. This often requires complicated medical regimens to maintain the organ and to treat the side effects of immunosuppressive medications. Patients need regular medical follow-up meetings to prevent or address complications, as they are at an increased risk for the development of other medical problems (Dew et al., 2009). Because SOT is a permanent change and requires medical management for the life of the patient, children who receive solid organ transplants face an added challenge of transitioning, often while transferring care. It is at this ecological interface between the patient, family, and the medical community where providers have a unique opportunity to utilize and help build components of family resilience over time to increase the chances of continued health and successful transition. How could the medical community of the patient support this transition? What type of education is needed, and when should it start? What would the patient's internal and external environment look like? How can the family successfully engage their protective mechanisms to develop a strong but flexible plan for adapting to the patient's independence?

Transition, as a process, has been defined as the "purposeful, planned movement of adolescents and young adults with chronic physical and medical conditions from child-centered to adult-oriented health-care systems" (Blum, Garell, Hodgman, Jorissen, Okinow, Orr, & Slap, 1993), whereas the actual event in which patients move from pediatric centers to adult care centers is typically called "transfer." The transition process usually begins long before the actual transfer to an adult center and continues for some time after transfer. The process is meant to prepare the patient for the changes in health-related functioning she will likely encounter both personally and when interacting with providers, and to establish successful methods of sustained health and health care through adulthood. This is indeed a critical process to ensure a smooth and successful transition because the differences between pediatric and adult-based care are great. Mistakes or lapses in professional and self-administered care are not just expensive but can be costly or even fatal.

Differences between pediatric medical centers and adult medical centers that must be navigated by patients and caregivers include patient–provider expectations and the medical support structure itself. While being cared for at a pediatric care center, the primary caregivers assume responsibility for making sure medication is administered consistently. Caregivers also accept responsibility for consistently ordering and obtaining refills in a timely fashion. In contrast, adult care centers assume that their patients are capable of self-management and expect them to reliably get their own medication refills, unless they are identified as nonindependent adults. They are also assumed to adhere to the medication regimen regardless of supervision or reminders (McDiarmid, 2013). Adult patients are expected to schedule their own follow-up appointments at a time they believe to be suitable, which entails planning ahead, and are held responsible to attend follow-up clinic visits. Failure to adhere places them at risk of being dropped as a patient due to missed appointments (Betz & Redcay, 2005; Dovey-Pearce, Hurrell, May, Walker, & Doherty, 2005).

Undeniably, the process of transition is one that poses significant family risk and vulnerability. A family resilience framework highlights key processes that influence the adaptation of all members of the family unit and their relationships. It focuses on family strengths rather than family deficits and how those strengths can be amplified while minimizing risk and vulnerability in the face of adversity (Walsh, 2003). It attends to shifts in the developmental process over time, with recognition and acknowledgement that family interactions are dynamic and responsive to emerging issues and changing priorities. As such, its application to the transition process involved for SOT recipients has implications for understanding this key issue of development while highlighting the unique challenges associated with transition in chronic medical care.

The differences in pediatric and adult medical structures are not restricted to the nature of patient–provider interactions. The nature of the appointment/meeting is also different. In adult-based centers, visits tend to be shorter while the physician reviews instructions fairly quickly, expecting the patient to be able to comprehend and remember them. The patient is also expected to have sufficient knowledge about the nature of his/her condition and to come prepared with questions (Bell et al., 2008). In comparison, at pediatric care centers, most of the conversation is directed towards caregivers with responsibility for the care of the patient being placed on them. The patient is usually peripherally involved in the visit, they are often talked about rather than directly addressed and indeed, can be referred to in the third person. The caregivers are assumed responsible for scheduling follow-up meetings, for reporting changes in medical conditions, and for bringing the patient to the clinic at the appointed time.

Another difference between pediatric care and adult care is the availability, ease of access, and maintenance of health insurance. While many families that have a child with a significant health disability will usually qualify for Medicaid and Social Security Income (SSI), the process of maintaining eligibility becomes more difficult as young adulthood approaches. Additionally, the health care landscape changes frequently and sometimes rapidly, even in public sector insurance such as Medicaid and Medicare, which greatly increases the risk of lost coverage. This can lead to patients simply not refilling medications, not obtaining crucial lab work, and not coming to necessary appointments due to cost burden (Baughman et al., 2015; Olson, Tang, & Newacheck, 2005; Shepherd, Locke, Zhang, & Maihafer, 2014). Even upon transfer to their own health insurance policies, young adults must learn how to read, understand, and maintain financial responsibility for their share of medical expenses. They must also renew their policies on time or risk losing coverage.

The timing of transfer from a pediatric-based center to an adult-based center is often subjective and often a reflection of institutional bias. Patients 18 years and older are classified as adults and are transplanted in adult centers. Pediatric patients transplanted prior to the age of 18 may no longer be allowed admission to their center once they reach 18, while other centers may raise the age to 21 or beyond. The differences appear to be based on a lack of consensus regarding when and how to initiate the transition process, as well as how to measure if the patient and family are ready. Some studies claim transition beginning earlier in adolescence may be better (Bell et al., 2008; Lerret et al., 2012) whereas in actual practice, the transfer seems to be taking place when the patient is much older, specifically after 21 years of age (Annunziato et al., 2011; Annunziato et al., 2010). In either case, the majority of professionals are in agreement that the timing of the transition should be individualized and tailored to the patient's neurological condition and cognitive abilities, as well as the family's socioeconomic status (Bell et al., 2008).

It is generally agreed that the transition process should begin sometime before the actual transfer to adult care centers, and include follow-up after the transfer. Common practice is to ensure that the patient is stable 6 months prior to the transfer, without any gaps in psychological functioning or health insurance (Annunziato et al., 2011). Studies have been conducted to assess and improve the success of the transition process. The National Survey of Children with Special Health Care Needs (NS-CSHN; http://mchb.hrsa.gov/cshcn05/MI/NSCSHCN.pdf) was conducted by the Centers for Disease Control and Prevention's National Center for Health Statistics in 2009–2010. Authors surveyed a sample of 17,114 families who had children with special health care needs to evaluate the success of the transition process. The results demonstrated that overall, a paltry 40% of youth with special health care needs met the national transition outcome. However, when evaluated for specific component measures, 78% address the issue of taking increased responsibility for self-care, 59% discuss changing health care needs, 44% of pediatric care providers discuss transitioning to adult care providers with their patients, and only 35% discuss maintaining health insurance (McManus et al., 2013). Factors that negatively impacted the likelihood of meeting the standards set by the national transition outcome study included chronic conditions that significantly impacted physical activities and emotional or behavioral problems. Not only were children less likely to meet national standards, but they were also less likely to be encouraged to take on greater responsibility over time for their self-care by family or by medical team partners. This study seems to show that the majority of youth entering young adulthood with special health care needs are not receiving adequate preparation for transitioning from their pediatric health care providers.

6.3 Elements of Transition

There are at least four tasks that must be accomplished during transition to maximize the likelihood of positive medical outcomes. First, the pediatric patient must become more knowledgeable and feel more empowered in the management of his or her medical life, with increasing motivation and commitment to follow medical recommendations. Second, caregivers and providers must engage in an active and careful process of helping the patient take increasing control under supervision. Third, the community must ensure that access to health care is maintained until the patient is ready to self-advocate and do what is necessary to retain health coverage, establish an ability to pay, and ensure access to services and medicine. Last, the psychosocial needs of the patient, relative to development and chronic health maintenance self-management, must be understood and met as well as possible. This process must happen in the presence of supports, as there is strong proof that with active teamwork, transplant patients can successfully navigate their self-management and continue stable medical care as adults.

The necessity of this supported process is based on research demonstrating that failure to transition and transfer safely has resulted in greater than 40% graft loss (irreversible loss of organ function) in kidney transplants for patients aged 17–24 (Van Arendonk et al., 2013). However, the outcome of transition can be positive if caregivers demonstrate resilience and adapt positively to the chronic nature of the patients' health and quality of life, and medical team members provide tools in an effective, patient-and-family-centered way. The stressors of independence and increased risk may lead to positive family stress responses, which may activate an adaptive change such as parental help with the patient's mastery of health knowledge and participation in care.

6.3.1 Knowledge and Empowerment

When a patient of any age is going through pretransplant evaluation and education, assessment of understanding of the transplant process and posttransplant requirements is often a part of the commitment to care process that teams want families to endorse (Lefkowitz, Fitzgerald, Zelikovsky, Barlow, & Wray, 2014). This is due in part to the scarcity of solid organs available for transplantation, as well as the incredible costs associated with procuring, transplanting, and managing those organs over time. Additionally, medical problems can initially be very silent, having no symptoms or developing slowly such that subtle changes in physical functioning may not be noticed. Teams regularly review blood lab work, radiographic studies, growth, and development as well as clinical and physical changes to identify problems early. If families or patients do not commit to lifelong medical maintenance then, by the time medical problems are recognized, it may be too late to save the graft, or the patient's life.

The responsibilities encompassed within the commitment to care and associated with pre- and posttransplant management have the clear potential to create anxiety in caregivers and patients. It is clear that a family's adaptive system would be activated at the time a chronic illness diagnosis is made. During early childhood and into adolescence, the caregivers utilize family control systems to help the patient manage symptoms, procedures, and lifestyle recommendations made by the medical team. However, during transition, the necessary supports for a shift in understanding must interact with the family's adaptive and control systems to help empower the patient. Research shows that overly rigid and authoritarian parenting systems are maladaptive and tend to result in reduced patient autonomy and self-esteem as well as reduced family satisfaction (Henry, Morris, & Harrist, 2015). An example of this might be a patient who is not mindful and "listening" to functions of his body as it relates to transplant functioning, and so is passive about medical symptoms. He is more likely to not speak to the physician directly because his caregiver always asks questions of the physician and answers questions from the physician for him. After transition, when this patient is a young adult and living independently, he may continue in this pattern of passivity and enter a medical crisis because he never had to take ownership of his medical management and communicate thoroughly with his providers.

On the contrary, family control systems that set clear rules and limits for all family members and allow all members to voice their opinions when developmentally appropriate have been shown to be high functioning family structures. Such families tend to be good at decision-making and problem-solving and all together more resilient to added stressors (Henry et al., 2015). They are likely more open to team training and supervising increased self-management on the part of the patient. Additionally, empowerment means helping the patient learn mindful attention to physical processes in general and symptoms that may relate to transplant functioning. Once the patient is aware, this process can empower and help the patient find a voice in the clinic conversations so she can both answer and ask questions related to her medical functioning and planning. Families who utilize more flexible control methods and are less intrusive tend to foster more positive outcomes, and medical team members are encouraged to engage the caregivers to help safely create flexibility around this control. This process presents a challenge and sometimes risk based on the flexibility of the control system, but when team members engage in supportive ways, they join the system and help move both patient and caregivers forward, adding positive adaptation to the family system.

6.3.2 Increasing Comanagement and Shift in Responsibility

During adolescence, many patients and caregivers begin to wrestle with the issue of who is responsible for daily management of medications and expected health-related behavior, such as diet, fluid intake, temperature regulation, rest, and activity level, all of which may affect the body, the organ graft, and the immune system (Dew et al., 2009). Some caregivers may decide that the problems of conflict and authority struggles outweigh the benefits of medical stability in trying to ensure the adolescent patient takes prescribed medication, and let the patient manage without supervision. In addition, active youth and family schedules increase the risk of missed medication due to hectic early morning schedules, or after-school sports or social activities, making a clear case for a planned shift in management of daily responsibilities (Annunziato et al., 2008).

At a minimum, most transplant patients typically take at least 1–2 immunosuppressive medications twice daily. Some patients may take medications for preexisting conditions, while others may require additional daily medications due to secondary conditions resulting from immunosuppressive medications, such as diabetes or hypertension. Coupled with activities of daily living, even highly motivated adolescents will occasionally take medications late or forget altogether. This raises the likelihood of inadvertent medical complications. Furthermore, many patients may be intentionally nonadherent due to feeling depressed, psychologically fatigued, or defeated by medical routine and willing to risk potential problems to avoid the time medication adherence costs them or the negative side effects of taking the medications (Dobbels et al., 2010; Dobbels, Van Damme-Lombaert, Vanhaecke, & DeGeest, 2005; Fredericks, 2009). Thus, it may come as no surprise that studies have shown that graft loss during this vulnerable transfer time is shockingly high. In one study, 8 out of 20 young adult kidney transplant patients lost their grafts within 36 months of transferring to an adult kidney transplant program (Watson, 2000). This disturbingly high number was replicated in a national study where 42.4% of patients receiving a kidney transplant at any age prior to age 17, lost their grafts between the ages of 17 and 24 (Van Arendonk et al., 2013). A likely reason for these losses is inadequate self-management due to lack of transition during the transfer to adult-based medical management.

The answer to this concern, logically, is training and slow empowerment of the patient in taking on more responsibility—for keeping track of medications as they get low, creating and following a medication organization system, and reliably taking the correct amounts of medications on time. Providers, working with parents, can create a learning and responsibility plan, through education (which can empower adaptation positively, or challenge the control system) and developmentally sound shifts in responsibility (like supervised medication planning and mutual alarms with parental check-in on medication taking). By the time the young adult patient takes primary responsibility, the goal would be full fidelity to the medication regimen as well as good communication with the team when problems arise.

6.3.3 *Maintaining Medical Access and Care Coordination Through Transition and Transfer*

Another aspect of transition of care for solid organ transplant patients that has very little research history is that of insurance security. Many, if not most, solid organ transplant patients need some amount of public insurance (Medicaid or Medicare) to help cover their transplant-related expenses, due to the catastrophically high cost of medication and presurgical, surgical, and follow-up care http://www.transplantliving.org/before-the-transplant/financing-a-transplant/the-costs/). Even if private insurance covers the entire cost of transplant services and medication, the patient at some point will be required to switch insurance or work to keep benefits active, and policies can be complicated and confusing. As part of transition planning a social worker or financial coordinator who is trained in the complexities of insurance can help teach the whole family about the patient's role and responsibilities (Olson et al., 2005). Even though the goal is to help the patient avoid loss of coverage, this additional support can be either challenging or beneficial to the family and patient based on the family's established coping pattern.

A care coordinator, whose job is to ensure the young adult patient obtains an adult provider and fully establishes care with the adult center, can also be a helpful addition to the transition process. "Loss to follow-up" occurs when the patient appears to have insurance and sets appointments but then fails to come to follow-up medical appointments. In one study, Chaturvedi and others (2009) found that attendance at follow-up visits dropped significantly from pediatric clinics to adult clinics on the same patients (Chaturvedi, Jones, Walker, & Sawyer, 2009). Discomfort with the difference in patient–provider interactions, sudden moves, or loss of insurance coverage and inadequate psychosocial support during the change from pediatric to adult clinics all comprise possible causes for this. The benefit to families of a navigator who can provide education, solve problems, and empower the patient in the transition process is clear, but to families with rigid structures this can present a threat, a challenge, or a point of simply ignoring help. Resilient families with a resource orientation and flexible learning approach will make use of this support as part of their set of tools and human connections in an adaptive way.

6.3.4 Supporting the Patient's Psychosocial Needs During Transition

Transplant patients moving through adolescence and young adulthood often have psychosocial stressors unique to those with chronic illness and subsequently may require additional support. Although psychosocial needs and risk factors for chronically ill patients have been well studied (Blum, 1992; Olsson, Walsh, Toumbourou, & Bowes, 1997), how they affect transition periods has not. Feelings of social isolation from perceived or real stigma caused by chronic illness can affect how motivated a patient is to show up for appointments, take medications, and communicate medical concerns. Although some research supports the benefit of a peer and family relational support approach (Kelly, 2003; Ollson et al., 1997), a meta-analysis of research studies spanning 70 years in this area suggested further study of the relationship between specific types of social support and improved medical adherence and functioning is needed (DiMatteo, 2004). Interestingly, some research indicates that parental feelings of anxiety may be more prominent than anxiety expressed by the patient, and patients may weather the transfer process psychosocially better than caregivers (Fredericks et al., 2011). Nevertheless, assessment of the patient's psychosocial functioning and access to formal (clinic-based) and informal (relational) supports is a helpful component of care during transition. Taken together, the potential risks and barriers to stable adult health that transitioning patients face provide a strong argument for structured and active assistance, and patients themselves agree with much of the concern about transition needs. In a study of over 1000 adolescents being treated for chronic conditions, Van Staa, Jedeloo, van Meeteren, and Latour (2011) found that transition readiness was most helped by patients feeling able to manage their daily regimen and feeling positive about medical life after transfer to the adult service, among many other factors.

6.3.5 Insights from Promising Transition Programs

As transition to adult services for pediatric solid organ transplant recipients has emerged as a critical health care issue for long-term health and survival, recommendations to facilitate the transition process and transfer of care have been outlined (Bell et al., 2008; Bell & Sawyer, 2010). Included among these recommendations was an emphasis on the education and preparation of patients and their caregivers for transfer of care. A written transition plan, developed in close collaboration with the patient and his or her family, and a checklist of milestones or tasks that the patient should achieve prior to transfer along with a standardized assessment of transition readiness were suggested. Additionally, the designation of a transplant coordinator, increased collaboration between pediatric and adult care teams, and communication with primary care providers regarding the unique needs of patients with chronic disease or illness were recommended.

The recommended transition process components have the potential to confer additional benefit on family resilience by emphasizing increased knowledge, empowerment and enhanced communication. For example, in a study by Lerret et al. (2012), 35 pediatric liver transplant coordinators and 24 adult liver transplant coordinators were surveyed regarding their perceptions of essential components for the transition of patients from pediatric to adult care. Both pediatric and adult transplant coordinators felt the transition process should be standardized or formalized, and identified "knowledge of medications, independence, self-responsibility for medication administration, and compliance" (p. 255) as important issues to address during the process of transition. Both pediatric and adult transplant coordinators also emphasized communication. They highlighted the importance of ensuring accurate medical information through written records and patient knowledge. In another study by McCurdy et al. (2006), 17 young adults, who had received a solid organ transplant and underwent the transition process, participated in focus groups regarding their experience with the transfer of care. Feedback from these participants indicated that a transition orientation program at the adult center, including a tour of medical facilities, and a mentorship program to help new transfers would be beneficial. Additional preparation for the shift in responsibility and clearer communication regarding adult transplant team members' expectations of them were also deemed important. Participants were also "adamant about needing detailed information about organ-specific procedures, consequences of risky behaviors, medications, and related side effects" (p. 313). In the context of these guidelines, programs and services are being designed and implemented to address barriers to transition and to facilitate success. Despite the recent emphasis on this issue and the paucity of research in this area, there are some promising approaches or models to transition that may lay the foundation for future programming in this area.

The utilization of a transition coordinator to serve as a bridge from adolescent to adult health care has demonstrated potential in promoting positive outcomes among patients and families. For example, Annunziato et al. (2013) evaluated medication adherence in transplant patients transitioning to adult care with and without the involvement of a designated transition coordinator. The transition coordinator met patients prior to the transfer of care during their routine medical visits and worked with patients on issues regarding self-management. The transition coordinator facilitated patients' final visits in their pediatric care center and subsequently met with patients during their adult clinic visits at least once following the transition. The transition coordinator was available throughout the transfer process to address questions and concerns as the process progressed. The authors found that patients working with the transition coordinator demonstrated improved medication adherence before and after transfer of care compared to patients who received standard care.

There has been increasing interest in the role of transition clinics in mitigating factors that contribute to poor transition across subspecialties. The nature and reach of these services, however, can take a variety of forms. Of central importance is the opportunity for the providers to communicate regarding their shared patients and the opportunity for the patient to meet their adult health care provider through their pediatric care team. This can be accomplished through a single visit where the pediatric clinic team member accompanies the patient to his or her first office visit in the adult care center or a member of the adult care team meets the patient in the pediatric clinic prior to their transfer of care. Transfer of care can also be accomplished through fully shared or jointly operated adolescent–adult subspecialty clinics (Annunziato et al., 2014; Bell et al., 2008; Rosen, 2004).

While these transition clinics have increased in clinical practice, there are few studies that have established their utility or effectiveness in terms of measurable outcomes. Results, however, are promising. In one study, Chaturvedi et al. (2009) found that nine of eleven kidney transplant patients who participated in their transfer of care process, which involved attendance at a transition clinic where adolescents met with a designated transition adult nephrologist, remained clinically stable 1 year after transplant. Another study by Prestidge, Romann, Djurdjev, and Matsuda-Abedini (2012) involved the referral of patients 16 years and above to a multidisciplinary transition clinic until their formal transfer of care. The authors found that compared to a pretransition clinic group, patients attending the transition clinic demonstrated significantly less adverse outcomes with more stable allograft function and no allograft loss or death.

Another study by Harden et al. (2012) described a clinic in which patients aged 15–18 years are seen jointly by nephrologists and renal transplant nurses from pediatric and adult clinics, in preparation for the formal transfer of care to adult services. Additionally, patients are seen in a dedicated young adult clinic to facilitate transition and interaction between young adult patients. No transplant failures were observed in the group of patients who underwent the integrated transition process while several patients in the comparison group, who did not participate in the integrated process, exhibited adverse transplant outcomes. While these results suggest that transition clinics can facilitate the successful transfer of care, more empirical work is necessary. Additional research regarding the development of these clinics or other models of care intended to facilitate transition and research evaluating the implementation and outcomes of these programs are needed.

6.4 Implications for Understanding Family Resilience and Future Policy and Practice

While these promising program components appear to improve medical outcomes of young adult transplant patients through the transition to adult care, no one has yet undertaken a systematic analysis of the intersection between family resilience and transplant medical care. Outside the area of transplant medicine, however, other areas of research have begun to do this. Kichler and Kaugars (2015) describe the application of positive development principles to interventions to foster family resilience as an area of potential growth in the existing literature. They discuss positive development interventions as distinct types as outlined by Tolan (2014):

> "First, social competence promotion interventions focus on supporting learnable skills necessary for successful negotiation of social challenges within relationships and groups. Second, social and emotional learning interventions build skills to manage emotions, including self-control and awareness. Third, positive youth development intervention efforts include enhancing settings and organizations that support individual capabilities both psychologically and socially. Finally, positive psychology interventions emphasize growth of character traits and behavioral practices to improve well-being and focus on life satisfaction (e.g. mindfulness), but not through instilling skills or competencies (p. 1)."

Overall, researchers argue that a positive development framework supplements a resilience framework in two ways, first by clarifying protective factors that may mitigate existing risk factors and protect patients from the negative effects of stress, and second, by emphasizing promotive factors. They describe promotive factors as those key skills and/or processes that enhance patient's or family's functioning and support overall healthy functioning independent of the presence of risk factors (Kichler & Kaugars, 2015). Kichler and colleagues (2013) describe this type of framework in the context of a multifamily group intervention for children and adolescents with Type 1 Diabetes and their caregivers. Their intervention was an enhanced modification of Behavioral Family Systems Therapy for Diabetes (BFST-D, Wysocki et al., 2000). BFST-D is a multicomponent, family-based intervention that has been shown to have positive impacts on family functioning and treatment adherence for youth with insulin dependent diabetes mellitus (IDDM). Carpenter, Price, Cohen, Shoe, and Pendley (2014) modified BFST-D by offering treatment in a group format, shortening treatment duration, and focusing on the communication skills and problem-solving skills training components of BFST-D. The authors also enhanced BFST-D to include additional emphasis on facilitating promotive factors. Findings from this study revealed that patients who actively participated in intervention had improved clinical outcomes at posttreatment (lower HbA1c). Thus, this type of program, which combines both resilience and positive development frameworks, may be particularly suited for transition programs, which require strengthening both patient and family functioning in order to successfully navigate the transition period.

6.5 A Final Word

One consideration not heretofore discussed is the fact that no pediatric patients are able, based on the ethical understanding of informed consent with respect to their developmental status as minors, to fully consent to the world in which they find themselves, full of procedures, medications, surgeries, and monitoring. They did not choose their diagnosis, and they did not, at least initially, choose their treatments. While caregivers and medical experts who take the patient through transplant clearly agree that the best outcome for the patient is that she is functioning well postsurgically with a grafted solid organ, the pediatric patient matures to the point where all of the decisions and daily requirements are on her shoulders. The goal of adequate transition education, monitoring, and safe transfer is that she, too, lives in such a way that she feels it has all been worth it. The medical community's responsibility, then, is to create, support, evaluate, and continuously improve this process for her. More research is needed to prove the medical community is honoring the system into which it has raised her. The components of promising transition care models, namely education and empowerment, patient assumption of comanagement and responsibility, safe management of the transfer and psychosocial support, all involve interaction of the team with the family system, and dynamic interaction with the functional adaptations the family has made. Through teaching and teach-back methods, the team provides positive tools; through shift in responsibility, the team can help lower anxiety and provide scaffolding for change; through safe management of the transfer, the team becomes an active part of the control system; and through psychosocial support, the provider can act as a temporary helper for functioning. The future of good medical care for this population who has received the rare and extraordinary gift of transplant lies in understanding and working best within the set of strengths and challenges of the patient's family ecology.

Discussion Questions

1. You have been asked to conduct a focus group of pediatric patients who will transition to an adult facility in the near future. What questions will you ask the group?
2. What would you advise the parents of a patient soon to be transitioned, and how would you explain their new role? How involved should the parents be in the transition process, and at what patient age do you think you should start?
3. How would you address a patient's concerns about making the transition to an adult facility?
4. What sorts of innovative and meaningful methods of information delivery do you think would be useful with this population?

5. Imagine that you are counseling a couple whose 17-year-old son is in the hospital following serious complications from a gap in medication, which occurred when they allowed the son to go on a spring break trip and he missed several doses. The couple is distraught that their son will soon be transitioning to adult care, and fear for the stability of his transplant as well as his life. They question how it can be ethical to allow him to manage his own health care when his first attempt went so poorly. How would you start working with this couple? What are your own values and beliefs in this situation, and how would you manage them effectively?
6. As children age and become directors of their own health care decisions, this can include decisions about end-of-life care and ceasing life-saving medication. Discuss your own concerns and values about being a part of a medical team that would require you to assess an adolescent wishing to discontinue life-saving interventions. What methods would you use?

References

Annunziato, R.A., Baisley, M.C., Arrato, N., Berton, C., Henderling, F., Arnon, R., & Kerkar, N. (2013). Strangers headed to a strange land? A pilot study of using a transition coordinator to improve transfer from pediatric to adult services. The Journal of Pediatrics, 163, 1628–33. doi:10.1016/j.jpeds.2013.07.031

Annunziato, R., Emre, S., Shneider, B. L., Dugan, C., Aytaman, Y., McKay, M. M., et al. (2008). Transitioning health care responsibility from caregivers to patient: A pilot study aiming to facilitate medication adherence during this process. Pediatric Transplantation, 12, 309–315. doi:10.1111/j.1399-3046.2007.00789.x

Annunziato, R. A., Freiberger, D., Martin, K., Helcer, J., Fitzgerald, C., & Lefkowitz, D. S. (2014). An empirically based practice perspective on the transition to adulthood for solid organ transplant recipients. Pediatric Transplantation, 18, 794–802. doi:10.1111/petr.12359

Annunziato, R. A., Hogan, B., Barton, C., Miloh, T., Arnon, R., Iyer, K., et al. (2010). A translational and systemic approach to transferring liver transplant recipients from pediatric to adult-oriented care settings. Pediatric Transplantation, 14, 823–829. doi:10.1111/j.1399-3046.2010.01348.x

Annunziato, R., Parkar, S., Dugan, C., Barsade, S., Arnon, R., Miloh, T., et al. (2011). Brief report: Deficits in health care management skills among adolescent and young adult liver transplant recipients transitioning to adult care settings. Journal of Pediatric Psychology, 36, 155–159. doi:10.1093/jpepsy/jsp110

Baughman, K. R., Burke, R. C., Hewit, M. S., Sudano, J. J., Meeker, J., & Hull, S. K. (2015). Associations between difficulty paying medical bills and forgone medical and prescription drug care. Population Health Management, 18(5), 358–366. doi:10.1089/pop.2014.0128. Epub 2015 Apr 9.

Bell, L. E., Bartosh, S. M., Davis, C. L., Dobbels, F., Al-Uzri, A., Lotstein, D., et al. (2008). Adolescent transition to adult care in solid organ transplantation: A consensus conference report. American Journal of Transplantation, 8, 2230–2242. doi:10.1111/j.1600-6143.2008.02415.x

Bell, L. E., & Sawyer, S. M. (2010). Transition of care to adult services for pediatric solid-organ transplant recipients. Pediatric Clinics of North America, 57, 593–610. doi:10.1016/j.pcl.2010.01.007

Betz, C. L., & Redcay, G. (2005). Dimensions of the transition service coordinator role. Journal for Specialists in Pediatric Nursing, 10, 49–59. doi:10.1111/j.1744-6155.2005.00010.x

Blum, R.W.M., Garell, D., Hodgman, C.H., Jorissen, T.W., Okinow, N.A., Orr, D.P., & Slap, G.B. (1993). Transition from child-centered to adult health-care systems for adolescents with chronic conditions: A position paper of the society for adolescent medicine. Journal of Adolescent Health, 14, 570–576.

Blum, R. W. (1992). Chronic illness and disability in adolescence. *Journal of Adolescent Health. 13*, 364–368. doi:10.1016/1054-139X(92)90029-B

Carpenter, J. L., Price, J. E. W., Cohen, M. J., Shoe, K. M., & Pendley, J. S. (2014). Multifamily group problem-solving intervention for adherence challenges in pediatric insulin-dependent diabetes. *Clinical Practice in Pediatric Psychology, 2*, 101–115.

Chaturvedi, S., Jones, C. L., Walker, R. G., & Sawyer, S. M. (2009). The transition of kidney transplant recipients: A work in progress. *Pediatric Nephrology, 24*, 1055–1060. doi:10.1007/s00467-009-1124-y

Dew, M. A., Dabbs, A. D., Myaskovsky, L., Shyu, S., Shellmer, D., DiMartini, A. F., et al. (2009) Meta-analysis of medical regimen adherence outcomes in pediatric solid organ transplantation *Transplantation, 88*, 736–746. doi:10.1097/TP.0b013e3181b2a0e0

DiMatteo, M. R. (2004). Social support and patient adherence to medical treatment: A meta-analysis. *Health Psychology, 23*, 207–218. doi:10.1037/0278-6133.23.2.207

Dobbels, F., Ruppar, T., De Geest, S., Decorte, A., Van Damme-Lombaerts, R., & Fine, R. N. (2010) Adherence to the immunosuppressive regimen in pediatric kidney transplant recipients: A systematic review. *Pediatric Transplantation, 14*, 603–613. doi:10.1111/j.1399-3046.2010.01299.x

Dobbels, F., Van Damme-Lombaert, R., Vanhaecke, J., & DeGeest, S. (2005). Growing pains: Non-adherence with the immunosupressive regimen in adolescent transplant recipients. *Pediatric Transplant, 9*, 381–390.

Dovey-Pearce, G., Hurrell, R., May, C., Walker, C., & Doherty, Y. (2005). Young adults' (16–25 years) suggestions for providing developmentally appropriate diabetes services: A qualitative study. *Health and Social Care in the Community, 13*, 409–419. doi:10.1111/j.1365-2524.2005.00577.x

Fredericks, E. M. (2009). Nonadherence and the transition to adulthood. Supplement: ILTS/AASLD transplant course: Long-term outcomes of adult and pediatric liver transplantation. *Liver Transplantation, 14*, S63–S69.

Fredericks, E. M., Dore-Stites, D., Lopez, M. J., Well, A., Shieck, V., Freed, G. L., et al. (2011). Transition of pediatric liver transplant recipients to adult care: Patient and parent perspectives. *Pediatric Transplantation, 15*, 414–424. doi:10.1111/j.1399-3046.2011.01499.x

Harden, P. N., Walsh, G., Bandler, N., Bradley, S., Lonsdale, D., Taylor, J., et al. (2012). Bridging the gap: An integrated paediatric to adult clinical service for young adults with kidney failure. *British Medical Journal, 344*, e3718. doi:10.1136/bmj.e3718

Henry, C. S., Morris, A. S., & Harrist, A. W. (2015). Family resilience: Moving into the third wave. *Family Relations, 64*, 22–43. doi:10.1111/fare.12106

Kelly, D. (2003). Strategies for optimizing immunosuppression in adolescent transplant recipients: A focus on liver transplantation. *Paediatric Drugs, 5*, 177–183. doi:10.2165/00148581-200305030-00004

Kichler, J. C., & Kaugars, A. S. (2015). Commentary: Applying positive development principles to group interventions for the promotion of family resilience in pediatric psychology. *Journal of Pediatric Psychology*, 1–2. doi:10.1093/jpepsy/jsu115

Kichler, J. C., Kaugars, A. S., Marik, P., Nabors, L., & Alemzadeh, R. (2013). Effectiveness of groups for adolescents with type 1 diabetes mellitus and their parents. *Families, Systems & Health, 31*, 280–293. doi:10.1037/a0033039. Epub 2013 Aug 19.

Lefkowitz, D. S., Fitzgerald, C. J., Zelikovsky, N., Barlow, K., & Wray, J. (2014). Best practices in the pediatric pretransplant psychosocial evaluation. *Pediatric Transplantation, 18*, 327–335. doi:10.1111/petr.12260

Lerret, S. M., Menendez, J., Weckwerth, J., Lokar, J., Mitchell, J., & Alonso, E. M. (2012). Essential components of transition to adult transplant services: The transplant coordinators' perspective. *Progress in Transplantation, 22*, 252–258. doi:10.7182/pit2012110

McCurdy, C., DiCenso, A., Boblin, S., Ludwin, D., Bryant-Lukosius, D., & Bosompra, K. (2006). There to here: young adult patients' perceptions of the process of transition from pediatric to adult transplant care. *Progress in Transplantation, 16*, 309–316.

McDiarmid, S. V. (2013). Adolescence: Challenges and responses. *Liver Transplantation, 19*(Suppl 2), S35–S39. doi:10.1002/lt.23740

McManus, M., Pollack, L. R., Cooley, W. C., McAllister, J. W., Lotstein, D., Strickland, B., et al. (2013). Current status of transition preparation among youth with special needs in the United States. *Pediatrics, 131*, 1090–1097. doi:10.1542/peds.2012-3050

Moore, F. D., Birtch, A. G., Dagher, F., Veith, F., Krisher, J. A., Order, S. E., et al. (2006). Immunosuppression and vascular insufficiency in liver transplantation. *Annals of the New York Academy of Sciences, 120*, 729–738. doi:10.1111/j.1749-6632.1964.tb34765.x

Olson, L. M., Tang, S. S., & Newacheck, P. W. (2005). Children in the United States with discontinuous health insurance coverage. *The New England Journal of Medicine, 353*, 382–391. doi:10.1056/NEJMsa043878

Olsson, C. A., Walsh, B., Toumbourou, J. W., & Bowes, G. (1997). Chronic illness peer support. *Australian Family Physician, 26*, 500–501. Retrieved from http://europepmc.org/abstract/med/9170665

Prestidge, C., Romann, A., Djurdjev, O., & Matsuda-Abedini, M. (2012). Utility and cost of a renal transplant transition clinic. *Pediatric Nephrology, 27*, 295–302. doi:10.1007/s00467-011-1980-0

Rolland, J.S., & Walsh, F. (2006). Facilitating family resilience with childhood illness and disability. *Current Opinion in Pediatrics, 18* (5), 527–38.

Rosen, D. S. (2004). Transition of young people with respiratory diseases to adult health care. *Paediatric Respiratory Reviews, 5*, 124–131. doi:10.1016/j.prrv.2004.01.008

Shapiro, E.R. (2002). Chronic illness as a family process: A social-developmental approach to promoting resilience. *Journal of Clinical Psychology, 58* (11), 1375–84.

Shepherd, J. G., Locke, E., Zhang, Q., & Maihafer, G. (2014). Health services use and prescription access among uninsured patients managing chronic diseases. *Journal of Community Health, 39*, 572–583. doi:10.1007/s10900-013-9799-1

Starzl, T. E., Groth, C. G., Brettschneider, L., Penn, I., Fulginiti, V. A., Moon, J. B., et al. (1968). Orthotopic homotransplantation of the human liver. *Annals of Surgery, 168*, 392–415. Retrieved from http://www.pubmedcentral.nih.gov/articlerender.fcgi?artid=1387344&tool=pmcentrez&rendertype=abstract

Starzl, T. E., Iwatsuki, S., Van Thiel, D. H., Gartner, J. C., Zitelli, B. J., Malatack, J. J., et al. (2010). Evolution of liver transplantation. *Hepatology, 2*, 614–636. doi:10.1002/hep.1840020516

Starzl, T. E., Marchioro, T. L., Rowlands, D. T., Kirkpatrick, C. H., Wilson, W. E., Rifkind, D., et al. (1964). Immunosuppression after experimental and clinical homotransplantation of the liver. *Annals of Surgery, 160*, 411–439. Retrieved from http://www.pubmedcentral.nih.gov/articlerender.fcgi?artid=1408795&tool=pmcentrez&rendertype=abstract

Starzl, T. E., Marchioro, T. L., Vonkaulla, K. N., Hermann, G., Brittain, R. S., & Waddell, W. R. (1963). Homotransplantation of the liver in humans. *Surgery, Gynecology & Obstetrics, 117*, 659–676. Retrieved from http://www.pubmedcentral.nih.gov/articlerender.fcgi?artid=2634660&tool=pmcentrez&rendertype=abstract

Tolan, P. (2014). Future directions for positive development intervention research. *Journal of Clinical Child and Adolescent Psychology, 43* (4), 686–94.

Van Arendonk, K. J., James, N. T., Boyarsky, B. J., Garonzik-Wang, J. M., Orandi, B. J., Magee, J. C., et al. (2013). Age at graft loss after pediatric kidney transplantation: Exploring the high-risk age window. *Clinical Journal of the American Society of Nephrology, 8*, 1–8. doi:10.2215/CJN.10311012

Van Staa, L., Jedeloo, S., van Meeteren, J., & Latour, J. M. (2011). Crossing the transition chasm: Experiences and recommendations for improving transitional care of young adults, parents and providers. *Child: Care, Health and Development, 37*, 821–832. doi:10.1111/j.1365-2214.2011.01261.x

Walsh, F. (2003). Family resilience: A framework for clinical practice. *Family Process, 42*(1), 1–18. doi:10.1111/j.1545-5300.2003.00001.x

Watson, R. (2000). Non-compliance and transfer from paediatric to adult transplant unit. *Pediatric Nephrology (Berlin, Germany), 14*(6), 469–472. doi:10.1007/s004670050794

Wysocki, T., Harris, M., Greco, P., Bubb, J., Danda, C. E., Harvey, L. M., et al. (2000). Randomized, controlled trial of behavior therapy for families of adolescents with insulin-dependent diabetes mellitus. *Journal of Pediatric Psychology, 25*, 23–33. doi:10.1093/jpepsy/25.1.23

Chapter 7
Fighting for the Forgotten: Risk and Resilience of Children and Families Involved with the Foster Care System

Deborah Shropshire, Amanda Williams, Lauren Burge, and Larissa Hines

This is the story of the health of children and youth who are in foster care. More than 400,000 US children are not safe in their own homes (AFCARS, July 2014). The majority of these children are neglected, coming from family situations that include inadequate food, unsafe living conditions, lack of appropriate supervision, parental mental health and substance abuse concerns, and domestic violence. Others have experienced physical or sexual abuse at the hands of adults who were responsible for their care. Within unsafe families, adversities tend to co-occur, such as substance use and neglect, as do harmful mental and physical health outcomes among children (Takayama, Wolfe, & Coulter, 1998). As a result, these children are removed from their family environment and placed in the foster care system, with the state serving as their guardian. The traumas experienced in the family of origin have significant and long-term impacts on the development of the young brain and can result in a variety of health problems that extend into adulthood. However, simple removal of the child(ren) from the abusive or neglectful family and placement in a home that is somehow "better" doesn't solve the problem, as the child protection systems that have been developed may cause additional trauma in the process and incur their own unique health and psychosocial deficits. Foster care placement is indicative of transgenerational family risk as it proxies for a host of family-level adversities, is a significant risk factor for poor outcomes during youth and

---

D. Shropshire, M.D., M.H.A. (✉)
Oklahoma Department of Human Services, University of Oklahoma College of Medicine, 1200 N. Childrens Avenue #12400, Oklahoma City, OK 73104, USA
e-mail: deborah-shropshire@ouhsc.edu

A. Williams, Ph.D.
University of Southern Mississippi, Hattiesburg, MS 39406, USA
e-mail: amanda.l.williams@usm.edu

L. Burge, M.D. • L. Hines, M.D.
University of Oklahoma College of Medicine, Oklahoma City, OK 73104, USA

adulthood, and places children's future offspring at risk—and these risks increase exponentially with multiple foster care placements (Cowal, Shinn, Weitzman, Stojanovic, & Labay, 2002; Shinn, Rog, & Culhane, 2005; Stott, 2012).

7.1 Child Protection in the United States

At the time the United States was founded, the responsibility for child protection fell squarely on the shoulders of a child's family. Rarely, the local police might become involved if family abuse was severe. In 1875, public outrage over the abuse and neglect of a 9-year-old child in New York City led private citizens to organize advocacy organizations whose focus was the protection of children (Myers, 2008). This effort spread throughout many cities across the country, and they influenced law enforcement, media, and the court system. The development of the juvenile court system around the turn of the twentieth century further enhanced society's awareness of child maltreatment. In the 1940s and 1950s, the medical community began to publish case reports of children found to have brain injuries associated with long-bone fractures (Caffey, 1946). A pediatrician, Dr. Henry Kempe published a landmark paper in 1962 identifying these injuries as the result of the "battered child syndrome" (Kempe, 1962). Because of this new understanding and awareness of abuse, especially physical abuse, federal legislation was introduced in 1962 instructing all states to develop child protection systems (Myers, 2008). The systems were instructed to include a mechanism to receive and investigate reports of suspected child abuse or neglect, and should work to protect these children. By 1974, every state had an identified child welfare agency. That year there were 60,000 reports of child abuse. By 1980, that number had increased to one million, and by 2000, the number of reports of child maltreatment to state child welfare systems topped three million. The number has stabilized over the past decade.

Upon receipt of a report of child abuse or neglect, the state makes a determination as to whether the concern is significant enough to warrant child welfare involvement. Many reports are screened out because the concerns expressed by the reporting party do not rise to the level of abuse or neglect, or because the information given is inadequate or duplicated. Once a report of maltreatment is accepted for investigation, a social services worker gathers information from the child, family members, and others who may have knowledge of the circumstances surrounding the allegation. They may also enlist the assistance of professionals such as physicians, nurses, or mental health providers to evaluate the child. At the conclusion of the investigation, the child welfare agency determines whether the family is providing adequate care for the child, and whether the child is unsafe. The agency may determine that no maltreatment has occurred and close the case. They may find family circumstances that warrant referral to local resources, such as food pantries or counseling, but may not require formal state involvement. For others, the concern for safety may be too great, and 250,000 children are placed in foster care annually (Child Welfare Information

Gateway, 2013). While in foster care, they enter shelters, emergency foster placements, foster homes, group homes, and unfortunately, some require short or long-term treatment at psychiatric facilities. The state's immediate goal is protection, but for more than half of the families involved, the ultimate goal is improvement of the home circumstances and reunification with biological families.

Once a child is placed in foster care, the child welfare agency, the juvenile court, and the birth family work together on a plan that will correct the household concerns. They also set a visitation schedule, which initially often involves brief supervised visits between parents and children, occurring weekly or monthly. Rarely, the abuse or neglect is so severe that the state moves to terminate the parental rights immediately. When the plan is in place, regular court hearings monitor the progress of the family. As the family situation improves, visitation frequency or length may increase, and direct supervision may not be required. Eventually, if all goes well, the child will return home. The process takes time, however, and the average length of stay in foster care is 13.4 months. Fifteen percent of children remain in custody for 3 or more years (Child Welfare Information Gateway, 2013). Unfortunately, despite the fact that reunification is the planned outcome in most child welfare involved cases, only about half of children in custody return to live with their birth parents. Others will be adopted, age out of foster care, enter guardianships with other caregivers, or run away.

Contact with biological parents while in foster care can be a stressful experience for youth and requires professional interventions surrounding those encounters (Terling-Watt, 2001). Interestingly, even when reunification is unsuccessful while a child is in foster care placement, they will often reconnect with their birth parents after they have aged out of the system (Avery, 2010). This emphasizes the importance of a family-centered approach to child welfare involving birth family members in the process of addressing pathologies and developing positive coping and relationship skills. Even if the child does not return to their family of origin, when they age out of foster care it is highly likely that they will become involved with their family members again, relationally or residentially, and if the adversities that caused the removal of the child in the first place are never addressed, they will continue to disrupt the youth's life into adulthood (Avery, 2010). Upon exiting foster care, many youth crave social connection and supportive relationships and those who are able to maintain relationships with their biological parents generally fare better over the long-term (Cushing, Samuels, & Kerman, 2014; Flower, Toro, & Miles, 2010, Scannapieco, Connell-Carrick, & Painter, 2007). However, it is unlikely that an "adult" switch is flipped once a youth becomes independent and they are instantly able to forge these strong, healthy ties with their families, regardless of their adverse histories (Arnett, 2007). Similarly, without any intervention it is unlikely their family of origin will have addressed all the risk factors that led to removal of their child (Cushing et al., 2014). There is a body of research linking relationships with both mental and physical health indicating the centrality of birth families, as well as foster families, in the mental and physical health services provided by the child welfare process.

7.2 Health Needs of Children in Foster Care

Children and youth arrive to foster care with significant physical health, mental health, and developmental needs. The reason for these needs is multifactorial and will be discussed further in this chapter, but without a doubt, children in foster care are one of the sickest pediatric populations in the United States. In fact, a 1995 United States General Accounting Office (USGAO), report stated that "as a group, children in foster care are sicker than homeless children and children living in the poorest sections of inner cities…"

Studies of the health of children in foster care suggest that up to 90% have some sort of health concern, and almost a third have three or more (Halfon, Mendonca, & Berkowitz, 1995). These health concerns stem from the following factors: (1) genetic and epigenetic disposition; (2) prenatal and birth conditions such as substance abuse and prematurity; (3) environmental conditions such as inadequate nutrition, poor parent–child interaction, inadequate health care, inadequate or unsafe living conditions, and physical or mental trauma; (4) routine childhood acute and chronic disease; and (5) the child's response to their environment, expressed as behavioral problems or high-risk behaviors. Each of these concerns, detailed below, has significant ties to the family of origin and likely contributed to the unsafe environment warranting child removal.

7.2.1 Genetics and Epigenetics

Many diseases and syndromes may be passed from one generation to the next through direct transmission of affected genes. Some genes may even have an influence over how resilient an individual is in the face of trauma. But the impact of inheritance is broader than just the direct impact of gene transmission. The field of epigenetics studies the impact of certain chemical markers that direct particular genes to turn "on" and other genes to turn "off." While the understanding of epigenetics is evolving, it seems clear that trauma in one generation can affect these markers, and the impact can be handed down to subsequent generations. If left unaddressed, these pathologies will continue to cycle across generations.

7.2.2 Prenatal and Birth Conditions

Substance abuse in pregnancy can result in a myriad of prenatal and postnatal health concerns. An estimated 400,000 children are exposed to alcohol or drugs annually, and some of these substances can have a direct impact on the developing fetus (Young et al., 2009). Also, mothers involved in substance abuse may have inadequate prenatal care, poor nutrition, and exposure to other risk factors such as domestic violence or other risk-taking behaviors and are at risk for premature delivery. Another risk for prematurity is young maternal age, and in the absence of an adequate support network, a very young parent may struggle to provide adequate care for the sometimes complex health needs of a premature infant, at times resulting in a safety risk to the child and ultimately child welfare involvement. Poor parent–child attachment within the first year of life has long-term implications for the child extending through adulthood and affecting their ability to positively parent their own offspring, potentially transmitting mental and physical health problems to the next generation (Fonagy, Steele, Moran, Steele, & Higgitt, 1993).

7.2.3 Environmental Conditions

Many environmental conditions may have an impact on the health of children in foster care. Inadequate nutrition may cause such conditions as failure to thrive and inadequate brain development. In some families, adequate nutrition is available but unpredictable, resulting in later food behaviors such as hoarding or overeating. A home environment may be unhealthy due to a lack of basic utilities such as water, electricity, or heat, impairing the family's ability to keep the space clean, appropriately handle waste products, and store perishable food. This may cause health risks for children such as exposure to spoiled food or environmental toxins. In addition, children may be exposed to infestations such as lice, scabies, or other insects. The level of stimulation in the environment can also have an effect on children. Studies suggest that sensory deprivation causes a lack of brain growth, less ability to problem solve, and an increase in mental health disorders, while overstimulation results in attention problems, poorer short-term memory, and greater risk-taking behavior.

Parent–child interaction plays a significant role in health and development as well. Children learn through joint attention, which occurs when the parent is actively engaged with the child during activities. An example of joint attention is when a parent and child look at the pictures in a book together, and the child points to a picture of a cow then looks at the parent to say "cow." The parent may then ask the child what sound the cow makes and then smile at the child awaiting the answer "moo." Another factor in development is the exposure of the child to activities or experiences. For example, fine motor skills are developed when the child is offered objects to manipulate, such as pegs in a pegboard or paper and scissors. Likewise, language is developed when parents talk to and read with their children. Social and environmental factors can negatively affect this. Children in lower socioeconomic homes hear 30 million fewer words by age 3 than their counterparts in homes that are more affluent (Hart, B. and Risley, T., 1995). This disparity results in significant language differences at the time of entry into school.

Extending beyond the dyadic parent–child relationship, the family as a systemic whole can affect a child's health. The family system, which includes a number of dynamic relationships (e.g., spouses, siblings, parent–child), is a child's first relational environment in which they learn about emotions, rules and hierarchies, family values and meanings, as well as standards for taking care of others and responding to stress (Henry, Morris, & Harrist, 2015). How families cope with and adapt to internal and external stressors, disruptions, and traumas impacts the health and well-being of individual family members as well as overall family functioning based on the positive or pathological nature of their feedback, reactivity, and escalation processes (Dishion & Kavanagh, 2003).

7.2.4 Routine Childhood Disease

Children in foster care are at least as likely as other children to develop acute or chronic health conditions. Such childhood maladies as ear infections, colds, and rashes are common. Chronic diseases such as Type I diabetes, allergic rhinitis, and asthma may also be present in high numbers; interestingly, some typical childhood illnesses such as asthma are even found with greater prevalence than the regular population, perhaps due in part to the impact of stress on the immune system (Halfon et al., 1995). Children in foster care may also experience constitutional symptoms, such as constipation, bedwetting, headaches, and stomachaches, which can be provoked by the anxiety of their situation. Some early risk factors for adult disease, such as hypertension and increased BMI, may also be present and have their origin in the abuse and neglect adversity the child has previously faced (Slopen, Koenen, & Kubzansky, 2014).

7.2.5 Behavioral Problems and High-Risk Behaviors

Behavioral problems such as Attention Deficit Hyperactivity Disorder, Oppositional Defiant Disorder, Posttraumatic Stress Disorder, attachment difficulties, depression, anxiety, and other mental health disorders are prevalent in significantly higher rates than in the general population, in perhaps as many as 60% of children in foster care. These disorders are often caused or exacerbated by the life circumstances a child or youth has experienced. Youth in foster care have a history of family abuse or neglect or were relinquished to state care to gain access to medical and behavioral interventions the birth family could not handle or afford (Bender, 2005). Once the child is in state custody, foster care placement can introduce new difficulties based on a number of factors such as child behavior, age, quality of foster care, and caseworker professionalism (Holtan, Handegård, Thørnblad, & Vis, 2013), which may result in multiple or disrupted transitions further aggravating youth behavioral problems. Youth in chaotic environments may develop risk-taking behaviors such as high-risk sexual behavior running away from foster homes, delinquent behavior, and experimentation with drugs or alcohol. As a result, they can develop associated health problems, such as sexually transmitted diseases, pregnancy, injuries related to violence, and drug or alcohol addiction.

7.2.6 Stressed Out

The role of stress in brain and immune function is a growing area of research and discussion (Shonkoff et al., 2012). Stress is defined as "the physical pressure, pull, or force exerted by one thing on another" (www.dictionary.com). Humans have a predictable biologic response to acute stress. The heart rate, blood pressure, and respiratory rate increase, the pupils constrict, blood is diverted away from the gastrointestinal tract and toward the heart and lungs, and organs used for regular resting activities are temporarily turned "off." The response is meant to help humans react to a dangerous or threatening situation, and it does this quite effectively by preparing our minds and bodies to be ready to fight or escape danger.

There is individual variation in what is perceived as "stressful." For example, an event like public speaking might be extremely stressful to one person, yet perfectly comfortable to someone else. Also, the body's response may vary from person to person. While the overall biology of the stress response is the same in all people, the situations that trigger it and the intensity of it may also vary among individuals, depending on their own genetic and biologic makeup as well as their own previous experiences. This is one reason why individuals who experience the same event may have very different reactions.

Repetti, Taylor, and Seeman (2002) explain how the family environment is a child's first context for risk or protection. Cascading risks, risk factors or disadvantages that accumulate across the life course, place youth on trajectories of positive or negative adaptation over time (Repetti et al. (2002), see also Masten & Cicchetti, 2010; Wickrama, Merten, & Wickrama, 2012). These cascading risks have biological underpinnings directly linked with physical stress responses that can become dysregulated (e.g., abnormal cortisol responses indicating heightened or diminished stress reactivity) as early as prenatal development (for full discussion of HPA/cortisol responses, see Repetti et al., 2002).

Not all stressful events are bad. Some stressors can be part of the normal developmental experience. For example, separating from parents to go to school is a common stressor, but it is generally good to learn how to function independently. Other stressors are extraordinary, but tolerable. These are generally not the normal developmental experiences that everyone has. An example might be surviving a house fire, a tornado, or a death in the family. These events are stressful, and they can certainly impact us deeply, but in the presence of healthy supports from friends, family, and our community, the events may be tolerable stressors and may even shape who we become in a positive way. However, exposure to parental substance abuse, domestic violence, and child abuse are atypical and toxic stressors. When these stressors occur, especially in high frequencies, and without the buffering presence of supportive adult relationships, the impact is poisonous (Johnson et al., 2013). The human body is not designed to live in a state of constant, toxic stress. It takes only milliseconds for cortisol to be released during a stress event; up to 8–10 hours are needed to rid the body of the effects of that cortisol, and fully return to a resting state. What happens, then, when the body experiences stress event after stress event in the same day? When cortisol is always circulating? When there is no resting? What happens when the protective factor of healthy relational support does not exist? Humans, especially children, become acutely and/or chronically ill.

7.3 Adult Health Outcomes

Thirty years ago Vincent Felitti was an internal medicine doctor who ran a clinic aimed at trying to help adults lose weight and be healthier. Many of his patients did well in the program, which focused on nutrition and exercise, but there were some patients who initially succeeded, only to drop out, gain weight, and return to their previous state of poor health. This is extremely frustrating for primary care physicians who are focused on improving health and preventing future problems. Dr. Felitti set about the business of understanding why this subset of patients was failing. He performed in-depth interviews with some patients, and as he listened to stories of eating habits, he also heard stories of substance abuse, depression, and relational difficulties. In searching for the beginning of all these dysfunctional behaviors, what he heard over and over again was the story of childhood abuse, neglect, abandonment, loss, and other toxic stressors. He identified ten childhood experiences that he called *Adverse Childhood Experiences* (*ACEs*), and a few years later he and the Centers for Disease Control launched a large study investigating the relationship of ACEs to adult health factors (Felitti et al., 1998) (Fig. 7.1).

Over 17,000 people completed a survey about their adverse experiences in childhood and current adult health indicators. Two-thirds had experienced at least one category of childhood adversity. One in five had experienced three or more adversities. And when that childhood trauma was matched against adult health disease, the results were startling. The more ACEs, the higher the rate of health behaviors such as overeating, smoking, excessive drinking, drug use, and high-risk sexual

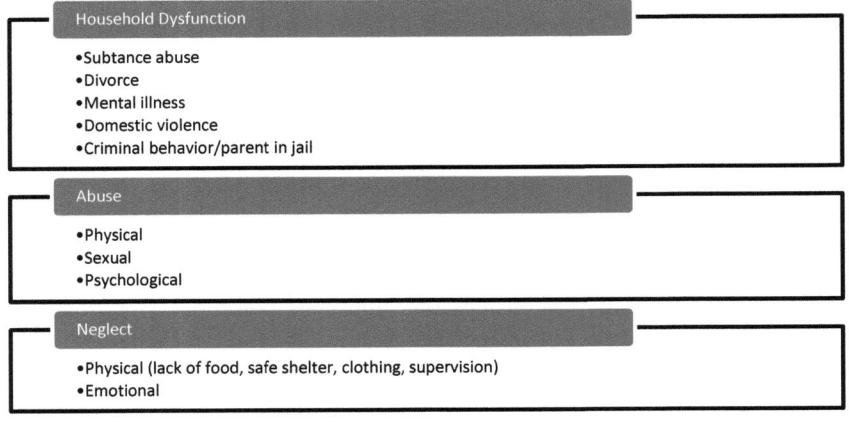

Fig. 7.1 Adverse Childhood Experiences (ACEs)

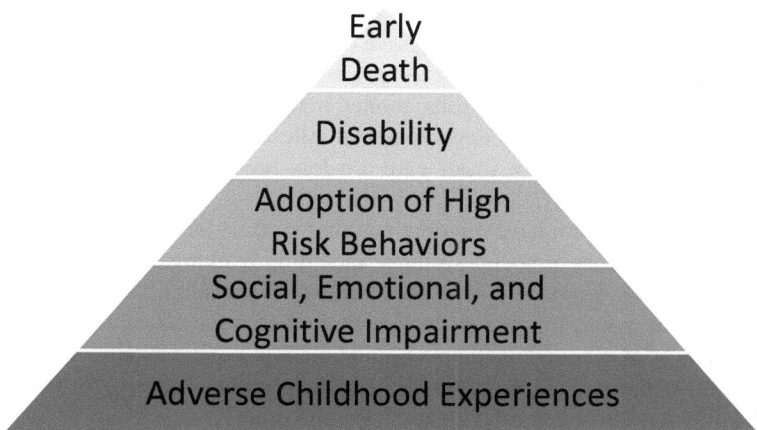

Fig. 7.2 Cascading risks associated with Adverse Childhood Experiences (ACEs)

behavior. In turn, participants with more ACEs had been diagnosed with chronic lung disease, ischemic heart disease, depression, and liver disease. They also had greater likelihood of suicide attempts, unwanted pregnancies, and domestic violence. In fact, being exposed to a lot of ACEs, or toxic stress, created risk for lifelong health and social problems, job and relational dysfunction, disability, and early death. These cascading risk factors are modeled in Fig. 7.2.

This information provides greater context for working with children who come into foster care from abusive or neglectful homes and sheds light on potential future outcomes based on their family histories. Even those children who seem relatively healthy often have three or more ACEs. This model suggests that in the absence of some sort of intervention, their adult lives will be plagued with health and social challenges.

7.4 Social Outcomes of Children in Foster Care

Child Welfare Systems attempt to find permanency for children in foster care. This permanency can come in the form of reunification with parents, adoption, or guardianship. However, when children turn 18 while in foster care (i.e., "age out"), most foster care systems no longer retain legal custody of them. Just as the expected health outcomes of children exposed to abuse or neglect are concerning so are their social outcomes.

A study of youth who turned 18 while in foster care found that one in five spent at least one night homeless during their first year on their own (Reilly, 2003). Half of these youth did not graduate from high school or complete a GED, which is not surprising given the previous information about education delays and the relative lack of support that extends beyond 18. Even though some resources may extend beyond age 18, often youth have a negative opinion of Child Welfare and choose to try life on their own. They, like most teens, are wildly unprepared to do this, having very little or no experience with jobs, money management, and accessing housing or transportation. These are all developmental milestones associated with emerging into adulthood that youth in foster care are less prepared for than their family-housed peers (Arnett, 2007).

A youth who does not have ongoing parental support faces very real challenges in navigating all kinds of social systems, including banking, housing, transportation, and education, to name a few. Their biological parents likely also struggle in these areas. The youth might also have a limited or nonexistent support network lacking mentors or other adults helping guide them in good decision making. Thus, they may make the same kinds of mistakes as their nonfoster peers, but without any sort of safety net leading to more devastating outcomes.

When the practical barriers to growing up are combined with histories of adversity stemming from birth families and foster care placements, it is clear how stressors, health risks, risky behaviors, and relational difficulties can endure. While striving to achieve developmental milestones associated with becoming an adult (work, intimacy, ideology; Arnett, 2007), youth with foster care backgrounds continue to bear the burden of the physical and mental health concerns their life circumstances loaded on them long after they have exited the system. At age 25, they typically have more mental health diagnoses than their peers, but less career success and are less likely to have health insurance, which limits or prevents access to appropriate and quality health care services to address their physical and mental health concerns.

Box 7.1. Implications for Practice
With over 30 years of experience supporting children and families in the child welfare system, including working in shelters and early intervention settings, I've gleaned a few insights that I'd like to share with professionals in the field. First, always remember that families—both biological and foster families—are doing the best that they can. Accept these families as they are, and refrain from judging those facing obstacles. Be sensitive to the notion that some families simply don't have the social support they need to effectively cope with normative and nonnormative stressors. Recognize the strengths of each family, and build on those.

Most children come into the child welfare system because of neglect; we do well to identify and provide resources to families prior to an incident of neglect. Potentially beneficial resources vary based on each family's needs; know your community partners, and be ready to offer referrals. That being said, I've learned that "it's only help when it's *what* you need, *when* you ask for it." In other words, a resource that you consider helpful might be contrary

> to what the family truly needs, or might be disregarded if it is offered out of sync with the family's perceived needs at that point in time. As such, I've found that it is essential to communicate clearly and respectfully with families. If you make your good intentions known, you will be accepted.
>
> Never lose sight of the fact that in the midst of multiple placements and transitions, it is *still the same child*, with unique interests, needs, and characteristics; that child wants to be home. I noticed that children who fare well in the shelter setting possess resilience characteristics such as good social skills, self-confidence, and the ability to 'connect' with others. If a child can connect with someone in the child welfare system—maybe even you—then it can 'tide them over' until their placement becomes permanent; don't underestimate the impact of your relationship with each child. Finally, as you work with families and children facing challenges, I'd strongly encourage you to *never count them out*.
>
> —Cyd Roberts, Child Welfare Professional

7.5 Barriers to Health Care Access and Delivery

As the guardian for children and youth in foster care, the state becomes responsible for providing health care services. The Federal Title IV-E program provides significant funding for foster care systems based on certain socioeconomic and other eligibility criteria of children entering state custody. In addition, the vast majority of children in foster care are eligible for Medicaid, which gives them access to health care services. For those who are undocumented and ineligible for Medicaid or have needs beyond what their state's Medicaid program may meet, the state child welfare/child protection agency may designate funds to meet these needs.

While financing may not be a significant barrier, many others do exist. Children in foster care often arrive in custody without anyone knowing an adequate health history. Caseworkers have very little training on obtaining medical information, and at the time of removal, the circumstances may be too chaotic to obtain the information anyway. Sometimes parents are not available to give medical information. Once a child is in custody, mobility can be a barrier to continuity of health care. Half of children in custody move at least once within the first six months, and among older children, a quarter move more than eight times while in custody (Wulczyn, Hislop, & Chen, 2007). Each move poses challenges in passing medical information, medications, and medical equipment from one place to the next. Also, the moves may be across town or across the state. This can disrupt the current relationship between the child and the health care provider, resulting in delays in establishing a new provider and obtaining appropriate appointments or referrals. The placement instability can be a serious barrier for children who have complex medical needs, a lot of ancillary services such as occupational or physical therapy, or a strong relationship with a provider.

Moving around can *cause* problems as well. Children who have frequent placement moves have greater difficulty with attachment, increased frequency of behavior problems, and decreased educational success. In fact, highly mobile students, those who move three or more times, are behind by one full grade level by the sixth grade. There are a number of reasons why children may move from one placement to another while in custody. Early placements usually occur in the immediate crisis of the child's removal from the home, so the first placement may be a shelter or emergency foster home, but may move quickly to a more stable home such as with a relative or traditional foster parent. Larger sibling groups are difficult to place in the same home because of space or resource limitations, so initially these brothers and sisters may find themselves scattered across several placements. It is a child welfare system goal to place siblings together, so as the case progresses, children may move from those initial placements to homes where they can be together. There are child and foster parent issues that might play a role in placement disruption as well. Children may have medical or behavioral problems that can be difficult to manage—sometimes impossible given a foster parent's level of training, ability, and number of other responsibilities. The foster parents may not have adequate support or respite and may become overwhelmed. In addition, they may also have their own personal stressors such as illness, moving, job changes, or relationship challenges that affect their ability to serve as a foster home. Whatever the cause, moving is both a common experience and a troublesome one.

7.6 Delivering Health Care to Children in Foster Care

In 1988 the Child Welfare League of America developed general standards for health care delivery for foster children. Nearly 20 years ago the American Academy of Pediatrics (AAP) convened the Task Force on Health Care for Children in Foster Care, a multidisciplinary group charged with developing more specific guidance for primary care providers on the health management of children and youth in foster care. Several principles underpin the recommendations, including the following: (1) children in foster care must have a medical home, (2) children in foster care need comprehensive health care services, (3) children in foster care have more intensive service needs than the general population, and (4) health care intervention should include preventive educational and mental health services and health care management across multiple disciplines (Task Force on Health Care for Children in Foster Care, 2005).

A medical home is a medical practice that has certain characteristics. The practice should be accessible and family-centered, and should provide care that is coordinated, compassionate, comprehensive, and continuous over time. In addition, a medical home for children in foster care needs to have professionals who recognize the unique challenges that these children face as well as the willingness to engage the others who are involved, such as child welfare, courts, foster, and birth parents. Given the potential for genetically linked mental and physical health challenges, the involvement (or awareness) of the youth's family of origin in the their treatment is key.

The AAP guidelines on foster health care set forth a schedule for routine health visits that is more robust than a typical well child schedule and include recommendations specific to a child navigating the foster care system. This includes gathering information from child welfare on the cause of custody and the current status of the case, more focus on trauma and ACE history, making placement recommendations to child welfare agencies that consider the needs of the child, and checking "goodness of fit" of the child and foster home, and systematically communicating with birth parents, foster parents, case workers, and the court on the health status and needs of the child. A summary of the AAP recommendations is provided in Figs. 7.3, 7.4, and 7.5.

Health Information Gathering at the Time of Removal
- health problems
- name of health care providers
- medications
- medical devices, including glasses, hearing aides or any other equipment needed

Initial Medical Screen
- within 24 hours of removal from home
- address any active health concerns
- review available health information
- recommend placement and followup plan

Fig. 7.3 American Academy of Pediatrics (AAP) recommendations for initial health evaluation

Ongoing Health Information Gathering
- complete medical history, including family history of illness/disease
- perinatal history for 0-6, including drug exposure
- developmental and trauma/behavioral health history
- psychosocial history, including ACE's, reason for placement, and status of siblings
- nutrition and education history

Comprehensive Health Assessment
- within 30 days of placement
- review complete health history
- physical exam and specialty referral for concerns
- developmental and trauma/behavioral screening and referral
- immunization review
- dental, hearing and vision screen
- lab studies as indicated

Fig. 7.4 American Academy of Pediatrics (AAP) recommendations for health stabilization

Follow-Up Assessment
- 30 days after comprehensive health assessment
- review health information, including referral reports
- identify interval problems that have surfaced
- physical exam
- assess "goodness of fit" with foster home
- update immunizations and screening
- determine follow-up schedule

Periodic Preventive Health Care
- frequency depends on age, health status, and social stability
- more frequent visits than non-foster children
- ongoing behavioral and developmental screening and referral

Discharge Encounter
- review conditions identified and treatment provided with new caregiver

Fig. 7.5 American Academy of Pediatrics (AAP) recommendations for health maintenance

7.7 Mental Health and Psychotropic Medication Use

As has been described, children who have been abused or neglected and ultimately been brought into foster care have experienced a number of potentially traumatic events. They may have ongoing relational loss or emotional trauma as well, as they may face blaming or rejecting behaviors by birth parents, separation from a family and community culture that is familiar, the ongoing uncertainty of being placed in foster care, multiple transitions, and even abuse or neglect while in foster care. They also likely did not have good role models for healthy interpersonal and family relationships. Their ability to process all these stressful events can be impaired by cognitive limitations or mental health conditions such as depression, anxiety, or posttraumatic stress disorder (PTSD).

Children in foster care should be screened upon entry and routinely for evidence of mental health concerns. Most children will require referral for further evaluation and treatment. Much like the medical home, mental health services for children in foster care should be provided by well-trained, experienced mental health professionals who understand childhood trauma as well as the unique nature of the stresses imposed by the foster care system. Detailed case information, family history and ongoing ties, relationships within foster care placements, and current behavior in the foster home and other environments such as school are vital pieces of information needed by the mental health professional. Continuity is also a must, since most mental health treatment occurs over time and requires a significant trust relationship between the caregivers, child, and mental health provider.

When possible, evidence-based mental health care treatment should be provided. *Parent–child interaction therapy* is a strategy for teaching caregivers how to connect with their young children and how to navigate challenging situations such as discipline. *Trauma-focused cognitive behavioral therapy* is a therapy that teaches the individual how to process their emotions and thoughts related to the traumatic experience. They are given the tools to alleviate overwhelming thoughts that can cause anxiety or depression and are taught to process thoughts and emotions in a more healthy way. *Family-centered interventions* (Dishion & Kavanagh, 2003) that involve or address the birth family as well as foster care parents and caseworker, and that can be delivered at multiple levels (family, school, community), can contribute to positive adaptation given the youth's accumulation of risks. Such an approach supports relationship and coping skills development that can benefit the youth currently and after they exit foster care. Coordinating services with youth, their foster family, and their birth family can be a sensitive, complicated, and difficult process; however, many youth do have contact with and involvement of their families during treatment (Southerland, Burns, Farmer, Wagner, & Simpson, 2014). There is a growing body of support for family-centered approaches to optimize youth outcomes in social services contexts (e.g., Kemp, Marcenko, Hoagwood, & Vesneski, 2009; Pennell, Edwards, & Burford, 2010) as well as health care contexts (See Council on Children With Disabilities and Medical Home Implementation Project Advisory Committee, 2014).

As part of their mental health treatment, the use of psychotropic medications in children in foster care is a complicated and controversial topic. The stressors encountered prior to and during foster care, combined with the lack of detailed information, and the discontinuity with adults in their lives and with health care providers, creates significant challenges. A 2011 study by the USGAO found that in the five states reviewed, children in foster care were prescribed psychotropic medications 2.7–4.5 times as often as children who were not in foster care. Similar disparities were found when considering the use of concurrent psychotropic medication. It is difficult to determine what the "right" rate should be, since almost all children in foster care have experienced significant loss and trauma, and are at much higher risk for developing mental health conditions that medications may treat. But these medications are not a magic bullet, and they do not come without significant risk for side-effects. It is important that the decision to start psychotropic medications occurs in the proper context: (1) the child should have routine health care being delivered in a medical home; (2) positive mental health screening should result in further evaluation by the appropriate pediatric-trained mental health professional; (3) a diagnosis should be supported by adequate information regarding the child's history and current behavioral function; (4) psychotropic medication should be part of a larger mental health plan that includes appropriate therapy, family and school intervention; (5) psychotropic medication should match the diagnosis, and should be initiated and monitored by a pediatric psychiatrist or, if possible, a pediatrician with significant experience and training in behavioral management; (6) providers should use the lowest dose needed to achieve stability; and (7) regular follow-up should review mental health and social changes as well as side-effects (www.aap.org). Ideally, pharmacological interventions facilitate the mental and physical therapies necessary to help the child learn coping skills and positively adapt in the uncertain and transitory foster care system, not simply dull the pain of their experiences.

7.8 Conclusion

Individual health is generally viewed as an individual issue, but resilience researchers promote a "whole community" approach understanding links between risk and protective factors at individual, family, school, and community levels to provide resources and foster healthy development, particularly among children (Khanlou & Wray, 2014, p. 75). There is also strong empirical support that resilience-focused approaches to improving mental and physical health are effective and have long-term benefits extending from childhood into adulthood (Khanlou & Wray, 2014). Approaches aimed at fostering resilience among youth faced with risks and hardships associated with family maltreatment and foster care placement are critical for their current health. However, family-level resilience interventions aimed at improving family relationships and restoring the family system to a higher level of functioning than when the child was removed are also important for the child's long-term development, mental and physical health, and contributions to the community as an independent and functioning adult (Boss, 2001).

Providing health care to children and youth in foster care is challenging work. Their story is one of childhood toxic stress, a complex child protection system that faces difficulties with stability and continuity and may even add to the trauma experienced by the children it is trying to protect, and an adult health and social prediction that is depressing. But, just as brokenness can transfer across generations, so can wholeness—even repaired wholeness from resilience-focused and family-centered foster care interventions. For the children in our care today, the future has not yet been written, and it is the opportunity of health care providers, child welfare systems, and the community at large to intervene, reconnect the broken strands of their lives, and change the ending of their family's story.

Discussion Questions

1. *For Health Sciences Students*: Physicians play a salient role in determining whether allegations of child abuse or neglect are substantiated by medical evidence. What challenges come with being in a position requiring you to provide information that has the potential to significantly affect the immediate future of the child (i.e., removal from the home) as well as affect the long-term outcomes of the child? Consider both ethical/professional challenges, as well as personal challenges (i.e., dissonant thoughts or feelings) that may emerge during the process. How do you go about addressing these challenges and resolving these issues?
2. *For Human Sciences Students*: Relationships are the heart of the classroom; strong teacher–child relationships and teacher–family relationships are essential for children's educational success. Brainstorm a list of challenges that teachers must address in order to nurture teacher–child relationships with children in foster care as well as teacher–family relationships with foster families. Do you

think teachers are adequately trained to meet the unique needs of children and adolescents in foster care as well as the families caring for them? If not, what do they need to know?
3. Design a longitudinal study to examine the outcomes of children in foster care. What physical health, mental health, and/or educational outcomes would you assess and why? What community partners would you need to engage in order to successfully implement your study?
4. Consider the authors' concluding appeal to service providers and the larger community to embrace the opportunity to "intervene, reconnect the broken strands of (children's) lives, and change the ending of their family's story." Using a *strengths-based approach*, strategize pathways to answer this call to action.

References

AFCARS Report. (2014). Retrieved from http://www.acf.hhs.gov/programs/cb
Arnett, J. (2007). Afterword: Aging out of care—Toward realizing the possibilities of emerging adulthood. *New Directions for Youth Development, 113*, 151–161. doi:10.1002/yd.207
Avery, R. (2010). An examination of theory and promising practice for achieving permanency for teens before they age out of foster care. *Children and Youth Services Review, 32*, 399–408. doi:10.1016/j.childyouth.2009.10.011
Bender, E. (2005). State seeks solution to foster care crisis. *Psychiatric News from the American Psychiatric Association, 40*(2), 8–58. doi:10.1176/pn.40.2.00400008. http://dx.doi.org/
Boss, P. (2001). *Family stress management: A contextual approach* (2nd ed.). Thousand Oaks, CA: Sage.
Caffey, J. (1946). Multiple fractures in the long bones of infants suffering from chronic subdural hematoma. *Radiology, 194*, 163–173.
Child Welfare Information Gateway. (2013). *Foster care statistics 2012*. Retrieved from https://www.childwelfare.gov/pubs/factsheets/foster.cfm
Council on Children with Disabilities; Medical Home Implementation Project Advisory Committee. (2014). Patient- and family-centered care coordination: A framework for integrating care for children and youth across multiple systems. *Pediatrics, 133*, e1451–e1460. doi:10.1542/peds.2014-0318
Cowal, K., Shinn, M. B., Weitzman, B. C., Stojanovic, D., & Labay, L. (2002). Mother-child separations among homeless and housed families receiving public assistance in New York City. *American Journal of Community Psychology, 30*, 711–730. doi:10.1023/A:1016325332527
Cushing, G., Samuels, G., & Kerman, B. (2014). Profiles of relational permanence at 22: Variability in parental supports and outcomes among young adults with foster care histories. *Children and Youth Services Review, 39*, 73–83. doi:10.1016/j.childyouth.2014.01.001
Dishion, T., & Kavanagh, K. (2003). *Intervening in adolescent problem behaviors: A family-centered approach*. New York, NY: Guilford.
Felitti, V. J., Anda, R. F., Nordenberg, D., et al. (1998). Relationship of childhood abuse and household dysfunction to many of the leading causes of death in adults: The Adverse Childhood Experiences (ACE) Study. *American Journal of Preventive Medicine, 14*, 245–258. doi:10.1016/S0749-3797(98)00017-8
Flowers, P., Toro, P., & Miles, B. (2010). Emerging adulthood and leaving foster care: Settings associated with mental health. *American Journal of Community Psychology, 47*, 335–348. doi:10.1007/s10464-010-9401-2
Fonagy, P., Steele, M., Moran, G., Steele, H., & Higgitt, A. (1993). Measuring the ghost in the nursery: An empirical study of the relation between parents' mental representations of

childhood experiences and their infant's security of attachment. *Journal of the American Psychoanalytic Association, 41*, 957–989. doi:10.1177/000306519304100403

Halfon, N., Mendonca, A., & Berkowitz, G. (1995). Health status of children in foster care. *Archives of Pediatric & Adolescent Medicine, 149*, 386–392. doi:10.1001/archpedi.1995. 02170160040006

Hart, B. and Risley, T. Meaningful Differences in the Everyday Experiences of Young American Children (1995). Paul H. Brookes Publishing Co. Healthy Foster Care America. (2016). (n.d.) Mental and behavioral health. Retrieved from, http://www.aap.org/en-us/advocacy-and-policy/aap-health-initiatives/healthy-foster-care-america/Pages/Mental-and-Behavioral-Health.aspx

Henry, C., Morris, A., & Harrist, A. (2015). Family resilience: Moving into the third wave. *Family Relations, 64*, 22–43.

Holtan, A., Handegård, B., Thørnblad, R., & Vis, S. (2013). Placement disruption in long-term kinship and nonkinship foster care. *Children and Youth Services Review, 35*, 1087–1094. doi:10.1016/j.childyouth.2013.04.022

Johnson, S. B., Riley, A. W., Granger, D. A., & Riis, J. (2013). The science of early life toxic stress for pediatric practice and advocacy. *Pediatrics, 131*, 319–327. doi:10.1542/peds.2012-0469

Kemp, S., Marcenko, M., Hoagwood, K., & Vesneski, W. (2009). Engaging parents in child welfare services: Bridging family needs and child welfare mandates. *Child Welfare, 88*, 101–118. http://lynx.lib.usm.edu/login?url= http://earch.ebscohost.com/login.aspx?direct=true&db=c8h&AN=2010318523&site=ehost-live

Kempe, C. H., Silverman, F. N., Steele, B. F., Droegemueller, W., & Silver, H. K. (1962). The Battered Child Syndrome. *Journal for the American Medical Association, 181*, 17–24.

Khanlou, N., & Wray, R. (2014). A whole community approach toward children and youth resilience promotion: A review of resilience literature. *International Journal of Mental Health and Addiction, 12*, 64–79. doi:10.1007/s11469-013-9470-1

Masten, A., & Cicchetti, D. (2010). Developmental cascades. *Development and Psychopathology, 22*, 491–495. doi:10.1017/S0954579410000222. http://dx.doi.org.lynx.lib.usm.edu/

Myers, J. E. B. (2008). A short history of child protection in America. *Family Law Quarterly, 42*(3), 449–463.

Pennell, J., Edwards, M., & Burford, G. (2010). Expedited family group engagement and child permanency. *Children and Youth Services Review, 32*, 1012–1019. doi:10.1016/j.childyouth. 2010.03.029

Reilly, T. (2003). Transition from care: Status and outcomes of youth who age out of foster care. *Child Welfare, 82*, 727–746. http://lynx.lib.usm.edu/login?url=http://search.ebscohost.com/login.aspx?direct=true&db=c8h&AN=2004187339&site=ehost-live

Repetti, R., Taylor, S., & Seeman, T. (2002). Risky families: Family social environments and the mental and physical health of offspring. *Psychological Bulletin, 128*, 330–366. doi:10.1037/0033-2909.128.2.330. http://dx.doi.org.lynx.lib.usm.edu/

Scannapieco, M., Connell-Carrick, K., & Painter, K. (2007). In their own words: Challenges facing youth aging out of foster care. *Child and Adolescent Social Work Journal, 24*, 423–435. doi:10.1007/s10560-007-0093-x

Shinn, M. B., Rog, D. J., & Culhane, D. P. (2005). *Family homelessness: Background research findings and policy options*. Washington, DC: U.S. Interagency Council on Homelessness.

Shonkoff, J. P., Garner, A., & The Committee on Psychosocial Aspects of Child and Family Health, Committee on Early Childhood, Adoption, and Dependent Care, & Section on Developmental and Behavioral Pediatrics. (2012). The lifelong effects of early childhood adversity and toxic stress. *Pediatrics, 129*, e232–e246. doi:10.1542/peds.2011-2663

Slopen, N., Koenen, K. C., & Kubzansky, L. D. (2014). Cumulative adversity in childhood and emergent risk factors for long-term health. *Journal of Pediatrics, 164*, 631–638. doi:10.1016/j.jpeds.2013.11.003

Stott, T. (2012). Placement instability and risky behaviors of youth aging out of care. *Child and Adolescent Social Work Journal, 29*, 61–83. doi:10.1007/s10560-011-0247-8

Stress. (n.d.). Retrieved from www.dictionary.com

Southerland, D., Burns, B., Farmer, E., Wagner, H., & Simpson, A. (2014). Family involvement in treatment foster care. *Residential Treatment for Children & Youth, 31*, 2–16. doi:10.1080/0886571X.2014.878586

Takayama, J., Wolfe, E., & Coulter, K. (1998). Relationship between reason for placement and medical findings among children in foster care. *Pediatrics, 101*, 201–207. doi:10.1542/peds.101.2.201

Task Force on Health Care for Children in Foster Care. (2005). *Fostering health: Health care for children and adolescents in foster care*. New York, NY: American Academy of Pediatrics.

Terling-Watt, T. (2001). Permanency in kinship care: An exploration of disruption rates and factors associated with placement disruption. *Children and Youth Services Review, 23*, 111–126. doi:10.1016/S0190-7409(01)00129-3

US Government Accountability Office. (1995). Foster care: Health needs of many young children are unknown and unmet. Retrieved from http://www.gao.gov/archive/1995/he95114.pdf

US Government Accountability Office. (2011). Foster children: HHS guidance could help states improve oversight of psychotropic medications. Retrieved from http://www.gao.gov/assets/590/586570.pdf

Wickrama, T., Merten, M., & Wickrama, K. A. S. (2012). Early community influence on young adult physical health: Race/ethnicity and gender differences. *Advances in Life Course Research, 17*, 25–33. doi:10.1016/j.alcr.2012.01.001

Wulczyn, F., Hislop, K., & Chen, L. (2007). *Foster care dynamics 2000-2005: A report from the multistate foster care data archive*. Chicago, IL: Chapin Hall Center for Children at the University of Chicago.

Young, N. K., Gardner, S., Otero, C., Dennis, K., Chang, R., Earle, K., et al. (2009). *Substance-exposed infants: State responses to the problem*. Rockville, MD: Substance Abuse and Mental Health Services Administration. HHS Pub. No. (SMA) 09-4369.

Chapter 8
Strengthening Families Facing Breast Cancer: Emerging Trends and Clinical Recommendations

Merle Keitel, Alexandra Lamm, and Alyson Moadel-Robblee

Breast cancer affects not only patients but their family members and close friends as well, with family members reporting significant stress (Lund, Ross, Petersen, & Groenvold, 2014). Diagnosis and subsequent treatment can introduce considerable tension into the family. Disruptions in family functioning, perhaps more so than the illness itself, are responsible for decreased social and psychological well-being (Lavee, McCubbin, & Olson, 1987). The Family Adjustment and Adaptation Response (FAAR) Model (McCubbin & Patterson, 1983) conceptualizes the impact of chronic illness on a family as a function of the resources the family possesses, how the family members perceive the illness, and their ability to manage it (McCubbin & Patterson, 1983). The model recognizes that families who have the capacity to be flexible can adapt to a chronic stressor such as breast cancer by reallocating roles, changing their perceptions, and enhancing their resources. These

---

M. Keitel, Ph.D. (✉)
Counseling & Counseling Psychology, Fordham University,
113 West 60th Street, New York, NY 10023, USA
e-mail: mkeitel@fordham.edu

A. Lamm
Fordham University, Bronx, NY 10458, USA
e-mail: alamm@fordham.edu

A. Moadel-Robblee, Ph.D.
Albert Einstein College of Medicine, 1300 Morris Park Avenue, Bronx, NY 10461, USA
e-mail: alyson.moadel@einstein.yu.edu

© Springer International Publishing Switzerland 2017
G.L. Welch, A.W. Harrist (eds.), *Family Resilience and Chronic Illness*,
Emerging Issues in Family and Individual Resilience,
DOI 10.1007/978-3-319-26033-4_8

resilient families are able to successfully navigate the breast cancer experience by capitalizing on their strengths and reducing their vulnerabilities. A strong marriage and potential *social support* from friends, coworkers, and their religious communities are examples of protective factors. Vulnerability factors include low socioeconomic status, inadequate insurance, distance from extended family, and limited childcare options (cited in Henry, Morris, & Harrist, 2015).

This chapter focuses on how to support partners of breast cancer patients and the couple subsystem, because when the couple is stable, the entire family system functions better. It is particularly important to include intimate partners in treatment because they have been found to be equally or even more depressed and anxious than the patients (Grunfeld et al., 2004; Keitel, Zevon, Rounds, Petrelli, & Karakousis, 1990). According to Wagner, Bigatti, and Storniolo (2006), spouses of women with breast cancer scored lower on general health, mental health, and vitality than spouses of women without health concerns. Men are particularly vulnerable because they tend to have less developed social support networks. In fact, their wives tend to be their primary source of support. When their wives are ill, however, they hesitate to ask them for support, and thus can become emotionally isolated (Ell, Nishimoto, Mantell, & Hamovitch, 1988).

Medical family therapy utilizes a biopsychosocial system model where therapists and health care professionals work collaboratively to treat individuals with medical problems and their families (Tyndall, Hodgson, Lamson, White, & Knight, 2014). The interdisciplinary team is tasked with assessing the psychosocial aspects of the illness (e.g., individual strengths and barriers), and other stressors, which often involve the family (Tyndall et al., 2014). Such a collaborative approach has been found to benefit health care providers, patients, and their partners. Oncology professionals and staff are relieved to have the medical family therapist on-site to provide information, support, and hope to patients and their families. Among the benefits to patients and their families are less emotional suffering, greater hope, and improved clarity about the cancer experience (Sellers, 2000). Medical family therapists can help couples communicate openly and support one another, which leads to better coping and family functioning.

Family therapy with all family members included may not be realistic or effective for families facing breast cancer. One prominent obstacle is that family members often hide their true emotions from one another out of fear that expressing themselves will cause further suffering (Davey, Gulish, Askew, Godette, & Childs, 2005). Family members need a space to speak freely given that emotional expression has been linked with positive psychological outcomes (Stanton et al., 2000). Other logistical barriers include insurance coverage and coordination of schedules, which can be especially complicated when children are in school and family members work.

While weekly family therapy may not be ideal, individual support for patients and their partners and couples interventions have been found to help families cope more effectively (Breitbart et al., 2012; Badr & Krebs, 2013; Davey et al., 2005; Zahlis & Lewis, 2010). Clinicians can counsel couples on how to support each other and how to approach their children to improve family functioning during this stressful time.

8.1 Literature Review

Breast cancer is the second most prevalent cancer among American women after skin cancer, with one in eight women in the USA (12%) developing invasive breast cancer (ACS, 2014). According to the American Cancer Society, 14% of all cancer diagnoses are breast cancers; almost a quarter of a million new cases of *invasive breast cancer* (stages I–IV) and over 62,000 new cases of noninvasive early stage cancer (*ductal carcinoma* in situ) will be diagnosed in the USA in 2014. Only 0.05–1% of individuals diagnosed with breast cancer are men, but the incidence is rising (Ruddy & Winer, 2013). Breast cancer is the most prevalent cancer in African American and Hispanic women. Although Caucasian women are diagnosed at higher rates, African American and Hispanic women, on average, are diagnosed with more advanced disease. The risk of developing breast cancer increases with age. It is most commonly diagnosed in women ages 55–64, with a median age of 61 (ACS, 2014). Fortunately, fewer women are dying from breast cancer due to earlier detection, increased awareness and screening, and improved treatment. As of 2014, there are more than 2.8 million breast cancer survivors in the USA. These statistics are dramatic but when you consider all the close family members that also are affected, the numbers are all the more staggering.

According to a report by the American Cancer Society (2014), breast cancers are categorized by where the cells grow; e.g., carcinomas start in the lining of the breast tissue; adenocarcinomas grow in the glandular tissue; and sarcomas grow in the muscle, fat or connective tissue. They are further classified by proteins on the cancer cells that signal whether the cancers grow in a particular hormonal environment, i.e., estrogen, progesterone, or have too much of a growth-promoting protein (i.e., HER2/Neu). The most common type of breast cancer affecting 80% of those diagnosed is invasive ductal carcinoma, which starts in the milk ducts. Triple negative breast cancers are those that are not estrogen, progesterone, or HER2 positive. This form of breast cancer tends to be more aggressive and is more likely to affect younger women and African American and Latina women. Five-year relative survival rates vary with stage of disease and are estimated as follows: I (100%), II (93%), III (72%), IV (22%). While only 10% of breast cancers are linked to genetic mutations, and fewer than 15% of those diagnosed have a family history of breast cancer, up to 46% of women overestimate their risk (Herman & Herman, 2013).

8.1.1 Cancer Caregiving: Burdens and Benefits

Intimate partners of individuals with breast cancer often assume a caregiving role. The general cancer caregiving literature, reported below, is based primarily on male patients and female caregivers (typically Caucasian, middle-aged, female partners). Please note that this caregiver profile is not necessarily true for more diverse samples. Certainly, the caregiving literature specific to breast cancer provides a window into the often overlooked experiences of male caregivers.

Caregiving is most consuming during the first 2 years after diagnosis and at *terminal stages* (National Alliance for Caregiving, 2012). After 2 years, about a third of family member caregivers are still having difficulty coping with their own distress as well as the distress of the patient, in addition to dealing with lifestyle changes and a lack of information and tangible support (Kim, Kashy, Spillers, & Evans, 2010). Five years after diagnosis, 21% of caregivers still needed help coping with the patients' mental state, and 12% of caregivers reported *emotional distress*, a stressed relationship with the patient, and concerns about the adequacy of their health insurance (Kim et al., 2010). It is clear that individuals who provide extensive care but do not have adequate support are at risk for poor *quality of life* and high distress (Printz, 2011). This distress most likely results from worrying about their loved one's future, dealing with disrupted family functioning, and experiencing challenges managing everyday tasks. In a review of the research on cancer caregiving, Stenberg, Ruland, and Miaskowski (2010) found that many family caregivers have elevated levels of anxiety, sexual problems, sleep disturbance, and fatigue. Caregivers who are particularly vulnerable to distress include women, younger individuals, employed caregivers, and those with lower socioeconomic status (Kim & Given, 2008).

While caregiver burden and burnout have received increased and deserved attention in the professional literature, as intimated in the findings above, caregiving also appears to provide positive rewards such as enriched relationships and improved *self-esteem*. The concept of benefit finding, or post-traumatic growth, refers to positive psychological growth as a result of struggling with a challenging life event, with individuals reporting increased appreciation for and purpose in life, improved relationships, and enhanced spirituality. This phenomenon has been well-documented in cancer patients (Jim & Jacobsen, 2008), and there is growing evidence, that family members of cancer patients not only appreciate their relationships more but also adapt better (Kim, Schulz, & Carver, 2007).

Another benefit of cancer caregiving is the "teachable moment" that a cancer diagnosis can bring; that is, an event that can increase awareness and thereby mobilize an individual towards positive behavior change. While cancer patients often exhibit health-promoting behavior change such as smoking cessation, increased physical activity, and improved dietary practices, families of cancer patients have also been shown to improve their lifestyle, albeit to a lesser extent (Humpel, Magee, & Jones, 2007).

In an ongoing study of 46 ethnically diverse breast cancer patients and their caregivers in a low SES community in the Bronx, NY, Moadel (unpublished) found that changes for the better outweighed changes for the worse on 12 of the 16 items on the Bakas Caregiving Outcomes Scale (Bakas & Champion, 1999). Self-esteem, relationships between the patient and family members, and roles in life demonstrated particularly positive outcomes. On the other hand, caregiving exerted a heavy toll on emotional well-being, financial well-being, social time, and energy (see Fig. 8.1).

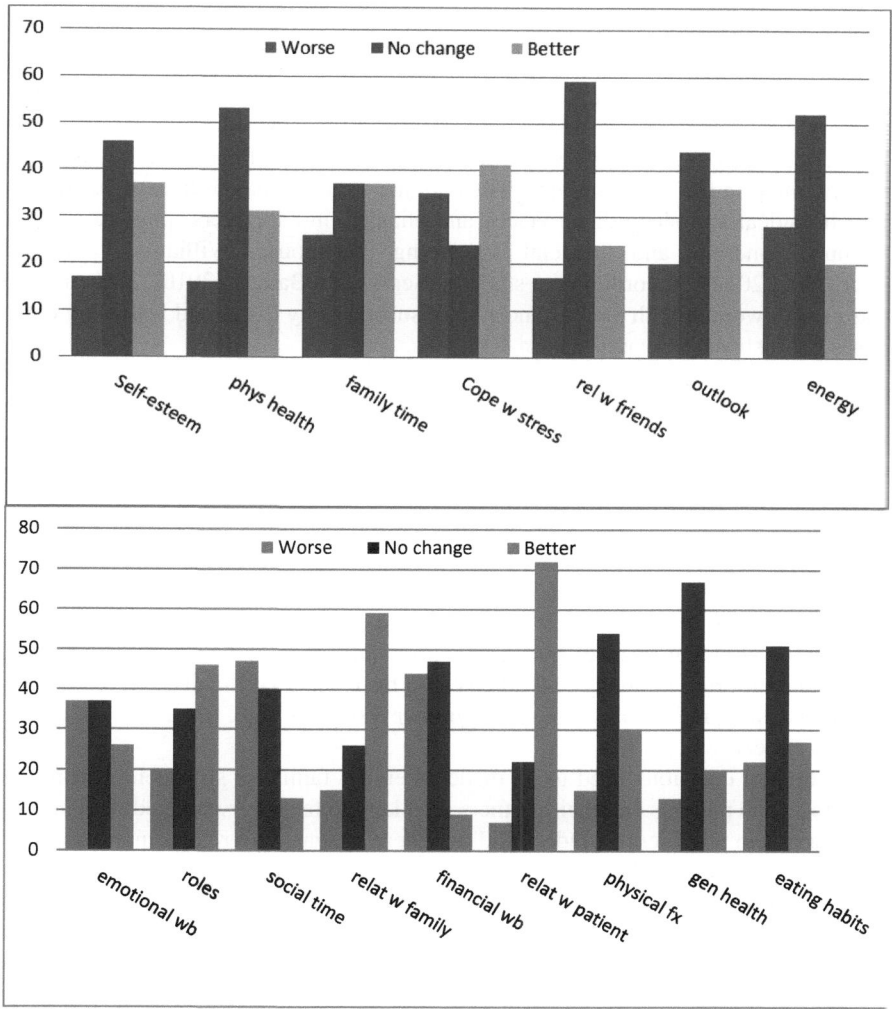

Fig. 8.1 Bakas caregiving outcomes of breast cancer caregivers in the Bronx, NY ($n=46$)

8.1.2 Phases of the Breast Cancer Experience

Breast cancer is not a single entity but a process that encompasses diagnosis, treatment (surgery, chemotherapy, and/or radiation), post-treatment, and potentially recurrence and end of life. The challenges at each phase require different interventions (Keitel, Kopala, & Potere, 2003). Each of these phases is discussed below with an eye toward implications for family functioning.

8.1.3 Diagnosis

In the 6–24 months after diagnosis, partners of breast cancer patients consult their doctors significantly more often, with both somatic and psychosocial problems (Heins et al., 2013), and cite worry about their partner's illness as the reason for seeking help in the first 6 months. The diagnostic period has been associated with psychological and sleep disturbances and changes in caregivers' physical health, immune function, and financial well-being (Northouse, Williams, Given, & McCorkle, 2012). According to a study by Segrin and Badger (2010), 25% of male partners of women with breast cancer were substantially distressed following diagnosis but distress decreased within 10 weeks.

Partners need assistance with a myriad of issues at this time, and these may differ according to the family's developmental stage. When cancer strikes a family at an early life stage (under 50), the diagnosis can be particularly devastating. Patients and their partners are typically preparing for or establishing their career, and perhaps raising a young family. A serious illness is not expected and anxiety is high. What if their loved one dies; how will they raise the children alone? How and what do they tell the children? How will they manage work and still provide support to their partner and children? In contrast, when cancer is diagnosed after retirement age, it is more normative to be ill. Partners and patients may have a peer group to consult with to identify excellent medical providers, understand treatment logistics, and feel comforted knowing individuals who have survived the disease. While it is still distressing, individuals often have greater resources (e.g., time, medical coverage) to cope.

Treatment decisions need to be made when the family is still reeling from the diagnosis and patients and their partners are likely to feel overwhelmed. It is important for health providers to understand that there are vast differences in individuals' preferences regarding their desire for information (Steginga, Occhipinti, Wilson, & Dunn, 1998) and involvement in making treatment decisions. Some patients want information but prefer that their physicians make the treatment decisions. Information can be a great antidote to anxiety arising from uncertainty, and although not all uncertainty can be removed, family members of individuals with early stage breast cancer may be reassured by the encouraging statistics (Keitel & Kopala, 2000). Alternatively, other individuals become overwhelmed with too much information and prefer to defer to their doctors. Patients and their partners also may differ in how much detail they prefer. Health professionals can help by being responsive to family members' unique needs.

In addition to receiving sufficient information, other methods such as relaxation techniques, yoga, meditation, and/or exercise can help family members reduce their anxiety during this period (Keitel & Kopala, 2000). All family members should be encouraged to engage in some type of self-care activity and to enlist the help of a wider support network so they have the time to do so. Couples will need guidance on how much to disclose to the children. Taking their cues from the children seems to be a wise course of action. It is important to stay calm, and respond honestly and in language that children understand (Keitel & Kopala, 2000). Greening (1992) reported that children who receive clear information and are given an opportunity to express their reaction adjust better. Children can pick up tension in the family and telling them that nothing is going on is likely to increase their anxiety. Their fantasies about what is happening may be worse than the reality.

8.1.4 Treatment

Yabroff and Kim (2009) reported that spouses/partners provide an average of 8 h of care per day during active treatment. Less educated individuals and those with lower annual incomes ($20,000 or less) spent more time providing care than did college educated and wealthier individuals. Spouses who carry the family health insurance plan may work more hours for fear of losing employment and thus health insurance coverage. Below, we describe how breast cancer affects partners during treatment.

8.1.5 Mastectomy

Rowland and Metcalfe (2014) conducted a systematic review of men's experiences of their partner's *mastectomy*. Numerous studies found that men prioritized their spouse's health over their physical appearance (Holmberg, Scott, Alexy, & Fife, 2001; Marshall & Kiemle, 2005). Marshall and Kiemle (2005) reported that men were more worried about their partner's reaction to losing a breast than their own reaction. Most men report that their partner's absent breast or scarring did not affect their emotional or sexual relationship (e.g., Hilton, Crawford, & Tarko, 2000; Hoga, Mello, & Dias, 2008). Some men, however, do experience lower sexual desire for their partner post-mastectomy (Holmberg et al., 2001) and/or are anxious about damaging the reconstructed breast (Marshall & Kiemle, 2005). In a more recent study by Andrzejczak, Markocka-Maczka, and Lewandowski (2012) couples reported reduced satisfaction with their sex life. Almost 75% of couples had reduced sexual activity. Most men felt uncomfortable discussing changes to their wives' body because they feared upsetting them and were also unsure how to respond to their partners' diminished feelings of femininity due to altered *body image* (Zahlis & Shands, 1991).

When a family is in an early life stage, recovering from a mastectomy can be extremely challenging because the patient requires bed-rest and cannot lift anything heavy for at least 4 weeks. Younger women often opt for breast reconstruction, which entails numerous follow-up appointments and a lengthy recovery. This puts all caregiving responsibilities on partners who may be working and are also trying to cope with their fear about their partner's health. Partners have many competing responsibilities at a time in which they are already depleted. Due to gender socialization, male caregivers often have difficulty acknowledging distress and vulnerability and seeking help. Without additional support, their distress is likely to escalate.

At a later life stage when there are fewer responsibilities, partners have less to juggle (e.g., work, childcare) and may also have adult children who volunteer to help. Adult children and close friends who are retired can provide both emotional and tangible support.

Interventions for partners of women undergoing mastectomy include: (a) helping them communicate with their partners about body image; (b) encouraging them to share their experiences with other partners in support groups, and (c) providing information about mastectomy, *reconstructive surgeries*, and the potential impact on their partners (Hilton et al., 2000; Rowland & Metcalfe, 2014).

> **Box 8.1. A Personal Reflection**
>
> Our mother, Kathy, was diagnosed with breast cancer when she was 50 years old, with a second primary cancer, ovarian, when she was 56 and with a third primary cancer, duodenal, when she was 64. The duodenal cancer took her life after spending almost a year in the hospital and a skilled nursing facility. Of course, at the time we didn't know what a "primary cancer" was. We didn't know that that meant the cancers were all new and unrelated. There was so much we didn't know. Finding out that a loved one has cancer is entering a foreign world with an unknown culture and language you must learn quickly to survive. We suddenly needed to make life changing decisions that depended on our knowing words like redaction, lymph nodes, j tubes, skilled nursing, OT, LTC, and hospice. We are a college educated family and we have an uncle who is a doctor. Surely, if anyone could make sense of the medical world our family had a chance. We were no match. It was overwhelmingly stressful, confusing, lonely and terrifying. We depended on each other as a family but also found that the stress brought out the worst in us at times. We feared we would lose not only our mother but our relationships as well.
>
> There were hundreds of medical professionals, social workers and therapists involved in my mother's care. Some were wonderful and some nearly destroyed us. The difference was the good ones listened to our questions even if they had heard the same questions a million times from other families (this was the first time we were going through this.) They spent time allaying our fears even when they were busy, would act as a translator of the unknown culture and language of the medical world, and they took care of the family as well as the patient. The ones who made things more difficult seemed to have an attitude that suggested that my mother was not worthy of their time because she was not likely to live. Devastating. Her surgeon told us he didn't bother to check if the tumor had spread to her pancreas because she was going to die anyway. He said it like "well, duh" but it was a bomb going off in our world.

A second surgeon told my mother, "this will take your life." No preparation. No soft place to fall. No talking to the family beforehand so we could help prepare her. No acknowledgment of what we were doing to try to save her life. Just "you are going to die" and then he left us alone to pick up the pieces. She didn't know the cancer would take her life; she thought chemo was giving her a chance. We all did. And she wasn't dying right that minute. So what now? Is there no emotional support available for patients and their families? We were fighting for her life, for our mother, for our hero who had always fought for us. Who cares if her arm is swelling due to her lymph node removal from her breast cancer surgery when she is dying of another tumor? Well, we cared. We cared if she hurt or she was suffering or what it could mean. Admittedly, we focused on the things we could see and understand and we wanted them fixed. Maybe that's the hallmark of an annoying family, but what care would you demand for your loved one? We continue to pray for the patients who had no one to speak for them.

As I am writing this it is almost a year since my mother's passing. I still miss her every day and I still cry most days. It is a good time, though, to look back on the epic journey at the end of her life and thank those who helped us through the most difficult experience my family and my mother had ever faced. No family can be emotionally prepared for an experience like this but we are happy to say that we have ultimately grown closer to each other. We will be eternally grateful to the countless kind souls who supported us throughout that difficult time regardless of the ultimate destination.

—Jamie Alexander, teacher and caregiver

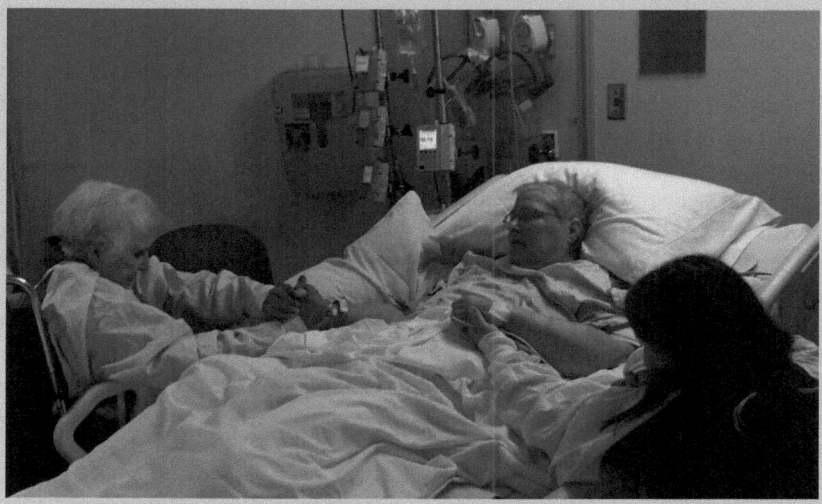

My mother, with her mother and my sister.

8.1.6 Chemotherapy and Radiation

Chemotherapy can last from a few months to a few years depending on the regimen and response to treatment. Many patients experience nausea, vomiting, diarrhea, fatigue, hair loss, memory loss, infection, and mouth and throat sores when undergoing chemotherapy. Further, chemotherapy-induced premature menopause affects many breast cancer survivors and can result in hot flashes, mood swings, sexual impairment, infertility-related distress, and poor body image (Rosenberg et al., 2014). *Radiation* generally involves daily treatment for 6 weeks. Side effects of radiation may include skin irritation, pain, fatigue, and less commonly, low white blood cell count, and difficulty breathing. Despite these significant side effects and the need for family members to provide care during active treatment, much less research has been conducted on the experience of family caregivers during chemotherapy and radiation. One *qualitative study* of caregivers of cancer patients receiving chemotherapy (i.e., Ream et al., 2013) indicated that caregiving was stressful, emotionally draining, and time consuming. One man caring for his sister even said he wanted to "run away" (Ream et al., 2013). It can be very difficult for family members to tolerate watching their loved ones suffer the side effects of chemotherapy as they are often more distressing than the physical impact of the disease itself. Given and colleagues (1993) found that caregivers (primarily spouses of chemotherapy patients) were more affected by patients' mental states (i.e., depression) than their physical status.

At first, partners may question how to best support their loved one during treatment. Family members, particularly partners, may feel guilty and helpless watching their loved one suffer. When one's partner is depressed, exhausted, and nauseated, it is common to feel at a loss for words that would provide comfort. Words may feel inadequate because they do not spare their loved ones from the side effects of treatment. The most they can do is to be physically present and emotionally available. This may be especially difficult for men because they are socialized to take action and solve problems. For example, Carlos, 55 years old, is very devoted to his wife Lena who is undergoing a third round of chemotherapy. Lena wants physical and emotional closeness with her husband but Carlos grew up in a culture in which men were expected to be stoic. This disconnect between Carlos and Lena is causing tension in their marriage because she feels isolated and he feels guilty for not knowing how to meet her emotional needs. As a result, both partners are withdrawing from each other. They are also struggling with role shifts that are necessary during the treatment phase. Lena is having difficulty relinquishing control of household duties because being a homemaker is an integral part of her identity. Carlos blocks Lena from doing housework because he thinks she needs to rest. Lena feels useless and lost and Carlos is struggling to balance work and domestic responsibilities.

Recommendations for how to support partners during treatment include: (a) emphasizing improved communication with health professionals such as advocating for more convenient appointments and asking for education on drugs and strategies for reducing negative *side effects* (Tamayo, Broxson, Munsell, & Cohen,

2010); (b) helping partners identify ways of supporting the patient and still making time for themselves; (c) encouraging partners to express their sadness and helplessness if and when the patient has debilitating side effects from chemotherapy; (d) providing guidance on when to assume additional roles and responsibilities and when to relinquish them as patients recover.

8.1.7 Post-treatment and Recurrence

According to Meyerowitz, Christie, Stanton, Rowland, and Ganz (2012), the period after their wives' medical treatment can be difficult for husbands because they may expect that life will quickly return to normal and it does not. Men who had more realistic expectations for this time period were better adjusted, which implies that health professionals should educate them on what to expect. Once patients are determined to be cancer free, distress levels in caregivers tend to approximate those in the general population (Romito, 2013). Unfortunately, not all cancer patients remain cancer free.

Recurrence is often more stressful than the initial diagnosis (Given & Given, 1992). Family members of women with breast cancer report significant impairments in their own emotional well-being (Northouse et al., 2002). Family caregivers should be included in treatment to help counteract the negative effects on their mental health, and to enable them to continue as effective caregivers (Northouse et al., 2002). Recommendations for helping couples during recurrence include: (a) encouraging them to use coping strategies that have proven effective in the past; (b) facilitating frank and open discussions about their fears and validating those feelings; (c) challenging common distortions that may arise at this time such as "three strikes and you're out."

8.1.8 Advanced Disease

Caregivers of terminal patients and those who are *bereaved* have the highest levels of distress (Romito, Goldzweig, Cormio, Hagedoorn, & Andersen, 2013). Grunfeld et al. (2004) studied 89 caregivers of women with advanced breast cancer in Canada where over half of the caregivers were male spouses or partners. Almost 70% of caregivers had their work adversely affected, particularly during the terminal period. Some caregivers (5%) had to quit their job or decline advancement, and a large proportion lost work hours or used personal days and holidays to fulfill their caregiving responsibilities. Perceived *caregiver burden* and depression increased as patients' ability to care for themselves declined. According to Hasson-Ohayon, Goldzweig, Braun, and Galinsky (2009), spouses of women with advanced breast cancer reported more psychological distress than patients. Spouses also received less support from family and friends than did patients. This is particularly problematic because support from friends was the support they most desired. In this study, religious/spiritual beliefs were positively correlated with distress in patients and spouses; however, other research shows religion and spirituality to be beneficial (e.g., Balboni et al., 2010). Conceptions of a punishing God, however, tend to be associated with anger toward God and more distress (Exline, Park, Smyth, & Carey, 2011). Similarly, differing beliefs, values, and approaches regarding end-of-life care have been noted among diverse cultural groups (Crawley, Marshall, Lo, & Koenig, 2002). When family members have different treatment goals than patients, tensions increase. Loved ones often want to expend all options to extend survival, whereas patients may have reached their limits with medical intervention and want to stop treatment. Having open and direct discussions with both the patient and family about treatment goals, advanced directives, and *palliative care* options early on is an important way to facilitate family adjustment and coping during this stage.

Advanced disease in young women is particularly devastating because it is not expected at this life stage. Partners fear becoming single parents and may not know how to speak with their children about the seriousness of the illness. Caregivers with children are likely to want help navigating what and how much to tell their children and how to respond to their children's questions.

Learning that an elderly family member has advanced stage cancer is still devastating, but it is more normative. Older couples tend to have experience with other families in which one partner has advanced cancer or has passed away. A therapist can be instrumental in helping the couple to get support from adult offspring or other extended family members at this time to reduce potential social isolation and garner tangible support.

8.2 Emerging Trends: Under-Researched Populations

8.2.1 Racial-Ethnic Minority Populations and Cultural Beliefs

A major trend in the demographics of the USA is rapidly growing ethnic diversity with minorities now 37% of the population, projected to comprise 57% in 2060 (CDC, December 12, 2012). Specifically, the Hispanic population will triple to 30%; African Americans will rise to 15%, and non-Hispanic whites will drop to 43% of the US population. Breast cancer is the most prevalent female cancer among these major ethnic groups (DeSantis, Ma, Bryan, & Jemal, 2014). Moreover, both Hispanic and African American women are at increased risk for more advanced disease at diagnosis, and recent trends suggest younger age at diagnosis for African Americans (DeSantis et al., 2014; Haile et al., 2012). One's response to and experience with caregiving can be significantly influenced by cultural beliefs about cancer, medical treatment, and disease disclosure (Daher, 2012). In many cultures, cancer is still seen as the "dread" disease that connotes a death sentence even when the prognosis is positive. In fact, one Jamaican patient disclosed to one of the authors (AMR) that *cancer in my country is like leprosy; people avoid you and it's best not to tell anyone.*

As such, stigma and secrecy around the diagnosis can exist whereby patients do not disclose the disease to other family or friends (Henderson, Davison, Pennebaker, Gatchel, & Baum, 2002), which can compound isolation and caregiver burden. Fearing that patients would suffer because of knowledge of their disease, family members may also withhold the diagnosis from patients (Mitchell, 1998; Orona, Koenig, & Davis, 1994), which places full burden of caregiving and medical decision making on the caregiver. *Medical mistrust*, bred by historical medical research abuses with ethnic minorities, is also part of the cultural fabric of many ethnic groups, and can result in reduced medical help-seeking behavior (Bickell, Weidmann, Fei, Lin, & Leventhal, 2009). Fatalism, or the belief that events are predetermined and inevitable, is a common belief among African American and Hispanic patients (Chavez, Hubbell, Mishra, & Valdez, 1997; Powe & Finnie, 2003). Believing that what happens to their loved one "is in God's hands" may be comforting and help mitigate guilt, blame, or stress, but can also present further barriers to appropriate medical treatment (Franklin et al., 2007). Clearly, it is important to understand the meaning of illness and treatment among family members to ensure they are receiving the support and education they need to provide optimal care to both themselves and the patient.

8.2.2 Male Breast Cancer Patients and Their Families

Another area that requires further attention in the cancer literature is the experience of family members of men with breast cancer. Breast cancer is significantly more prevalent in women, so the majority of research has focused on female patients and their family members. However, men are often diagnosed with breast cancer at a more advanced stage and have worse prognoses than women (Gnerlich et al., 2011). More specifically, African American men living in non-metropolitan areas have particularly poor outcomes including higher mortality rates (Crew et al., 2007; Klein, Ji, Rea, & Stoodt, 2011; O'Malley, Prehn, Shema, & Glaser, 2002).

While it is established that family members of cancer patients of both genders experience psychological distress, no research has specifically studied female partners of men with breast cancer (Northouse, Katapodi, Song, Zhang, & Mood, 2010). We do not know if the interventions that have been found to be effective for female patients and their families are also effective for male patients and their families. Future research should focus on interventions for male patients and their family members.

8.2.3 Sexual Orientation and Breast Cancer

A Williams Institute review conducted in April 2011 found that nearly 4% of American adults identify as lesbian, gay, bisexual and/or transgendered (LGBT); a figure that translates to approximately nine million adult Americans (Gates, 2014). It is established that gay women are diagnosed with breast cancer at higher rates than heterosexual women (Brown & Tracy, 2008). Explanations for this finding are that gay women are more likely to be obese and/or use drugs and alcohol, all risk factors for cancer (Aaron et al., 2001; Boehmer & Bowen, 2009). Some studies also suggest that gay women are less likely to receive preventive screenings than heterosexual women (Brandenburg, Matthews, Johnson, & Hughes, 2007; Hart & Bowen, 2009). This may be in part because of a *heterosexist* focus in the medical community (Hutchinson, Thompson, & Cederbaum, 2006).

Gay women with breast cancer regularly develop feelings of traumatic stress, anxiety, and low *self-efficacy* (Fobair et al., 2002). Despite higher prevalence of breast cancer and greater distress, the experience of lesbian caregivers is unexplored. The minimal research on lesbian caregivers of women with breast cancer has demonstrated that these women are at risk for emotional distress because their partners' physicians and family members commonly fail to support them (Matthews, 1998).

8.3 Implications

8.3.1 *Implications for Family Resilience*

Although 7% of marriages end in the aftermath of a breast cancer diagnosis (Lichtman, 1982), many marriages remain the same or grow stronger after facing breast cancer (Lichtman, Taylor, & Woods, 1987). Taylor-Brown, Kilpatrick, Maunsell, and Dorval (2000) reported that most marital relationships remain stable after breast cancer and that breakdown is most likely in those relationships with preexisting difficulties. Clinicians should inquire about the marital relationship because the stress of cancer tends to exacerbate problems in a marriage. The public perception that partners abandon women with breast cancer is a misconception that must be challenged because it unnecessarily escalates stress for women who are diagnosed. The sexual impact of cancer treatment, particularly related to *iatrogenic menopause*, premature menopause due to surgical removal of or medical damage to both ovaries, and body image distress, can stress the marital relationship if education and communication around these issues are absent.

Patients and their partners experience cancer together and thus it is important to understand how they interact. Belcher et al. (2011) found that daily support provided by the patient with early stage breast cancer to her spouse enhanced relationship intimacy even when spouses did not report receiving the support. Likewise, spouses who provided support to the patient enhanced relationship intimacy. Intimate relationship satisfaction has been associated with improved mental health in couples facing breast cancer (Segrin, Badger, Sieger, Meek, & Lopez, 2006). Counselors should communicate to couples the benefits of the patient supporting her partner, as typically the emphasis is on the partner supporting the patient.

Experience with illness in their families of origin influences how partners cope with illness (Rolland, 1994), and differences in coping strategies can affect marital satisfaction (Keitel et al., 1990; Ptacek, Ptacek, & Dodge, 1994). In some families, illness is not discussed and the patient is expected be strong and stoic. In other families, the ill person is catered to and nurtured. If partners have very different perspectives about how to care for someone who is ill, this may cause tension in the relationship. According to Kraemer, Stanton, Meyerowitz, Rowland, and Ganz (2011), women are more satisfied with their marriages when their male partners use *approach-oriented* rather than *avoidant coping*. Generally, congruent coping strategies are associated with greater relationship satisfaction.

There is debate about whether couples interventions should encourage the nonpatient partners to take an active or supportive role in patient care. Active partners are highly involved and the couple makes health care decisions collectively. Supportive partners are less personally involved and act more like a "coach" who comforts the patient and helps him/her acquire new coping skills (Badr & Krebs, 2013, p. 1691). A recent *meta-analysis* revealed that cancer patients with supportive partners had better psychological outcomes (Badr & Krebs, 2013). However, active and supportive partners were equally ineffective in improving the patient's physical health, the partner's psychological well-being, and the couple's relationship (Porter, Baucom, Keefe, & Patterson, 2012; Porter et al., 2009). The authors encourage future researchers to establish whether supportive or active partners lead to better outcomes under varying conditions including, but not limited to, stage at diagnosis, prognosis, and social support.

8.3.2 Implications for Practice

A strong *therapeutic alliance* is critical to successful outcomes (Falkenström, Granström, & Holmqvist, 2013) because clients must feel safe to share their feelings (Elliott, Bohart, Watson, & Greenberg, 2011). When therapists actively listen and are perceived as more empathic, treatment is judged to be more credible (Dowell & Berman, 2013). Therapists who can tailor their approaches to meet the specific needs of patients and family members will be more effective. A one size fits all approach will not be as effective as tailoring treatment given different needs, personalities, values, and cultural beliefs.

8.3.3 Couples Interventions

The last decade has witnessed a surge of research on couples-based interventions to improve psychological well-being in cancer patients and their partners. It is well established that interpersonal factors play an important role in a cancer patient's psychological health (Badr & Krebs, 2013). Relationship discord, due to lack of communication, *empathy*, and attentiveness, has been linked to diminished psychological well-being in women with breast cancer (Pistrang & Barker, 1995). Interventions most often have specifically targeted intimate partners, because breast cancer patients indicate that their partners are their greatest source of support (Pistrang & Barker, 1995).

Badr and Krebs (2013) conducted a meta-analysis evaluating the efficacy of couples interventions for cancer patients. Most studies targeted couples in which one partner had breast or prostate cancer. Overall, the meta-analysis revealed that couples interventions effectively increased quality of life for both the patient and partner. Couples are helped only under certain conditions. For example, certain couples interventions improved quality of life only in individuals who had dysfunctional relationships, heightened levels of cancer-related stress, or ineffective communication skills (Badr & Krebs, 2013). Future research should explore factors that make couples more or less appropriate candidates for couples interventions.

Most of the interventions were adapted from established *marital therapy* or *cognitive behavioral therapy* (*CBT*) approaches. While CBT usually consists of 8–12 sessions, most of the couples interventions lasted at most six sessions (Badr & Krebs, 2013). It was not realistic for patients in active cancer treatment to attend more sessions. We do not yet know how many couples sessions are optimal.

Research by Baucom, Kirby, and Kelly (2010) suggests that couples interventions should be tailored specifically to each dyad. If the couple's predominant issue is relationship discord, then traditional couples counseling may be most effective. If the couple's primary concern is cancer, a *psycho-educational intervention* about the disease and how it affects relationships may be more suitable.

8.3.4 General Treatment Recommendations

1. Do not make assumptions. The most distressed individuals are not always the ones with family members with advanced disease or the most severe treatment side effects. How family members subjectively appraise the situation is much more relevant than the objective medical facts. Empathize with the worry and anxiety rather than trying to reassure the family member that everything is going to be fine. When people hear the word cancer, they are likely to be frightened even when their loved one has an excellent prognosis. If you validate the emotions your client is expressing and your client feels heard, it is likely that he or she will be better able to actually integrate encouraging medical news.
2. There is no one right way to cope. Help family members share what has helped them cope with other stressful events in their lives and encourage those coping strategies. For some people distraction is helpful, others seek social support, spirituality and prayer. Some coping strategies such as the use of substances or alcohol have generally been found to be ineffective, although in a crisis or when waiting for test results, a mild sedative prescribed by a physician can help.

3. Respect cultural beliefs. Consider cultural factors when exploring strategies that could be helpful. In many cultures, spirituality and religion are primary coping mechanisms. When women with breast cancer view God as benevolent and involved in their lives, they tend to see cancer as less of a threat and more of an opportunity to grow (Gall & Cornblatt, 2002). This needs to be investigated in family members, but our clinical experience tells us that it may be true for them as well. Mental health professionals who understand their clients' spiritual and religious beliefs can help them draw on these strengths and also minimize negative religious interpretations (e.g., my family member's illness is a punishment from God so I must be a terrible person).
4. Incorporate adult offspring. Treatment for breast cancer usually requires meeting with multiple doctors including oncologists, surgeons, radiologists, and other specialists. These appointments can be overwhelming for older patients and their partners who do not see or hear well or have memory difficulties. Adult offspring can be particularly useful during this time by attending appointments, taking notes, and participating in treatment decisions. This additional support can help take the pressure off the patient and his or her partner during a time in which they may not be cognitively prepared to make life or death treatment decisions. Additionally, for families who do not speak proficient English, adult children may be able to translate at medical appointments.
5. Be flexible. Remember that breast cancer is a process not a single event. Interventions that are helpful during the crisis of diagnosis are not necessarily helpful during active treatment, post-treatment or recurrence. Be flexible about when, where, and how you see family members. When family members are employed, they are not necessarily free to come during traditional appointment hours. You may need to visit the hospital room or the outpatient clinic where the patient is getting treated.
6. Manage expectations. It is crucial to manage expectations about treatment and its outcomes. Negative events are more psychologically detrimental when they are unexpected (Welkenhuysen, Evers-Kiebooms, & Decruyenaere, 2001), therefore, health professionals should prepare families about what to expect during all phases of the cancer experience. Without this preparation, family members often turn to the Internet for information which tends to be confusing and overwhelming (Sandham & Harcourt, 2007). It is important to help cancer patients and their families understand how diagnosis will impact their daily routine. Preparing family members for responsibilities they may be expected to assume can help them plan so they do not have to sacrifice other important parts of their life. Additionally, realistic optimism is considered beneficial for cancer patients, even those who are at the end stages of the disease (Twycross, 1997). Be honest with your patients and their families; encourage optimism but do not give false hope.
7. Help caregivers understand their children's reactions. Mental health professionals can help parents identify how they want to handle interactions with their children and how to evaluate whether their wishes are in the children's best interest. Sharing information about developmental stages can help parents

understand their children's possible reactions. In other words, if an adolescent daughter carries on with her normal school and social life, parents can interpret this as indifference and feel wounded. Reframed as a way for the daughter to cope and also continue with a developmentally appropriate lifestyle may help parents understand her behavior in a new way.

8. Help partners make efficient use of their time. Partners are swamped with responsibilities and exploring time management strategies can yield significant benefits. For the technologically sophisticated, establishing a website for posting updates on the patient can be an efficient way for partners to communicate with family and friends. An alternative is establishing an email list for sending updates that can minimize the time involved in making or responding to individual phone calls. Less time informing others can enable partners to spend more time with the patient, on *self-care*, and/or connecting with those who they find most comforting.

9. Help family caregivers seek additional support if needed. Therapeutic factors present in support groups include *universality, normalizing*, and an opportunity to vent about feelings not appropriately directed to the person who is ill. Support groups also provide opportunities for family members to learn a variety of tips, some of which include navigating the health care system, alternative and *complementary remedies*, insurance, and nutrition.

10. Treat couples as a unit. It is important to recognize that both partners and patients can benefit from professional intervention. When treated together, even better outcomes can be achieved than through individual treatment. Not all aspects of quality of life improve via couples treatment but diminished caregiver burden, lower distress and anxiety, improved coping ability and confidence as caregivers, and better marital and family relationships are likely outcomes (Badr & Krebs, 2013). When caregivers are stable, they are able to provide more optimal care to the patient.

8.3.5 Case Vignette

Camila, a 46-year-old Dominican wife and mother of two teenage girls, was diagnosed with stage III breast cancer. She met and married Juan in the Dominican Republic when she was 22, and soon after migrated to the USA along with extended family. While Camila and Juan fell into traditional cultural and gender roles (she focused on family and home life, he on wage-earning), they had a strong and affectionate marriage buoyed by a deep spiritual faith that helped balance Juan's emotional and often "machismo" style of relating. When Camila found the breast lump, she prayed and shared the news first with her sister, a nurse. She waited a few days before telling her children, aging parents, and Juan because she feared their reactions. After Juan's tears dried, his anger emerged and he insisted that Camila seek religious healing rather than medical care. A family discussion ensued, and through more tears and moments of rage, he agreed to consult with a family friend who was a doctor. Each step of the breast cancer experience was a similar dance in which Juan would erupt in pained anger. He felt helpless to prevent his wife from losing her breast, her hair, her "superwoman" stature, and potentially her life. Eventually, he would concede to Camila's wishes and allow the family to intervene. One of the biggest challenges to their marriage was the lack of regular sexual intimacy they enjoyed prior to the diagnosis due to Camila's body image distress and hormonal changes. It was only when a nurse asked about sexual changes, that Camila broke down and shared this secret for the first time. This opened the door to Camila and Juan seeking counseling as a couple. In counseling, they learned to communicate more openly, draw from their faith, and allow their children and extended family to share the experience with them.

8.4 Conclusions

We have accrued substantial knowledge about Caucasian female breast cancer patients and their families; however, we lack information on racial-ethnic minority families, and families of male and lesbian individuals with breast cancer. It is important to examine the various factors that may influence the experience of caregiving. These findings will allow for new interventions to reduce psychological distress in these populations. One obstacle for recruiting diverse research samples is that cancer centers are not always centrally located. To attract diverse samples, Badr and Krebs (2013) suggested developing online interventions that would be significantly more accessible for many family members especially those with physical disabilities or financial struggles that make it difficult to travel. It is also important to recruit at places of worship or other locations in the community. Researchers may wish to investigate how health-related behaviors of the partner influence physical and psychological outcomes of the patient. Future studies might explore how couples interventions for cancer populations impact coping skills, caregiver burden, and symptom management (Badr & Krebs, 2013; Baucom, Kirby, & Kelly, 2010).

Breast cancer can challenge family resilience, and family resilience can be discovered and strengthened through the experience of breast cancer. In the words of Ralph Waldo Emerson, "when it is dark enough, you can see the stars." As clinicians, by meeting our patients and their partners individually and together, we have a chance to help them not only survive but thrive as a family after cancer and throughout the course it takes. We have learned that it is not the circumstances that are most important to adaptation, but the perspective. Therapists can play a critical role in finding the inner resources each family possesses to promote a resilient lens. Furthermore, although empirically supported treatments for couples facing cancer have been found to improve patients' and partners' mental and physical health including decreased patient mortality, they are rarely offered (Northouse et al., 2012). All families can benefit from receiving accurate and sufficient information and emotional and tangible support. Medical professionals cannot do it alone; therapists and counselors should be part of an interdisciplinary team providing care to individuals with breast cancer and their families. In sum, we hope that this chapter offers a helpful road map for strengthening families.

Acknowledgments Thanks to Molly Brawer, Hannah Clarke, Gabrielle Schreyer, Chana Krupka, Eleanor Smith, and Kristen Lipari for initial library research, feedback on drafts of the manuscript, and assistance with the development of the discussion questions.

Discussion Questions

1. If you were to counsel a woman with advanced stage breast cancer, what types of interventions and approaches might you use and why?
2. How would you tailor your treatment of an individual who is undergoing a mastectomy alone versus an individual who must also receive chemotherapy? What other factors would weigh in on your treatment of these individuals?
3. What questions might you ask a couple about their relationship if the wife had been battling cancer for the past year?
4. What cultural factors might be relevant at diagnosis?
5. How might you engage and support the male partner of a breast cancer patient, who can only periodically attend medical visits with his wife due to work and childcare demands?
6. How would you address a young couple's concerns about sexual intimacy and fertility prior to starting chemotherapy?
7. How might you work with a couple where the partner and patient have very different styles of coping? For example, one may cope through minimizing the threat and the other by wanting to emote and process the anxiety s/he is experiencing.
8. How might spiritual/religious factors act as a facilitator or barrier to coping in the face of breast cancer at different stages?
9. If a couple facing breast cancer has underage children, how would you approach counseling this family?
10. A distraught breast cancer patient comes to you for counseling upon her partner abruptly leaving due to not "being able to take it anymore." How would you work with them from a family resiliency model?

References

Aaron, D. J., Markovic, N., Danielson, M. E., Honnold, J. A., Janosky, J. E., & Schmidt, N. J. (2001). Behavioral risk factors for disease and preventive health practices among lesbians. *American Journal of Public Health, 91*, 972–975.

American Cancer Society. (2014). *Cancer facts and figures*. Atlanta, GA: American Cancer Society. Last accessed August 21, 2014.

Andrzejczak, E., Markocka-Maczka, K., & Lewandowski, A. (2012). Partner relationships after mastectomy in women not offered breast reconstruction. *Psycho-Oncology, 22*, 1653–1657. doi:10.1002/pon.3197

Badr, H., & Krebs, P. (2013). A systematic review and meta-analysis of psychosocial interventions for couples coping with cancer. *Psycho-Oncology, 22*, 1688–1704. doi:10.1002/pon.3200

Bakas, T., & Champion, V. (1999). Development and psychometric testing of the Bakas Caregiving Outcomes Scale. *Nursing Research, 48*, 250–259. doi:10.1097/00006199-199909000-00005

Balboni, T., Paulk, M., Balboni, M., Phelps, A., Loggers, E., Wright, A., et al. (2010). Provision of spiritual care to patients with advanced cancer: Associations with medical care and quality of life near death. *Journal of Clinical Oncology, 28*, 445–452. doi:10.1200/JCO.2009.24.8005

Baucom, D. H., Kirby, J. S., & Kelly, J. T. (2010). Couple-based interventions to assist partners with psychological and medical problems. In K. Hahlweg, M. Grawe-Gerber, & D. H. Baucom (Eds.), *Enhancing couples: The shape of couple therapy to come*. Boston, MA: Hogrefe.

Belcher, A. J., Laurenceau, J. P., Graber, E. C., Cohen, L. H., Dasch, K. B., & Siegel, S. D. (2011). Daily support in couples coping with early stage breast cancer: Maintaining intimacy during adversity. *Health Psychology, 30*, 665–673. doi:10.1037/a0024705

Bickell, N. A., Weidmann, J., Fei, K., Lin, J. J., & Leventhal, H. (2009). Underuse of breast cancer adjuvant treatment: Patient knowledge, beliefs, and medical mistrust. *Journal of Clinical Oncology, 27*, 5160–5167. doi:10.1200/JCO.2009.22.9773

Boehmer, U., & Bowen, D. J. (2009). Examining factors linked to overweight and obesity in women of different sexual orientations. *Preventive Medicine, 48*, 357–361. doi:10.1016/j.ypmed.2009.02.003

Brandenburg, D. L., Matthews, A. K., Johnson, T. P., & Hughes, T. L. (2007). Breast cancer risk and screening: A comparison of lesbian and heterosexual women. *Women's Health, 45*, 109–130. doi:10.1300/J013v45n04_06

Breitbart, W., Poppito, S., Rosenfeld, B., Vickers, A. J., Li, Y., Abbey, J., et al. (2012). Pilot randomized controlled trial of individual meaning-centered psychotherapy for patients with advanced cancer. *Journal of Clinical Oncology, 30*, 1304–1309. doi:10.1200/JCO.2011.36.2517

Brown, J. P., & Tracy, J. K. (2008). Lesbians and cancer: An overlooked health disparity. *Cancer Causes and Control, 19*, 1009–1020. doi:10.1007/s10552-008-9176-z

CDC. (2012, December 12). *U.S. Census Bureau projections show a slower growing, older, more diverse nation a half century from now*. Retrieved from http://www.census.gov/newsroom/releases/archives/population/cb12-243.html

Chavez, L. R., Hubbell, F. A., Mishra, S. I., & Valdez, R. B. (1997). The influence of fatalism on self-reported use of Papanicolaou smears. *American Journal of Preventive Medicine, 13*, 418–424.

Crawley, L. M., Marshall, P. A., Lo, B., & Koenig, B. A. (2002). Strategies for culturally effective end- of-life care. *Annals of Internal Medicine, 136*, 673–679. doi:10.7326/0003-4819-136-9-200205070-00010

Crew, K. D., Neugut, A. I., Wang, X., Jacobson, J. S., Grann, V. R., Raptis, G., et al. (2007). Racial disparities in treatment and survival of male breast cancer. *Journal of Clinical Oncology, 25*, 1089–1098. doi:10.1200/JCO.2006.09.1710

Daher, M. (2012). Cultural beliefs and values in cancer patients. *Annals of Oncology, 23*, 66–69. doi:10.1093/annonc/mds091

Davey, M., Gulish, L., Askew, J., Godette, K., & Childs, N. (2005). Adolescents coping with mom's breast cancer: Developing family intervention programs. *Journal of Marital Family Therapy, 31*, 247–258. doi:10.1111/j.1752-0606.2005.tb01558.x

DeSantis, C., Ma, J., Bryan, L., & Jemal, A. (2014). Breast cancer statistics, 2013. *CA: A Cancer Journal for Clinicians, 64*, 52–62. doi:10.3322/caac.21203

Dowell, N. M., & Berman, J. S. (2013). Therapist nonverbal behavior and perceptions of empathy, alliance, and treatment credibility. *Journal of Psychotherapy Integration, 23*, 158–165. doi:10.1037/a0031421

Ell, K. O., Nishimoto, R. H., Mantell, J. E., & Hamovitch, M. B. (1988). Psychological adaptation to cancer: A comparison among patients, spouses, and non-spouses. *Family Systems Medicine, 6*, 335–348.

Elliott, R., Bohart, A. C., Watson, J. C., & Greenberg, L. S. (2011). Empathy. *Psychotherapy, 48*, 43–49. doi:10.1037/a0022187

Exline, J. J., Park, C. L., Smyth, J. M., & Carey, M. P. (2011). Anger toward God: Social cognitive predictors, prevalence and links with adjustment to bereavement and cancer. *Journal of Personality and Social Psychology, 100*, 129–148. doi:10.1037/a0021716

Falkenström, F., Granström, F., & Holmqvist, R. (2013). Therapeutic alliance predicts symptomatic improvement session by session. *Journal of Counseling Psychology, 60*, 317–328. doi:10.1037/a0032258

Fobair, P., Koopman, C., DiMiceli, S., O'Hanlan, K., Butler, L. D., Classen, C., et al. (2002). Psychosocial intervention for lesbians with primary breast cancer. *Psycho-Oncology, 11*, 427–438. doi:10.1002/pon.624

Franklin, M., Schlundt, D., McClellan, L., Kinebrew, T., Sheats, J., Belue, R., et al. (2007). Religious fatalism and its association with health behaviors and outcomes. *American Journal of Health Behavior, 31*, 563–572. doi:10.5993/AJHB.31.6.1

Gall, T. L., & Cornblatt, M. W. (2002). Breast cancer survivors give voice: A qualitative analysis of spiritual factors in long-term adjustment. *Psycho-Oncology, 11*, 524–535.

Gates, G. J. (2014). *LGB families and relationships: Analyses of the 2013 National Health Interview Survey*. UCLA School of Law: Williams Institute. Retrieved from http://williamsinstitute.law.ucla.edu/wp-content/uploads/lgb-families-nhis-sep-2014.pdf

Given, B., & Given, C. W. (1992). Patient and family caregiver reaction to new and recurrent breast cancer. *Journal of the American Medical Women's Association, 47*, 201–206.

Given, C. W., Stommel, M., Given, B., Osuch, J., Kurtz, M. E., & Kurtz, J. C. (1993). The influence of cancer patients' symptoms and functional states on patients' depression and family caregivers' reaction and depression. *Health Psychology, 12*, 277–285.

Greening, K. (1992). The "Bear Essentials" program: Helping young children and their families cope when a parent has cancer. *Journal of Psychosocial Oncology, 10*, 47–61. doi:10.1300/J077v10n01_05

Gnerlich, J. L., Deshpande, A. D., Jeffe, D. B., Seelam, S., Kimbuende, E., & Margenthaler, J. A. (2011). Poorer survival outcomes for male breast cancer compared with female breast cancer may be attributable to in-stage migration. *Annals of Surgical Oncology, 18*, 1837–1844. doi:10.1245/s10434-010-1468-3

Grunfeld, E., Coyle, D., Whelan, T., Clinch, J., Reyno, L., Craig, C., et al. (2004). Family caregiver burden: Results of a longitudinal study of breast cancer patients and their principal caregivers. *Canadian Medical Association Journal, 170*, 1795–1801. doi:10.1503/cmaj.1031205

Haile, R. W., John, E. M., Levine, A. J., Cortessis, V. K., Unger, J. B., Gonzales, M., et al. (2012). A review of cancer in U.S. Hispanic populations. *Cancer Prevention Research, 5*, 150–163. doi:10.1158/1940-6207.capr-11-0447

Hart, S. L., & Bowen, D. J. (2009). Sexual orientation and intentions to obtain breast cancer screening. *Journal of Women's Health, 18*, 177–185. doi:10.1089/jwh.2007.0447

Hasson-Ohayon, I., Goldzweig, G., Braun, M., & Galinsky, D. (2009). Women with advanced breast cancer and their spouses: Diversity of support and psychological distress. *Psycho-Oncology, 19*, 1195–1204. doi:10.1002/pon.1678

Heins, M., Schellevis, F., Rijken, M., Donker, G., Van der Hoek, L., & Koravaar, J. (2013). Partners of cancer patients consult their GPs significantly more often with both somatic and psychosocial problems. *Scandinavian Journal of Primary Health Care, 31*, 203–208. doi:10.3109/02813432.2013.861153

Henderson, B. N., Davison, K. P., Pennebaker, J. W., Gatchel, R. J., & Baum, A. (2002). Disease disclosure patterns among breast cancer patients. *Psychology & Health, 17*, 51–62. doi:10.1080/08870440290001520

Henry, C. S., Morris, A. S., & Harrist, A. W. (2015). Family resilience: Moving into the third wave. *Family Relations, 64*, 22–43. doi:10.1111/fare.12106

Herman, J. D., & Herman. S. M. (2013). Women's understanding of personal breast cancer risk: Does ethnicity matter? [Abstract]. *Journal of Clinical Oncology, 31*. Abstract retrieved from ASCO University database (Abstract No. 04).

Hilton, B. A., Crawford, J. A., & Tarko, M. (2000). Men's perspectives on individual and family coping with their wives' breast cancer and chemotherapy. *Western Journal of Nursing Research 22*, 438–459. doi:10.1177/01939450022044511

Hoga, L. A., Mello, D. S., & Dias, A. F. (2008). Psychosocial perspectives of the partners of breast cancer patients treated with a mastectomy: An analysis of personal narratives. *Cancer Nursing 31*, 318–325. doi:10.1097/01.NCC.0000305748.43367.1b

Holmberg, S. K., Scott, L. L., Alexy, W., & Fife, B. L. (2001). Relationship issues of women with breast cancer. *Cancer Nursing, 24*, 53–60. doi:10.1097/00002820-200102000-00009

Humpel, N., Magee, C., & Jones, S. C. (2007). The impact of a cancer diagnosis on the health behaviors of cancer survivors and their family and friends. *Support Care Cancer, 15*, 621–630. doi:10.1007/s00520-006-0207-6

Hutchinson, M. K., Thompson, A. C., & Cederbaum, J. A. (2006). Multisystem factors contributing to disparities in preventive health care among lesbian women. *Journal of Obstetric, Gynecologic, and Neonatal Nursing, 35*, 393–402. doi:10.1111/j.1552-6909.2006.00054.x

Jim, H. S., & Jacobsen, P. B. (2008). Posttraumatic stress and posttraumatic growth in cancer survivorship: A review. *Cancer Journal, 14*, 414–419. doi:10.1097/PPO.0b013e31818d8963

Keitel, M., & Kopala, M. (2000). *Counseling women with breast cancer*. Thousand Oaks, CA: Sage.

Keitel, M., Kopala, M., & Potere, J. (2003). Helping women negotiate the cancer experience. In M. Kopala & M. Keitel (Eds.), *Handbook of counseling women*. Thousand Oaks, CA: Sage.

Keitel, M., Zevon, M., Rounds, J., Petrelli, N., & Karakousis, C. (1990). Spouse adjustment to cancer surgery: Distress and coping responses. *Journal of Surgical Oncology, 43*, 148–153. doi:10.1002/jso.2930430305

Kim, Y., Kashy, D. A., Spillers, R. L., & Evans, T. V. (2010). Needs assessment of family caregivers of cancer survivors: Three cohorts comparison. *Psycho-Oncology, 19*, 573–582. doi:10.1002/pon.1597

Kim, Y., & Given, B. A. (2008). Quality of life of family caregivers of cancer survivors: Across the trajectory of the illness. *Cancer, 112*, 2556–2568. doi:10.1002/cncr.23449

Kim, Y., Schulz, R., & Carver, C. S. (2007). Benefit-finding in the cancer caregiving experience. *Psychosomatic Medicine, 69*, 283–291. doi:10.1097/PSY.0b013e3180417cf4

Klein, J., Ji, M., Rea, N. K., & Stoodt, G. (2011). Differences in male breast cancer stage, tumor size at diagnosis, and survival rate between metropolitan and nonmetropolitan regions. *American Journal of Men's Health, 5*, 430–437. doi:10.1177/1557988311400403

Kraemer, L. M., Stanton, A. L., Meyerowitz, B. E., Rowland, J. H., & Ganz, P. A. (2011). A longitudinal examination of couples' coping strategies as predictors of adjustment to breast cancer. *Journal of Family Psychology, 25*, 963–972. doi:10.1037/a0025551

Lavee, Y., McCubbin, H. I., & Olson, D. H. (1987). The effect of stressful life events and transitions on family functioning and well-being. *Journal of Marriage and the Family, 49*, 857–873. doi:10.2307/351979

Lichtman, R. R. (1982). *Close relationships after breast cancer.* Unpublished doctoral dissertation, University of California, Los Angeles, CA.

Lichtman, R. R., Taylor, S. E., & Woods, J. (1987). Social support and marital adjustment after breast cancer. *Journal of Psychosocial Oncology, 5*, 47–74. doi:10.1300/J077v05n03_03

Lund, L., Ross, L., Petersen, M. A., & Groenvold, M. (2014). Cancer caregiving tasks and consequences and their associations with caregiver status and the caregiver's relationship to the patient: A survey. *BMC Cancer, 14*, 541. doi:10.1186/1471-2407-14-541

Marshall, C., & Kiemle, G. (2005). Breast reconstruction following cancer: Its impact on patients' and partners' sexual functioning. *Sexual and Relationship Therapy, 20*, 155–179. doi:10.1080/14681990500113310

Matthews, A. K. (1998). Lesbians and cancer support: Clinical issues for cancer patients. *Health Care for Women International, 19*, 193–203. doi:10.1080/073993398246368

McCubbin, H. I., & Patterson, J. M. (1983). The family stress process: The double ABCX model of adjustment and adaptation. *Marriage and Family Review, 6*, 7–3. doi:10.1300/J002v06n01_02

Meyerowitz, B. E., Christie, K. M., Stanton, A., Rowland, J. H., & Ganz, P. A. (2012). Men's adjustment after their partners' complete treatment for localized breast cancer. *Psychology of Men & Masculinity, 13*, 400–406. doi:10.1037/a0029245

Mitchell, J. L. (1998). Cross-cultural issues in the disclosure of cancer. *Cancer Practice, 6*, 153–160. doi:10.1046/j.1523-5394.1998.006003153.x

National Alliance for Caregiving (NAC) in Collaboration with AARP. (2012). Caregiving in the U.S. Retrieved from: http://www.caregiving.org/pdf/research/Caregiving_in_the_US_2009_full_report.pdf

Northouse, L. L., Katapodi, M. C., Song, L., Zhang, L., & Mood, D. W. (2010). Interventions with family caregivers of cancer patients: Meta-analysis of randomized trials. *CA: A Cancer Journal for Clinicians, 60*, 317–339. doi:10.3322/caac.20081

Northouse, L. L., Mood, D. W., Kershaw, T., Schafenacker, A., Mellon, S., Walker, J., et al. (2002). Quality of life of women with recurrent breast cancer and their family members. *Journal of Clinical Oncology, 20*, 4050–4064. doi:10.1200/JCO.2002.02.054

Northouse, L. L., Williams, A. L., Given, B., & McCorkle, R. (2012). Psychosocial care for family caregivers of patients with cancer. *Journal of Clinical Oncology, 30*, 1227–1234. doi:10.1200/JCO.2011.39.5798

O'Malley, C. D., Prehn, A. W., Shema, S. J., & Glaser, S. L. (2002). Racial/ethnic differences in survival rates in a population-based series of men with breast carcinoma. *Cancer, 94*, 2836–2843. doi:10.1002/cncr.10521

Oncology Nursing Society. (2015). Psychoeducation/psychoeducational interventions. Retrieved from https://www.ons.org/intervention/

Orona, C. J., Koenig, B. A., & Davis, A. J. (1994). Cultural aspects of nondisclosure. *Cambridge Quarterly of Healthcare Ethics, 3*, 338. doi:10.1017/S0963180100005156

Pistrang, N., & Barker, C. (1995). The partner relationship in psychological response to breast cancer. *Social Science and Medicine, 40*, 789–797. doi:10.1016/0277-9536(94)00136-H

Porter, L. S., Baucom, D. H., Keefe, F. J., & Patterson, E. S. (2012). Reactions to a partner-assisted emotional disclosure intervention: Direct observation and self-report of patient and partner communication. *Journal of Marital and Family Therapy, 38*, 284–295. doi:10.1111/j.1752-0606.2011.00278.x

Porter, L. S., Keefe, F. J., Baucom, D. H., Hurwitz, H., Moser, B., Patterson, E., et al. (2009). Partner-assisted emotional disclosure for patients with gastrointestinal cancer: Results from a randomized controlled trial. *Cancer, 115*, 4326–4338. doi:10.1002/cncr.24578

Powe, B. D., & Finnie, R. (2003). Cancer fatalism: The state of the science. *Cancer Nursing, 26*, 454–467. doi:10.1097/00002820-200312000-00005

Printz, C. (2011). Cancer caregivers still have many unmet needs. *Cancer, 117*, 1331. doi:10.1002/cncr.26075

Ptacek, J. T., Ptacek, J. J., & Dodge, K. L. (1994). Coping with breast cancer from the perspectives of husbands and wives. *Journal of Psychosocial Oncology, 12*, 47–72. doi:10.1300/j077v12n03_04

Ream, E., Pederson, V. H., Oakley, C., Richardson, A., Taylor, C., & Verity, R. (2013). Informal caregivers' experience and needs when supporting patients through chemotherapy: A mixed method study. *European Journal of Cancer Care, 22*, 797–806.

Rolland, J. S. (1994). *Families, illness, and disability: An integrative treatment model*. New York, NY: Basic Books.

Romito, F., Goldzweig, G., Cormio, C., Hagedoorm, M., & Andersen, B. L. (2013). Informal caregiving for cancer patients. *Cancer, 119*, 2160–2169. doi:10.1002/cncr.28057

Rosenberg, S. M., Tamimi, R. M., Gelber, S., Ruddy, K. J., Bober, S. L., Kereakoglow, S., et al. (2014). Treatment-related amenorrhea and sexual functioning in young breast cancer survivors. *Cancer, 120*, 2264–2271. doi:10.1002/cncr.28738

Rowland, E., & Metcalfe, A. (2014). A systematic review of men's experiences of their partner's mastectomy: Coping with altered bodies. *Psycho-Oncology, 23*, 963–974. doi:10.1002/pon.3556

Ruddy, K. J., & Winer, E. P. (2013). Male breast cancer: Risk factors, biology, diagnosis, treatment, and survivorship. *Annals of Oncology, 24*, 1434–1443. doi:10.1093/annonc/mdt025

Sandham, C., & Harcourt, D. (2007). Partner experiences of breast reconstruction post-mastectomy. *European Journal of Oncology Nursing, 11*, 66–73. doi:10.1016/j.ejon.2006.05.004

Segrin, C., & Badger, T. A. (2010). Psychological distress in different social network members of breast and prostate cancer survivors. *Research in Nursing & Health, 33*, 450–464. doi:10.1002/nur.20394

Segrin, C., Badger, T. A., Sieger, A., Meek, P., & Lopez, A. M. (2006). Interpersonal well-being and mental health among male partners of women with breast cancer. *Issues in Mental Health Nursing, 27*, 371–389. doi:10.1080/01612840600569641

Sellers, T. S. (2000). A model of collaborative healthcare in outpatient medical oncology. *Families, Systems, & Health, 18*, 19–33. doi:10.1037/h0091851

Stanton, A. L., Danoff-Burg, S., Cameron, C. L., Bishop, M., Collins, C. A., Kirk, S. B., et al. (2000). Emotionally expressive coping predicts psychological and physical adjustment to breast cancer. *Journal of Consulting and Clinical Psychology, 68*, 875–882. doi:10.1037/0022-006X.68.5.875

Steginga, S., Occhipinti, S., Wilson, K., & Dunn, J. (1998). Domains of distress, the experience of breast cancer in Australia. *Oncology Nursing Forum, 25*, 1063–1070.

Stenberg, U., Ruland, C. M., & Miaskowski, C. (2010). Review of the literature on the effects of caring for a patient with cancer. *Psycho-Oncology, 19*, 1013–1025. doi:10.1002/pon.1670

Tamayo, G. J., Broxson, A., Munsell, M., & Cohen, M. Z. (2010). Caring for the caregiver. *Oncology Nursing Forum, 37*, 50–57. doi:10.1188/10.ONF.E50-E57

Taylor-Brown, J., Kilpatrick, M., Maunsell, E., & Dorval, M. (2000). Partner abandonment of women with breast cancer. Myth or reality? *Cancer Practice, 28*, 160–164. doi:10.1046/j.1523-5394.2000.84004.x

Twycross, R. G. (1997). *Introducing palliative care*. Oxon, UK: Radcliffe Medical Press.

Tyndall, L., Hodgson, J., Lamson, A., White, M., & Knight, S. (2014). A review of medical family therapy: 30 years of history, growth, and research. In J. Hodgson et al. (Eds.), *Medical family therapy*. Switzerland: Springer International. doi:10.1007/978-3-319-03482-9_2

United States Census Bureau. (2000, 2004). Retrieved from http://factfinder.census.gov/

Wagner, C. D., Bigatti, S. M., & Storniolo, A. M. (2006). Quality of life of husbands of women with breast cancer. *Psycho-Oncology, 15*, 109–120. doi:10.1002/pon.928

Welkenhuysen, M., Evers-Kiebooms, G., & Decruyenaere, M. (2001). Perception of the breast cancer risk: When do overestimations and unrealistic optimism occur together? *Risk Management, 3*, 65–76. doi:10.2307/3867914

Yabroff, K. R., & Kim, Y. (2009). Time costs associated with informal caregiving for cancer survivors. *Cancer, 115*, 4362–4373. doi:10.1002/cncr.24588

Zahlis, E. H., & Lewis, F. M. (2010). Coming to grips with breast cancer: The spouse's experience with his wife's first six months. *Journal of Psychosocial Oncology, 28*, 79–97. doi:10.1080/07347330903438974

Zahlis, E. H., & Shands, M. E. (1991). Breast cancer: Demands of the illness on the patient's partner. *Journal of Psychosocial Oncology, 9*, 75–93. doi:10.1300/J077v09n01_04

Chapter 9
Fostering Resilience Among Older Adults Living with Osteoporosis and Osteoarthritis

Brenda J. Smith and Whitney A. Bailey

The USA is experiencing a dramatic demographic shift, resulting in a greater proportion of older adults than ever before (US Department of Health and Human Services, 2014). It is projected that those 65 years and older will comprise 20% of the US population by the year 2030, with the fastest growing segment being those 85+ years (Ortman & Velkoff, 2014). Eighty percent of adults over 65 live with one chronic condition and one in five lives with four or more chronic conditions (AARP, 2009). Medical technology enables individuals to live longer, which in turn can increase the likelihood of age-associated illnesses like cancer, cardiovascular disease, and musculoskeletal disease. The experience of exceptional longevity or living in excess of 100 years is increasingly common. Yet the quality of that life is wholly another matter. It is important to examine factors and strategies that contribute to living *well* despite having one or more chronic conditions.

Musculoskeletal problems are the most common cause of chronic disability among older adults. The two most prevalent musculoskeletal diseases of later life are osteoporosis and osteoarthritis (Office of the Surgeon General, 2004; Felson et al., 2000). By definition, osteoporosis is a chronic disease that affects the skeleton, characterized by a decrease in bone density in response to deterioration of the bone's microarchitectural structures. Left untreated, this deterioration of bone ultimately leads to increased bone fragility and a significant increase in fracture risk. Based on National Health and Nutrition Examination Survey III (NHANES III)

B.J. Smith, Ph.D. (✉)
Department of Nutriitional Sciences, Oklahoma State University,
420 Human Sciences, Stillwater, OK 74078, USA
e-mail: bjsmith@okstate.edu

W.A. Bailey, Ph.D.
Department of Human Development and Family Science,
Human Sciences 233, Stillwater, OK 74078, USA
e-mail: whitney.a.bailey@okstate.edu

© Springer International Publishing Switzerland 2017
G.L. Welch, A.W. Harrist (eds.), *Family Resilience and Chronic Illness*,
Emerging Issues in Family and Individual Resilience,
DOI 10.1007/978-3-319-26033-4_9

data, ten million Americans have osteoporosis and another 43 million are considered "at risk" due to osteopenia or low bone mass (Wright et al., 2014). The majority of individuals with osteoporosis are women. Consistent with the aging of the population in the USA, it is estimated that by 2020, one in two non-Hispanic women and one in five men over 50 years of age will experience an osteoporotic-related fracture (Office of the Surgeon General, 2004). Osteoarthritis is a progressive disease that targets synovial joint tissues, including articular cartilage, subchondral bone, ligaments, menisci, periarticular muscles, peripheral nerves, or the synovium. Nearly 27 million Americans have osteoarthritis and though it occurs in people of all ages, it is more prevalent in women and individuals aged 65 and older (Lawrence et al., 2008). Analogous to the anticipated increase osteoporosis, the incidence of osteoarthritis is expected to rise with the increasing number of older adults and associated risk factors.

The challenges associated with osteoporosis and osteoarthritis include living with chronic pain, restricted mobility (Greendale & Barrett-Connor, 2001; Laslett et al., 2012), financial strain (Hoerger et al., 1999), fear of falling, reliance on medicine, isolation, and threats to autonomy. Boss (2002) argued that individuals' ability to cope with challenges like these depend on five key factors. Attributional style, where a person is able to externalize the blame to explainable forces rather than internalizing it to unexplainable forces, is central to coping. Response style (distracting oneself vs. ruminating) enables a person to cope with day-to-day challenges associated with osteoarthritis and osteoporosis. Cognitive style (optimism vs. pessimism) is a key part of one's personality that has bearing on how they see an illness, respond to it, and ask for support. Social skills (connecting vs. isolating) and a person's approach to problem solving skills (seeking help from others vs. stoicism) all relate to how a person activates and receives the support network around them, which consequently leads to physical and psychological outcomes (Boss, 2002). Each of these feeds into the family system and its experience of resilience.

Those living with osteoarthritis and osteoporosis may need to rely on family members for support. Dependence on family members will likely be minimal early in the disease, but individuals may become increasingly reliant on caretakers if osteoporosis and osteoarthritis become more severe. For example, one in four patients who experience a hip fracture will become disabled in the following year and less than 50% will return to their pre-fracture status in terms of activities of daily living (ADL; Greendale & Barrett-Connor, 2001). Whether that support involves periodic visits or day-to-day care, family members are central to care of older loved ones. Research on the care of older family members has focused predominately on the implications for caregivers, with very little emphasis on the experiences of care recipients (Brosi, Ames, & Carolan, 2009). The lack of research on the implications of osteoporosis and osteoarthritis on family resilience, along with the dearth of research on older care recipients, demonstrates the need for further exploration of the impacts of these conditions on both individuals and families. This chapter examines the specific elements of individual and family resilience processes as they relate to the experiences of osteoporosis and osteoarthritis.

9.1 Review of Literature

Chronic musculoskeletal diseases such as osteoporosis and osteoarthritis can have devastating consequences. For the individual they often lead to limited mobility and chronic pain, which can challenge one's ability to live independently and compromise their quality of life (Greendale & Barrett-Connor, 2001; Laslett et al., 2012). The ensuing physical and psychological consequences can lead to a downward spiral in the individual's overall health and have serious social and economic ramifications (Office of the Surgeon General, 2004). The cost of treating osteoporotic fractures per case has been estimated at $40,000 and $25,000 for the hip and spine, respectively (Blume & Curtis, 2011). In comparison, direct medical costs associated with treating osteoarthritis have been estimated at approximately $13,000 per year (Gore, Tai, Sadosky, Leslie, & Stacey, 2011). Importantly, these estimates do not consider the cost of ongoing treatment of comorbidities and pain-related pharmacotherapy.

While these physical, psychological, social, and economic challenges undoubtedly impact the older adult suffering with osteoporosis or osteoarthritis, they can also test the resiliency of the family unit as a whole. Notably, when one member of a family lives with chronic pain, research has shown the family system adapts to care for that person's needs (Rosland, Heiser, & Piette, 2012). It is also shown that families adapt to take over functions that person is no longer able to perform (Evans & Lee, 2014). Further issues such as isolation, frustration, and fear have been linked to conflict in families experiencing chronic illness (Turner & Kelly, 2000). While the literature on chronic illness and its implications for families is vast, the literature addressing family resilience processes among families facing musculoskeletal conditions such as osteoporosis and osteoarthritis is limited. In order to more fully examine the factors that affect individual and family resilience, the next sections will examine the pathology, treatment options and factors associated with osteoporosis and osteoarthritis. We will conclude with recommendations for fostering resilience among families where one or more members suffer from these chronic and debilitating musculoskeletal conditions.

9.1.1 Understanding the Pathology of Osteoporosis and Osteoarthritis

In contrast to popular perception, bone is a dynamic tissue that is continuously responding to a variety of stimuli, including those of biomechanical, biochemical and hormonal origin. Bone's ability to adapt to stimuli is accomplished through the regulation of its cellular metabolic processes, termed bone remodeling. Bone remodeling results in the adult skeleton being replaced every 7–10 years. Like most metabolic processes, bone remodeling consists of both a catabolic and anabolic phase. The bone cells responsible for bone resorption, or the catabolic phase are

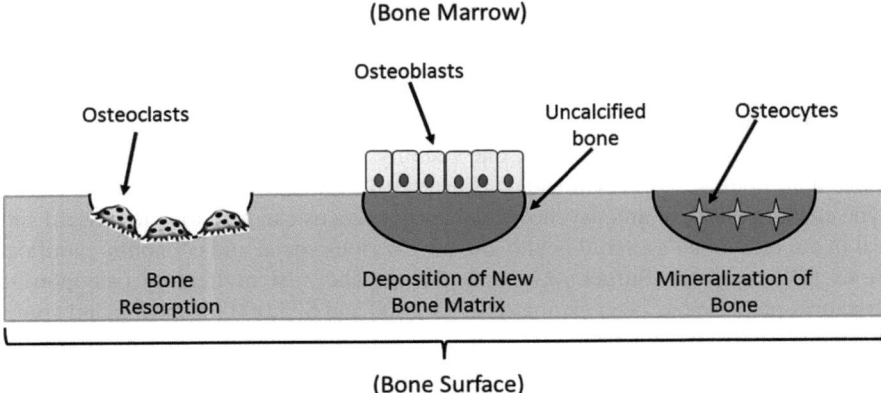

Fig. 9.1 Three major phases of bone remodeling that occur in the bone modeling unit (BMU) of the adult skeleton: (1) bone resorption by osteoclasts; (2) new bone protein matrix secretion by osteoblasts; and (3) mineralization of the bone matrix with some osteoblasts being entombed within the new bone and becoming osteocytes

known as osteoclasts, whereas bone cells responsible for bone formation or the anabolic phase are osteoblasts (Fig. 9.1). The balance of osteoclast and osteoblast activity within millions of bone modeling units (BMU) throughout the skeleton determines whether the net effect is bone acquisition, maintenance or loss.

Bone loss takes place across a large portion of the lifespan, beginning in the fourth or Primary osteoporosis, otherwise known as age-related osteoporosis, affects older adults and is Primary osteoporosis is the result of the cumulative effects of bone loss, combined with deterioration of bone microstructure as people age (Seeman, 2003). Primary osteoporosis is a major risk factor for osteoporotic fracture among older adults, but women are two to three times more likely than men to experience an osteoporotic fracture (Riggs, Khosla, & Melton, 2002).

Because of the rapid phase of bone loss that occurs during the first 5–10 years after menopause, the term "postmenopausal osteoporosis" is often used to describe age-related bone loss in women. Women, whose peak BMD is typically lower than men's, may lose as much as 5–10% of their denser, cortical bone and 20–30% of their trabecular bone which is found in the vertebra and ends of long bones (Riggs et al., 2002). Men's comparatively lower prevalence of osteoporotic fractures is primarily attributed to their higher peak BMD and their slower, more continuous rate of bone loss (Drake & Khosla, 2012).

The pathophysiology of osteoarthritis is not as well defined as that of osteoporosis. Understanding of osteoarthritis has been complicated due in part to questions of whether osteoarthritis is a single disease or a clinical end-point resulting from a number of different disease subtypes. Key features of the pathology include events occurring within the articulating cartilage of synovial joints. Cartilage is considered a poorly vascularized tissue, which slows its ability to repair (Lohmander, Lark, Dahlberg, Walakavits, & Roos., 1992; Buckwalter & Mankin, 1997). However, much

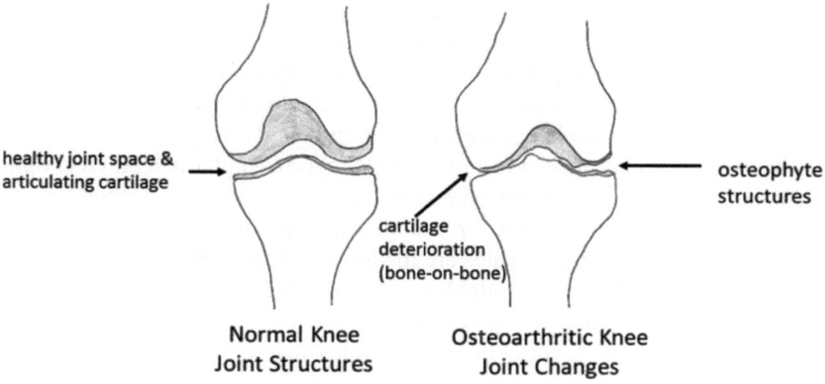

Fig. 9.2 Comparison on normal knee structures to the changes that occur as a result of osteoarthritis. Deterioration of the articulating cartilage can result in bone-on-bone contact and the development of boney structures known as osteophytes

like bone, the extracellular matrix of cartilage undergoes a remodeling process through which matrix components are degraded by matrix metalloproteinases (MMPs) and then growth factors stimulate the production of new matrix (Woessner & Gunja-Smith, 1991). Under normal circumstances the secretion of MMPs by synovial cells and chondrocytes is tightly regulated, but in osteoarthritis the production of proteases is greatly enhanced and the net effect is degradation of the cartilage (Poole, Ionescu, Swan, & Dieppe, 1994). This structural damage to the articulating cartilage leads to an inflamed joint that can have negative implications on boney structures and soft tissues surrounding the joint (Fig. 9.2).

The standard for clinical diagnosis of osteoarthritis is based on the evaluation of radiographic images using scoring schemes. These methods typically assess the presence of osteophytes, and the appearance of joint space narrowing, sclerosis, or joint deformity over time (Fig. 9.2). Common symptoms associated with osteoarthritis are pain, stiffness, and functional disability.

The most common joints affected by osteoarthritis are the knee, hand, and hip, with osteoarthritis of the knee and hand being the most prevalent. Patients may have a single joint affected by osteoarthritis, a few joints affected, or generalized osteoarthritis affecting multiple joints. Regardless of whether osteoarthritis affects one or multiple joints, it can be a debilitating disease.

9.1.2 Treatment Options for Osteoporosis and Osteoarthritis

The primary goals of osteoporosis and osteoarthritis treatments is to delay disease progression and to treat symptoms. Family members can have an important role in achieving both goals by supporting symptom management and positive lifestyle choices (Keefe et al., 1999). For example, as symptoms emerge and progress, family members are central to making home modifications, medical appointments, and finding resources. Another primary task of family members is to support medication management. However, the cost and time commitment of long-term treatment can have negative socioeconomic consequences on the family as well as the individual.

In the case of osteoporosis, most of the FDA-approved pharmacological options for osteoporosis are anti-resorptive therapies designed to prevent further bone loss. Only one pharmacological agent for anabolic therapy or reversal of bone loss is currently available. Bisphosphonates are the most widely prescribed class of osteoporosis medications. They are available in several forms (e.g., alendronate, risedronate, and zoledronate), each of which have different levels of potency and frequency of dosing. Regardless of the form, bisphosphonates bind to the mineralized hydroxyapatite of bone and impair bone resorption by osteoclasts. Compliance with oral, and typically more frequently administered, bisphosphonates is poor due to gastrointestinal irritation (Black et al., 2006). Additionally, more severe complications have been observed with the more potent bisphosphonates, including osteonecrosis of the jaw and atypical spiral fractures of the femur (Fleisher et al., 2013; Schlicher, Michaelsson, & Aspenberg, 2011); The newest anti-resorptive osteoporosis treatment is the human monoclonal antibody for ligand receptor activator of nuclear factor (RANKL) or Denosumab, which is anticipated to have fewer side effects than the bisphosphonates. The only treatment option available for patients with established osteoporosis and high risk of fracture is intermittent parathyroid hormone treatment or teriparatide. Although effective, this drug requires a daily injection regimen, is cost-prohibitive for most patients, and has been associated with serious side effects like gout and hypercalcemia (Black et al., 2003; Neer et al., 2001).

While most of the current treatment options for osteoporosis are aimed at preventing fracture, once a fracture occurs treatment attention is shifted to restoring the patient to pre-fracture functional status and promoting bone fracture healing (Cosman et al., 2014). Many of the conventional surgical approaches used by orthopedic surgeons may not be viable options in the osteoporotic patient. For example, vertebral fractures may not be repaired by standard pedicle screws and stabilization due to the compromised bone interface (Hu, 1997). Techniques such as vertebroplasty and kyphoplasty have been proposed as a reasonable alternative to more conventional fracture stabilization because they reduce pain, restore vertebral body height and correct some of the kyphotic deformity of the spine, while eliminating the need for major surgery (Gan et al., 2010; Shinn, Chin, & Yoon, 2009). Treatment of hip fractures typically involves surgery where the specific anatomical location and severity of the fracture determines the surgical procedure used. In some cases where the proximal end of the femur has been damaged, the end of the femur may be replaced with a prosthesis (i.e., partial hip replacement). In other cases a total hip replacement may be warranted, a procedure that involves replacing the proximal femur and the socket of the pelvis with a prostheses. In any case, patients undergoing repair of a hip fracture will need to undergo extensive rehabilitation that often requires months of physical and occupational therapy in either in-patient or out-patient facilities.

The treatment of osteoarthritis is aimed at reducing pain and joint inflammation while maintaining joint range of motion. Individuals who have mild-to-moderate pain may be able to treat with acetaminophen which has analgesic properties, but no anti-inflammatory effects. In contrast, nonsteroidal anti-inflammatory drugs (NSAIDs), which are available over-the-counter (e.g., ibuprofen and naproxen) and prescription medications that inhibit cyclooxygenase-2 (COX-2) have become a viable option for many patients. These drugs can be problematic due to their association with gastrointestinal distress, cardiovascular problems, liver and kidney damage (Trelle et al., 2011; Bhala et al., 2013). In severe cases in which the patient is not a good candidate for surgery, narcotics may be used to treat osteoarthritis pain. While these medications only relieve pain and suppress joint inflammation, physical therapy or occupational therapy may improve muscular strength and joint function. Maintaining physical activity is an important component of treatment for osteoarthritis. The magnitude of exercise benefits may be considered small to moderate; however, the effects are comparable to the benefits associated with analgesics and NSAIDs, but with fewer side effects (Bennell et al., 2014). Research shows that family caregivers and other members are central to helping older adults remain physically active (Schultz & Sherwood, 2008), while social isolation is a major risk factor for inactivity. Consequently, it is very important for family members to promote and participate in activities alongside older loved ones with osteoporosis and osteoarthritis.

In cases where osteoarthritis symptoms cannot be managed, more invasive options can be considered. The least invasive surgical option is arthroscopy for mild to moderate osteoarthritis. This procedure does not prohibit future surgical procedures, but recently the added benefit of arthroscopy has been questioned compared to the benefits of physical and pharmacological therapy (Kirkley et al., 2008). For active patients over the age of 60 years who want to continue an active lifestyle, osteotomy may be an option. Osteotomy is effective for osteoarthritis associated with misaligned hip or knee joints. Arthroplasty, also known as joint replacement surgery, is performed when other surgical approaches (e.g., arthroscopy and osteotomy) are not viable options. Return to full weight-bearing activity usually occurs between 1 and 3 months following physical therapy to restore range of motion and strengthening exercises.

As with any intensive period of therapy, the success of recovery for the osteoporosis and osteoarthritis patients, post-operatively is strongly influenced by the support provided. The role of family members in short and long term physical rehabilitation is well documented (Visser-Meily et al., 2006). Individuals are placed primary in the care of family members in lieu of or immediately following rehabilitation facility placement. In these situations, family members are the primary sources of transportation, emotional support, and coordination of medical visits and records. In fact, recent efforts by the American Association of Retired Persons (AARP) are leading many states to pursue caregiving related legislation. For example, Oklahoma passed the nation's first "CARE Act" where, upon discharge, hospital personnel are expected to identify and educate caregivers through both live demonstration and support materials. Similar legislation is taking hold in many other states and is evidence, in part, of the role that family members play in supporting those with acute and chronic conditions.

> **Box 9.1. Focus on Interdisciplinary Work**
> Osteoporosis presents many threats to individual and family resilience. Healthcare providers are frequently unfamiliar with the disease, its progression and alternative treatments. "When we attend healthcare appointments with members who have osteoporosis, the condition itself is rarely brought up by either the provider or the affected individual." Older adults know very little about the disease because it receives very little public health attention. Further, because there are no symptoms, it remains largely "invisible" to affected individuals and the people they share life with. "I had one member with osteoarthritis who loved to cook: it was her identity, her role in the family. So she would be in the kitchen preparing family meals, bending and twisting as needed, while being completely unaware that, at her stage of the disease, these activities could easily result in hip fracture. Likewise, her husband and adult children did not know the "mom's jobs" were a threat." When men are diagnosed, it can be even worse. "I had one member who really suffered because he had "a woman's disease" and everyone around him held tightly to the popular notion that "men are strong": so changing behavior was next to impossible."
>
> Poor public and professional understanding of osteoporosis, the fact that the disease itself is abstract (what does low bone density mean in day-to-day life) and doesn't have manifest symptoms, and common perception that it is a women's disease demands interdisciplinary work. Practitioners, like us, need practical strategies to help women and men age with dignity: how can mom retain her family identity as "chief meal preparer" while minimizing risks inherent in the activity? Or, how can dad retain his hobbies and passions like fishing or wood-working while minimizing risks of these activities? Public health education is needed to convey that osteoporosis affects both women and men, although women are more frequently affected. Marketing or communication strategies are needed to help make "brittle bones," the end product of osteoporosis, more concrete for the general population of older adults. Research is needed to identify new medicines and behavioral strategies to slow (or reverse) disease progression.
> —Case Management Team, Life Senior Services

9.2 Implications of Osteoporosis and Osteoarthritis on Individuals and Families

The literature on chronic illness and illness is vast, including research on cancers, dementias, hearing loss, strokes, among others (Grady, 2008; Yorgason et al., 2010). Yet the literature examining resilience processes among individuals who suffer from osteoporosis and osteoarthritis is limited. Research on resilience involves both individual and system attributes and spans several decades. While the applications of resilience to musculoskeletal diseases is limited, there is a broad base of literature as it applies to chronic illnesses, with an increased focus on aging in recent years (Johnston, Bailey, & Wilson, 2014).

Researchers (e.g., Fry & Keyes, 2011) have determined that positive health outcomes are associated with certain individual characteristics and coping strategies. Through research with samples facing one or more chronic conditions, scholars have identified personality traits like conscientiousness, and psychological resources such as optimism, hardiness, acceptance, and psychological flexibility as central elements of individual resilience. For example, individuals who scored higher on measures of optimism also reported higher expectations for positive outcomes from their chronic condition, and were more likely to actively try to overcome difficulties resulting from the condition. Those with higher scores on optimism reported a lower incidence of heart disease, faster recovery from cardiac procedures, lower likelihood of physical symptoms with HIV, and better coping was found among women with breast cancer (Trivedi et al., 2011). Those with higher optimism scores specifically used referencing, applying life lessons to their management of symptoms and the idea that their circumstances could be worse (Yorgason et al., 2010).

Although some can find meaning in their condition, chronic, progressive illnesses like osteoporosis and osteoarthritis can lead to disability and loss of functional status, which in turn impacts quality of life. Two of the major causal factors are chronic pain and limitations in mobility associated with bone and joint disease. Hip fractures are among the most devastating consequences of osteoporosis. Even among previously independent living individuals, many routine activities cannot be carried out following a hip fracture and only 50% will return to their pre-fracture status in terms of ADLs (Greendale & Barrett-Connor, 2001). In contrast, vertebral fractures seldom result in long-term care, but their negative effects on activities of daily living are essentially the same as those associated with hip fracture (Chrischilles, Butler, Davis, & Wallace, 1991). In severe cases limitations associated with fracture can increase the risk for more acute complications, including decubitus ulcers (i.e., pressure sores), pneumonia, and urinary tract infections. By comparison, joint pain associated with osteoarthritis is initially experienced during and after physical activity. However, as the disease progresses, pain becomes more constant and can occur with little movement or even at rest. Among older adults with osteoarthritis, pain is the strongest correlate of quality of life (Laslett et al., 2012). Ultimately, pain may not be controlled by analgesic agents, but if surgery is a viable option, arthroplasty and osteotomy often help patients with osteoarthritis experience improved quality of life for a number of years (Jones & Pohar, 2012; Tay et al., 2013).

It is important to note that the trajectory of osteoporosis and osteoarthritis is chronic and long-term, yet can include sudden onset injuries or complications. Individuals diagnosed with osteoporosis and osteoarthritis can experience social isolation, difficulty with activities of daily living, challenges with symptom ambiguity, fear of fractures, and battles associated with living with an "invisible" illness (Yorgason et al., 2010). For example, spine fractures are associated with a 20%

reduction in the quality of life in the first 12 months and a 15% reduction after 2 years (Tosteson et al., 2001). Even those who manage to remain living independently following a fracture typically experience a substantially reduced quality of life. Health-related quality of life is also decreased in patients with spine fractures, particularly those who have had repeated episodes (Cockerill et al., 2004). These data, combined with similar data from studies of osteoporosis, suggest that the negative impact of bone disease is substantial.

In addition to physical and quality of life challenges, patients with bone disease also bear significant financial expenses. Hoerger and colleagues estimated that 17% of the cost of managing osteoporosis is not covered by insurance (i.e., Medicare, Medicaid, or private coverage) (Hoerger et al., 1999). Patients and/or family members often bear some proportion of the average $2000 increase in direct medical expenses that occur in the year following a fracture (Gabriel et al., 2002). Furthermore, younger family members may experience reductions in earning power as they take time away from work to assist older patients during the time when care is needed (Brainsky et al., 1997); few studies to date have accounted for this type of lost productivity among individuals who must care for those who sustain fractures. However, significant research has been done on the economic implications of caregiving overall. The MetLife Mature Market studies have shown that approximately $50 billion a year is lost in productivity annually as a result of care to family members age 50+. Additionally, it is estimated that the economic value of caregiving (the measure of no cost care provided by family members) exceeds $250 billion. Increased medical bills coupled with a decrease in income often means that entire families may be unable to maintain their typical standard of living (West, Usher, & Foster, 2011).

The experiences of osteoarthritis and osteoporosis can present unique challenges for individuals and families in day to day life. A once active member may now be a sedentary bystander in family activities; couples may experience role reversals, communication breakdowns, and sexual and emotional dysfunction. There can be shifts in responsibilities and duties around the home with tasks such as cooking, cleaning, and yard maintenance. Rigid, traditional role socialization and gender roles may be challenged when roles need to be realigned (Boss, 2002). Long-held dreams or plans for the future may no longer be realistic which can lead to resentment and frustration within the family despite the concern held for the affected individual (West, Usher, & Foster, 2011). Feeling frustrated and overwhelmed with symptoms can lead to fear, anger, and uncertainty (Yorgason et al., 2010). A key contextual factor to this is the relative invisibility of the disease. While the limitations may be increasingly obvious to the family, the measurable signs of the illness are not. Added challenges exist when family members question or imply that the symptoms (namely pain) are less serious than reported. This can lead to a cycle of discouragement, self-doubt, and isolation for the person experiencing osteoarthritis or osteoporosis. Finally, research shows that fatalism, the belief that everything is determined by a higher power and that all events are predestined and cannot be avoided, can lead to feelings of powerlessness (Boss, 2002).

9.3 Resilience

For the purposes of this chapter, psychological resilience refers to the ability of an individual to cope, adapt to, and even overcome significant sources of stress. While individuals have the capacity for resilience, the contexts in which they develop and experience stressors significantly predict how resilience manifests. More specifically, the ability to adapt and be flexible relates not only to individuals but also to family and social systems, and we employ a families-as-systems approach when examining resilience among those experiencing osteoarthritis and osteoporosis (Henry, Morris, & Harrist, 2015).

9.3.1 Family Resilience

While individual characteristics are key to fostering resilience, family systems are the contexts in which resilience is experienced, nurtured, or resisted. Key family factors that are associated with resilience range from specific tasks (family communication skills) to resources (number of supportive members across various roles). Researchers (Black & Lobo, 2008; McCubbin & McCubbin, 1997) found that routines and traditions, those shared and embedded activities that promote family closeness, create a family culture that fosters family resilience. Similarly, shared spirituality and shared internal value systems enable families to jointly make meaning of an event (Black & Lobo, 2008; Unantenne, Warren, Canaway, & Manderson, 2013). For example, a family that has shared internal value systems will make sense of the diagnosis in similar ways ("this illness happened for a reason" or "this diagnosis has helped us draw closer") (Unantenne et al., 2013). Additionally, accord among family members frequently operationalized in terms of cohesion, nurturance, collaborative problem solving, consistent support, open emotional expressions, and appropriate use of humor is central to family resilience (Black & Lobo, 2008; Lowe & Henry, 2012; Trivedi et al., 2011). Finally, families that foster self-efficacy and a person's sense of control over the situation are more likely to contribute to family resilience. Therefore, families who keep family members with osteoporosis and osteoarthritis involved in health decisions, actively engaged in social activities, and empowered to exercise their opinions are more likely to demonstrate resilience.

The families-as-systems approach to osteoarthritis and osteoporosis requires consideration of the complex patterns of interaction that exist within families. This is critical to appreciating a family's collective meaning and response to a stressor like progression of chronic and disabling disease. Henry's and colleagues' new family resilience identifies several subsystems of family resilience. For the purposes of this chapter, family meaning systems and family maintenance systems are used to apply family resilience to osteoarthritis and osteoporosis.

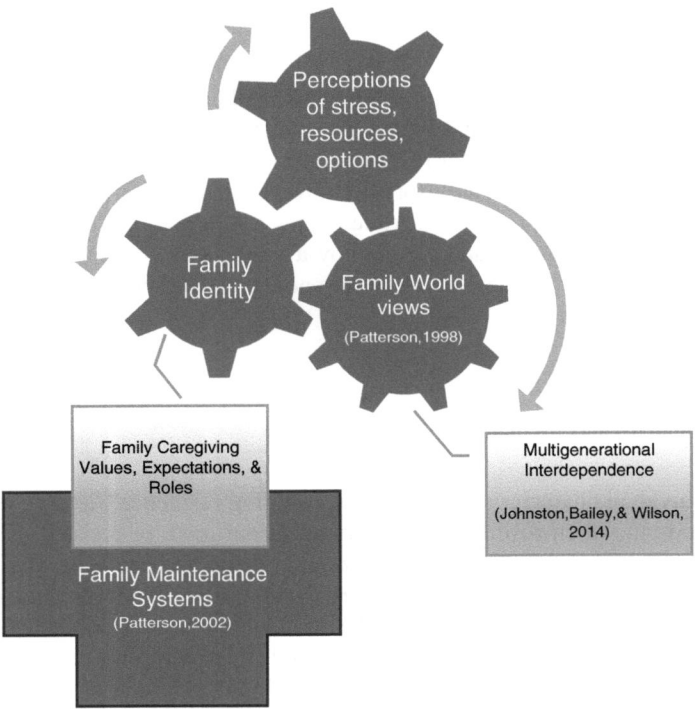

Fig. 9.3 Family meaning and family maintenance systems as they relate to aging families with osteoarthritis and osteoporosis (adapted from Henry et al., 2015)

Family meaning systems are critical to how family members respond to stressors, including a diagnosis of a musculoskeletal disease. The three main elements of family meaning systems—family world views, family identity, and perceptions—are interrelated and create a shared system of meaning that is essential to fostering family resilience (Henry et al., 2015). *Family maintenance systems* are central to how families carry out their social responsibility to loved ones as defined by society (see Fig. 9.3).

Family identity refers to the shared expectations and responses (e.g., practices) that serve as manifestations of what the family values. As applied to families where a member has been diagnosed with osteoarthritis or osteoporosis, issues of chronic pain, reduced mobility, and other aspects of these conditions increase individuals' reliance on others. Families with a clear identity organize themselves and respond in the form of supportive care through roles that range from indirect involvement to full-time care. With 80% of all care being provided by family members, as opposed to formal caregivers, research documents our overwhelming reliance on family caregivers. While many often associate increased reliance on others with negative outcomes, families can function in ways that foster individual and family resilience, despite an increase in chronic symptoms. "It is important to note that the pursuit of independence as defined by mainstream society (the ability to function outside of assistance from others) can create symptoms of anxiety and depression among older adults, therefore threatening individual and family resilience" (Johnston et al., 2014, p. 152). The family resilience model lends itself to the practice of interdependence rather than the dichotomy of independence (being able to do for oneself) vs. dependence (being reliant on others).

The *family maintenance system* represents the ways in which "families serve as a social institution expected to fulfill specific functions for the broader society" (Henry et al., 2015). Specific to older adults diagnosed with osteoarthritis or osteoporosis, this clearly links to the practice of family caregiving (see Fig. 9.2). In resilient families, members respond in ways that fill gaps left by other members of the system, including the macro systems of society. More specifically, gerontologists have long documented the inadequacy of support for older citizens, including significant shortages in geriatricians, gerontological nurses, social workers, and home health aides. Families are therefore expected to fill that gap, testing their skills, resources, and relationships. The caregiving literature depicts a clear picture of stress and risk among caregivers who support individuals with chronic illnesses (Gort et al., 2007). Many caregivers are more likely to serve in more than one caregiving role across their adult years, with one third of caregivers providing care to two or more elders at any one time (AARP, 2009). Women are not only more likely to be caregivers, they are also more likely to be care recipients themselves. And it is clear that while not exclusive to women, osteoarthritis and osteoporosis are more likely to affect older females.

9.4 Strategies for Fostering Resilience Among Individuals and Families Facing Osteoarthritis and Osteoporosis

Practitioners working with older adults with either osteoarthritis or osteoporosis should consider that the stress of these diagnoses presents in the form of chronic concern (condition progression, pain) coupled with the risk of immediate injury (fractures, falls). It is crucial that those working with these individuals understand the role of the family in short and long term support of their family member with osteoarthritis or osteoporosis. Professionals, be they medically or behaviorally focused, must focus on the challenges associated with these diagnoses, namely risk of isolation, invisibility of the illness, and reliance on others. It is important for practitioners to promote the family's ability to do the following:

1. Develop a shared narrative of the diagnosis (based on clear and accurate information; minimize false assumptions)
2. Facilitate positive communication (rooted in a balance between the needs of the person with osteoarthritis and osteoporosis and those of the family)
3. Map resources (personal, family, community)
4. Develop a care plan (who is who and who does what to support the individual and the family)

5. Create and support physical activity and dietary plans
6. Explore community education initiatives, such as a chronic disease self-management program

Individuals with OA and OP face a variety of challenges, some that are in line with other chronic diseases and yet others that are unique. Family systems are called upon by medical and social systems to tend to the needs of those with chronic illnesses, including osteoarthritis and osteoporosis. It is important for osteoarthritis and osteoporosis to be included in the research on chronic illnesses as they relate to family resilience. Further, scholars must begin to bridge knowledge gleaned from other chronic illnesses to the experiences of osteoarthritis and osteoporosis. Finally, as medical technology advances in the prevention and treatment of osteoarthritis and osteoporosis, family members and family resilience processes must be considered as part of the research, care plan, and response.

Discussion Questions

1. What does "family resilience" look like for an older adult with severe osteoporosis or osteoarthritis? How is this different from "effective coping"?
2. If there was no cure, what policy solutions exist for minimizing the burden of osteoporosis or osteoarthritis for the growing older adult population? What are the "costs" of these solutions and are these costs defensible?
3. Is a basic understanding of the pathophysiology of osteoporosis and osteoarthritis needed by a non-medical practitioner who works with older? Why or why not?
4. If you were to design an intervention to improve quality of life among older adults with osteoporosis or osteoarthritis,
   (a) what would you target (e.g., exercise, medication management, stress)?
   (b) how might you affect that target (e.g., create human support systems, offer non-human aids like reminders or behavioral contracting, professional oversight)?
   (c) how might key stakeholders (i.e., the older adult, his/her spouse, his/her adult child(ren), his/her health care provider) be affected by the requirements of intervention? Why?
   (d) How might key stakeholders be affected if the intervention was successful? Why?

References

American Association for Retired Persons (AARP). (2009). Chronic care—A call for action. Retrieved from http://www.aarp.org/health/medicare-insurance/info-03-2009/beyond_50_hcr.html

Bennell, K. L., Dobson, F., & Hinman, R. S. (2014). Exercise in osteoarthritis: Moving from prescription to adherence. *Best Practice & Research. Clinical Rheumatology, 28*(1), 93–117. doi:10.1016/j.berh.2014.01.009

Bhala, N., Emberson, J., Merhi, A., Abramson, S., Arber, N., Baron, J. A., et al. (2013). Vascular and upper gastrointestinal effects of non-steroidal anti-inflammatory drugs: Meta-analyses of individual participant data from randomised trials. *Lancet, 382*, 769–779. doi:10.1015/S0140-6736(13)60900-9

Black, D. M., Greenspan, S. L., Ensrud, K. E., Palermo, L., McGowan, J. A., Lang, T. F., et al. (2003). The effects of parathyroid hormone and alendronate alone or in combination in postmenopausal osteoporosis. *New England Journal of Medicine, 349*, 1207–1215. doi:10.1097/01.OGX.0000115856.54444.D6

Black, D. M., Schwartz, A. V., Ensrud, K. E., Cauley, J. A., Levis, S., Quandt, S. A., et al. (2006). Effects of continuing or stopping alendronate after 5 years of treatment: The Fracture Intervention Trial Long-term Extension (FLEX): A randomized trial. *Journal of the American Medical Association, 296*, 2927–2938. doi:10.1001/jama.296.24.2927

Black, K., & Lobo, M. (2008). A conceptual review of family resilience factors. *Journal of Family Nursing, 14*, 33–55. doi:10.1177/1074840707312237

Blume, S. W., & Curtis, J. R. (2011). Medical costs of osteoporosis in the elderly Medicare population. *Osteoporosis International, 22*, 835–844. doi:10.1007/s00198-010-1419-7

Boss, P. (2002). *Family Stress Management: A contextual approach* (2nd ed.). Thousand Oaks, CA: Sage Publications.

Brainsky, A., Glick, H., Lydick, E., Epstein, R., Fox, K. M., Hawkes, W., et al. (1997). The economic cost of hip fractures in community-dwelling older adults: A prospective study. *Journal of the American Geriatrics Society, 45*(3), 281–287.

Brosi, W.A., Ames, B.D., & Carolan, M.T. (2009). Decision making authority in caregiving relationships: Perceptions of mothers receiving care from adult daughters. Brazilian Journal of Home Economics, 20, 11–29.

Buckwalter, J. A., & Mankin, H. F. (1997). Articular cartilage, part 1: Tissue design and chondrocyte-matrix interaction. *Journal of Bone and Joint Surgery (American Volume), 79*, 600–611. Retrieved from http://jbjs.org/

Chrischilles, E. A., Butler, C. D., Davis, C. S., & Wallace, R. B. (1991). A model of lifetime osteoporosis impact. *Archives of Internal Medicine, 151*, 2026–2032. doi:10.1001/archinte.1991.00400100100017

Cockerill, W., Lunt, M., Silman, A. J., Cooper, C., Lips, P., Bhalla, A. K., et al. (2004). Health-related quality of life and radiographic vertebral fracture. *Osteoporosis International, 15*(2), 113–119.

Cosman, F., de Beur, S.J., LeBoff, M.S., Lewiecki, E.M., Tanner, B., Randall, S., Lindsay, R. (2014). National Osteoporosis Foundation Clinician's Guide to the Prevention and Treatment of Osteoporosis. Osteoporosis Int. 25(10), 2359–2381.

Drake, M. T., & Khosla, S. (2012). Male osteoporosis. *Endocrinology Metabolism Clinics of North America, 41*, 629–641. doi:10.1016/j.ecl.2012.05.001

Evans, D., & Lee, E. (2014). Impact of dementia on marriage: A qualitative systematic review. *Dementia, 13*, 330–349. doi:10.1177/1471301212473882

Felson, D. T., Lawrence, R. C., Dieppe, P. A., Hirsch, R., Helmick, C. G., Jordan, J. M., et al. (2000). Osteoarthritis: New insights. Part 1: The disease and its risk factors. *Annals of Internal Medicine, 133*, 635–646. doi:10.7326/0003-4819-133-8-200010170-00016

Fleisher, K. E., Jolly, A., Venkata, U. D., Norman, R. G., Saxena, D., & Glickman, R. S. (2013) Osteonecrosis of the jaw onset times are based on the route of bisphosphonate therapy. *Journal of Oral and Maxillofacial Surgery, 71*, 513–519. doi:10.1016/j.jms.2012.07.049

Fry, P. S., & Keyes, C. L. M. (2011). *New frontiers in aging: Life-strengths and well-being in late life*. Cambridge: Cambridge University Press.

Gabriel, S. E., Tosteson, A. N., Leibson, C. L., Crowson, C. S., Pond, G. R., Hammond, C. S., et al. (2002). Direct medical costs attributable to osteoporotic fractures. *Osteoporosis International, 13*(4), 323–330.

Gan, M., Yang, H., Zhou, F., Zou, J., Wang, G., Mei, X., et al. (2010). Kyphoplasty for the treatment of painful osteoporotic thoracolumbar burst fractures. *Orthopedic, 14*, 88–92. doi:10.3928/01477447-20100104-17

Gore, M., Tai, K. S., Sadosky, A., Leslie, D., & Stacey, B. R. (2011). Clinical comorbidities, treatment patterns, and direct medical costs of patients with osteoarthritis in usual care: A retrospective claims database analysis. *Journal of Medical Economics, 14*, 497–507. doi: 10.3111/13696998.2011.594347

Gort, A. M., Mingot, M., Gomez, X., Soler, T., Torres, G., Sacristán, O., et al. (2007). Use of the Zarit scale for assessing caregiver burden and collapse in caregiving at home in dementias. *International Journal of Geriatric Psychiatry, 22*, 957–962. doi:10.1002/gps.1770

Grady, C. L. (2008). Cognitive neuroscience of aging. *Annals of the New York Academy of Sciences, 1124*, 127–144. doi:10.1196/annals.1440.009

Greendale, G. A., & Barrett-Connor, E. (2001). Outcomes of osteoporotic fractures. In M. R. Feldman & J. Kelsey (Eds.), *Osteoporosis* (2nd ed., Vol. 1, pp. 819–829). San Diego: Academic.

Henry, C. S., Morris, A. S., & Harrist, A. W. (2015). Family resilience: Moving into the third wave. *Family Relations, 64*, 22–43. doi:10.1111/fare.12106

Hoerger, T. J., Downs, K. E., Lakshmanan, M. C., Lindrooth, R. C., Plouffe, L., Jr., Wendling, B., et al. (1999). Healthcare use among U.S. women aged 45 and older: Total costs and costs for selected postmenopausal health risks. *Journal of Women's Health & Gender-Based Medicine, 8*(8), 1077–1089.

Hu, S. (1997). Internal fixation in the osteoporotic spine. *Spine, 14*, S43–S48. doi:10.1097/00007632-199712151-00008

Johnston, J. H., Bailey, W. A., & Wilson, G. (2014). Mechanisms for fostering multigenerational resilience. *Contemporary Family Therapy, 36*, 148–161. doi:10.1007-s10591-012-9222-6

Jones, C. A., & Pohar, S. (2012). Health-related quality of life after total joint arthroplasty: A scoping review. *Clinics in Geriatric Medicine, 28*, 395–429. doi:10.1016/j.cger.2012.06.001

Keefe, F. J., Caldwell, D. S., Baucom, D., Salley, A., Robinson, E., Timmons, K., et al. (1999). Spouse-assisted coping skills training in the management of knee pain in osteoarthritis: Long-term followup results. *Arthritis Care and Research, 12*(2), 101–111.

Kirkley, A., Birmingham, T. B., Litchfield, R. B., Giffin, J. R., Willits, K. R., Wong, C. J., et al. (2008). A randomized trial of arthroscopic surgery for osteoarthritis of the knee. *New England Journal of Medicine, 359*, 1097–1107. doi:10.1056/NEJMoa0708333

Laslett, L. L., Quinn, S. J., Winzenberg, T. M., Sanderson, K., Cicuttini, F., & Jones, G. (2012). A prospective study of the impact of musculoskeletal pain and radiographic osteoarthritis on health related quality of life in community dwelling older people. *BMC Musculoskeletal Disorders, 13*, 168. doi:10.1186/1471-2474-13-168

Lawrence, R. C., Felson, D. T., Helmick, C. G., Arnold, L. M., Choi, H., Deyo, R. A., et al. (2008). Estimate of the prevalence of arthritis and other rheumatic conditions in the United States: Part II. *Arthritis & Rheumatism, 58*, 26–35. doi:10.1002/art.23176

Lohmander, L. S., Lark, M. W., Dahlberg, L., Walakovits, L. A., & Roos, H. (1992). Cartilage matrix metabolism in osteoarthritis: Markers in synovial fluid, serum, and urine. *Clinical Biochemistry, 25*, 167–174. doi:10.1016/0009-9120(92)90250-V

Lowe, P., & Henry, K. (2012). What factors impact the quality of life of elderly women with chronic illness: Three women's perspectives? *Contemporary Nursing, 41*, 18–27. Retrieved from http://www.tandfonline.com/

McCubbin, H., McCubbin, M., Thompson, A., Han, S., & Allen, C. (1997). Families under stress: What makes them resilient. *Journal of Family and Consumer Sciences, 89*(3), 2.

National Osteoporosis Foundation Clinician's Guide to the Prevention and Treatment of Osteoporosis. (2014) Version 1, 1–56.

Neer, R. M., Arnaud, C. D., Zanchetta, J. R., Prince, R., Gaich, G. A., Reginster, J. Y., et al. (2001). Effect of parathyroid hormone (1-34) on fractures and bone mineral density in postmenopausal women with osteoporosis. *New England Journal of Medicine, 344*, 1434–1441. doi:10.1097/00006254-200110000-00018

Office of the Surgeon General (US). (2004). *Bone health and osteoporosis: A report of the Surgeon General*. Rockville, MD: Office of the Surgeon General (US).

Ortman, J. M., & Velkoff, V. A. (2014). *An aging nation: The older population in the United States*. Retrieved April 19, 2015 from http://www.census.gov/prod/2014pubs/p25-1140.pdf

Poole, A. R., Ionescu, M., Swan, A., & Dieppe, P. A. (1994). Changes in cartilage metabolism in arthritis are reflected by altered serum and synovial fluid levels of the cartilage proteoglycan aggrecan, implications for pathogenesis. *Journal of Clinical Investigation, 94*, 25–33. doi:10.1172/JCI117314

Riggs, B. L., Khosla, S., & Melton, L. J., III. (2002). Sex steroids and the construction and conservation of the adult skeleton. *Endocrine Reviews, 23*, 279–302. doi:10.1210/edrv.23.3.0465

Rosland, A. M., Heiser, M., & Piette, J. D. (2012). The impact of family behaviors and communication patterns on chronic illness outcomes. *Journal of Behavioral Medicine, 35*, 221–239. doi:10.1007/s10865-011-9354-4

Schilcher, J., Michaelsson, K., & Aspenberg, P. (2011). Bisphosphonate use and atypical fractures of the femoral shaft. *New England Journal of Medicine, 364*, 1728–1737. doi:10.1056/NEJMoa1010650

Schultz, R., & Sherwood, P. R. (2008). Physical and mental health effects of family caregiving. *American Journal of Nursing, 108*, 23–27. Retrieved from http://ajnonline.com

Seeman, E. (2003). Invited review: Pathogenesis of osteoporosis. *Journal of Applied Physiology, 95*, 2142–2151. doi:10.1152/japplphysiol.00564.2003

Shin, J. J., Chin, D. K., & Yoon, Y. S. (2009). Percutaneous vertebroplasty for the treatment of osteoporotic burst fractures. *Acta Neurochirurgica, 14*, 141–148. doi:10.1007/s00701-009-0189-5

Tay, K. S., Lo, N. N., Yeo, S. J., Chia, S. L., Tay, D. K., & Chin, P. L. (2013). Revision total knee arthroplasty: Causes and outcomes. *Annals Academy of Medicine Singapore, 42*, 178–183. Retrieved from http://annals.edu.sg

Tosteson, A. N., Gabriel, S. E., Grove, M. R., Moncur, M. M., Kneeland, T. S., & Melton, L. J. 3rd. (2001). Impact of hip and vertebral fractures on quality-adjusted life years. *Osteoporosis International, 12*(12), 1042–1049.

Trelle, S., Reichenbach, S., Wandel, S., Hildebrand, P., Tschannen, B., Villiger, P. M., et al. (2011). Cardiovascular safety of non-steroidal anti-inflammatory drugs: Network meta-analysis. *BMJ, 342*, c7086. doi:10.1136/bmj.c7086

Trivedi, R. B., Bosworth, H. B., & Jackson, G. L. (2011). Resilience in chronic illness. In B. Resnick, L. P. Gwyther, & K. A. Roberto (Eds.), *Resilience in aging* (pp. 181–197). New York: Springer Publications.

Turner, J., & Kelly, B. (2000). Emotional dimensions of chronic care. *Western Journal of Medicine, 172*, 124–128. doi:10.1136/ewjm.172.2.124

Unantenne, N., Warren, N., Canaway, R., & Manderson, L. (2013). The strength to cope: Spirituality and faith in chronic disease. *Journal of Religion and Health, 52*, 1147–1161. doi:10.1007/s10943-011-9554-9

U.S. Department of Health and Human Services, Administration for Community Living, Administration on Aging. (2014). A profile of older Americans: 2014. Retrieved from http://www.aoa.acl.gov/Aging_Statistics/Profile/2014/docs/2014-Profile.pdf

Visser-Meily, A., Post, M., Gorter, J. W., Berlekom, S. B., Van Den Bos, T., & Lindeman, E. (2006). Rehabilitation of stroke patients needs a family-centered approach. *Disability & Rehabilitation, 28*, 1557–1561. doi:10.1080/09638280600648215

West, C., Usher, K., & Foster, K. (2011). Family resilience: Towards a new model of chronic pain management. *Collegian Journal, 18*, 3–10. doi:10.1016/j.colegn.201.08.004

Woessner, J. F., Jr., & Gunja-Smith, Z. (1991). Role of metalloproteinases in human osteoarthritis. *Journal of Rheumatology, 27*, 99–101. Retrieved from http://jrheum.org

Wright, N. C., Looker, A., Saag, K., Curtis, J. R., Dalzell, E. S., Randall, S., et al. (2014). The recent prevalence of osteoporosis and low bone mass based on bone mineral density at the femoral neck or lumbar spine in the United States. *Journal of Bone and Mineral Research, 29*, 2520–2526. doi:10.1002/jbmr.2269

Yorgason, J. B., Roper, S. O., Wheeler, B., Crane, K., Byron, R., Carpenter, L., et al. (2010). Older couple's management of multiple chronic illness. *Family System Health, 28*, 30–47. doi:10.1037/a0019396

Chapter 10
The Unfolding of Unique Problems in Later Life Families

Lee Hyer, Christine M. Mullen, and Krystal Jackson

"Aging is not for sissies" is a phrase now over 40 years old. The family at later life is systemically rich and, although similar to other ages, sufficiently different and complex to require a distinct understanding. On the one hand, it is growing: In 2011, there were 41.4 million adults ages 65 and older; 13.3% of the population, an increase of 18% since 2000 (Greenberg, 2012). The silver tsunami is under way. On the other, complexity is the norm as the possible numbers of morbidities, function problems, and system problems are prodigious.

Unless your target is pure biomarkers, discussing older adults requires the context of the family. If we are becoming a chronologically gifted society, then the variables related to families are worth studying. They also have changed. There is a gender gap, more racial and ethnic diversity, a gradient of health disparities that makes it difficult to simplify issues, a distinct mental health phenomenology, unique work and retirement issues, strange happenings like the existence of five-generation families, grand parenting and its many forms, widowhood, death and dying, as well as grief and hospice, the pesky prevalence of suicide, long term care and aging home models of increasingly variety, and dementia (the continuum of cognitive decline). Did we mention caregiving or the clear disparities between young old, and old, and oldest old (>84)? We hope the point is made that there is no one family type at later life; at some point, however, most deal with chronic and ineluctable loss or disease.

L. Hyer, Ph.D., A.B.P.P. (✉)
Mercer University Medical School & Georgia Neurosurgical Institute,
840 Pine Street Suite 800, Macon, GA 31201, USA
e-mail: lhyer@ganeuroandspine.com

C.M. Mullen, M.A. • K. Jackson, M.S.
Georgia Neurosurgical Institute, 840 Pine Street Suite 800, Macon, GA 31201, USA
e-mail: ChristineMarieMullen@gmail.com; krysstj31@gmail.com

© Springer International Publishing Switzerland 2017
G.L. Welch, A.W. Harrist (eds.), *Family Resilience and Chronic Illness*,
Emerging Issues in Family and Individual Resilience,
DOI 10.1007/978-3-319-26033-4_10

10.1 Literature Review

10.1.1 Later Life Problems

Where just age is concerned, we have had a sea change. In 1959, older people had the highest poverty rate (35%) followed by children (27%); by 2007, the proportion of older adults in poverty was just 10%. In fact, in 2007 older people in the middle income group made up the largest share of older people by category (33%) with those in the high income group up to 31% (Greenberg, 2012). Health ratings also were up. In 2008, 75% of people 65 or older rated their health as good, very good, or excellent; for 85 and older, these rates were still somewhat respectable at 66%. Life expectancy (the average number of years lived by a group of people born in the same year) along with a growing burden of chronic diseases also keeps rising (Peck, Hurwicz, Ory, Yuma, & Cook, 2010). We gained 3.8 years in two decades! If you are a male in the USA and 65, you can expect to live an average 18.5 years; if you are 85, you can expect 6.8 more years. Unfortunately for gains in life expectancy in the last decade, the time spent seriously sick is 1.5 years and time disabled has accrued by 2 years (Suthers, 2008).

Depression and anxiety are the two marker disorders at late life. Depression is a prevalent issue within this population (10–20%) that is typically under diagnosed and under treated (Haber, 2013). Its phenomenology also is distinct from other ages. "Real dysphoria," however, may be closer to 2%. Depression as a true disorder that is debilitating, not episodic and marginal in intensity, is clearly lower in prevalence. There are then varieties of the phenomenology of depression. Major, Minor, and Mixed Depression exist at late life. Annoyingly, subsyndromal depression (often defined as $\geq$ on the Center for Epidemiologic Studies Depression Scale (CES-D) but full MDD criteria are not met) is also a pervasive problem. In fact, 25% of dementias have a depression. All of these states are prevalent; all assert an influence on quality of life; and all (but depression in dementia) may segue to Major Depressive disorder at some point, if not handled when the symptoms are first noted. Most older patients do not solicit treatment.

In some ways anxiety disorders trump depression. They are the most common psychiatric illnesses in the USA with approximately 30% of the population experiencing anxiety-related symptoms in their lifetime (Kessler, Chiu, Demler, & Walters, 2005). Current rates of anxiety disorders extend to 10% with its symptoms actually doubling that number. This number is slightly less for older adults. Most anxiety problems occur earlier and continue in life (50–97%). Again as with depression, older adults with the core anxiety disorder, Generalized Anxiety Disorder (GAD), are more disabled, have worse quality of life, and demand a greater health care utilization than non-anxious groups (Porensky et al., 2009). Also GAD problems spread; 90% of older adults with GAD report dissatisfaction with sleep and the majority report depression. This is not unlike depression, affecting cognition and health.

Importantly simple prevalence rates at late life for any disorder are misleading because the "problems" extend into other life areas. The 2001–2003 National

Comorbidity Survey Replication, an epidemiological survey, found that approximately 25% of American adults meet criteria for at least one diagnosable mental disorder in any given year, and more than half report one or more chronic general medical conditions (Kessler et al., 2005). When mental and medical conditions co-occur, the combination is associated with elevated symptom burden, functional impairment, decreased length and quality of life, and increased costs. Adjustment by itself suffers just by getting older; at age 80, 60% of adults start having problems with ADLs. Cognition and function cohabit; ~40% of common variance is shared (Royall, Chiodo, Mouton, & Polk, 2007). More adjustment calamities ensue. Oh yes, the family is the essential context for all this.

Studies have also illustrated the fact that socioeconomic status and our living environment begin to play an even more significant role in our quality of life as we age, particularly with respect to the development of chronic diseases. Socioeconomic status predicts quality of life and general health better than perhaps any other researched factor. Lack of monetary resources, restricted access to quality healthcare, and environmental stressors add to the deterioration of older adults living in low-income environments. The practice of negative habits, such as lack of physical activity, poor diet, and smoking, also influences the onset of other chronic disorders, such as hypertension and diabetes, as well as mental health issues. Women and race especially report more health needs and disability in terms of functional limitations and report fewer economic resources (see Hyer, 2014). Again, in all of this, the family is the scaffold for the emergence of problems.

Recall too that psychiatric care is most often provided in a primary care clinic (PCC) context. Older adults seek mental health at lower levels (3–6% of all actual visits) as they see little connection between symptom and mental problems. Older adults do not use psychiatric clinics. In 2006, 79% of mental health care was addressed in PCC. Furthermore, only 15% complaints are clearly linked to a biological cause. Not surprisingly, if the default standard of care for older adults in the twenty-first century is the PCC, then the treatment of the moment is pharmacology, a truly blunt instrument with both helpful and harmful effects. Over a 20 year period, the percentage of Medicare enrollees diagnosed with depression who were treated with antidepressants rose from 53.7% to 67.1%. The percentage who received psychotherapy alone dropped to 10% from 16% (see Hyer, 2014).

Case Study
Joe and his wife present at a typical assessment and treatment session in a Primary Care Clinic. Joe has high blood pressure, diabetes, mild COPD, arthritis, and is now showing clear memory problems. Among these, his diabetes and blood pressure are concerns. Now he has failed a dementia screen. He is functioning to some extent by doing some housework, doing his medications (suspect), driving to small and well-known places, and can make small shopping trips with help. He can no longer handle his finances, his

(continued)

reading has stopped, and he is clearly forgetting input from wife and kids. He is now not taking his hypertension and diabetes medications.

Doctor: Any problems with the lapse in medication taking?
Patient: None

Wife: He just wants to be macho.
Patient: You know nothing. She just points to and exaggerates my weaknesses.

Doctor: Your BP was 170/100, a little high and you blood sugars are over 170.
Doctor: I feel fine. Anything else we need to do?
Wife rolls eyes.

Reaction: I am uncomfortable in such common settings. I am caught in the "family dynamics." It is, on the one hand, a tension between autonomy and beneficence; on the other, a family dynamic or personality issue under the dome of a degenerative disease. Each family member is playing a role. The role of Joe is to say—"Don't worry about me. I am making my choice;" the role of the wife is—"Let me take care of you and listen to other/good care." If the patient were from Japan or Thailand, the children would hold sway and the needs of the elder would be met, regardless of autonomy. Here roles are in play, the script from which each plays. If Joe switched roles, he was going to be a burden and selfish, weak if you will; if the wife switched, "OK, you win, we will just let what happens, happen," she would be uncaring.

This issue requires systemic thinking and intervention. A family dynamic is proponent here: This scenario has to play out with no agreement to have each feel complete and heard. This conflict also challenges the ethic-biased autonomy that accedes to the patient at all costs. In fact, the family needs to be considered. If we explore this situation from a family perspective and forget optimal care or autonomy for a second, then some clarity seems possible. Querying Joe about what his wife is thinking produces "She is trying to protect me." Querying her, she notes that he is prideful and this is quintessentially him. Again, it is Joe's role not to need help and her role to insist on helping. If the treatment is framed on what is best for Joe, it is rejected; framed as the reluctant acquisition of her wishes, it is more palatable. This issue then was not so much about individual autonomy as it was about a hybrid that met the needs of the family system, of each role. They needed to remain in mild friendly conflict over the management of suffering. In a sense the family was the patient. The intervention is systemic.

10.1.2 Family in Late Life

The transition to late adulthood comes with many decisions for the individual as well as the family. During this time, individuals progress into the last developmental state of the Erickson model, struggling with ego integrity versus despair. Most scenarios are filled with some debility. More than half of Medicare beneficiaries have five or more chronic illnesses (Bodenheimer, Chen, & Bennett, 2009; Paez, Zhoa, & Hwang, 2009; Thorpe & Howard, 2006). The majority of elderly are sick with their fatal chronic illness 3 years prior to their death (Lynn, Blanchard, Campbell, Jayes, & Lunney, 2001). The whole concept of the normal aging brain is now under review as there exists modal microbleeds, infarcts, white latter hyperintensities, and neuronal damage in well-functioning older adults. Normal aging is in flux; successful age is in doubt (Jeste & Palmer, 2013; Rowe & Kahn, 1997).

How does aging impact families? The family structure as a whole continues to shift from the previously conceived "nuclear" family to a more polysemous system due to increases in divorce, changes in gender roles, and a decrease in birth rates. Just by itself, the family structure can cause anxiety over the variability of its dependent members (Binstock, George, Cutler, Hendricks, & Schulz, 2006). Part of the equation in retaining autonomy in old age is the relationship between family networks and the service system, and particularly the extent to which families are supportive. The specific mix is related to three factors: family norms and care preferences; family culture that guides the level of readiness to use public services; and availability, accessibility, quality, and cost of services. Family care is substantial and there exists, often grudgingly, a collective responsibility through available public services.

Additionally, social support systems tend to dwindle in late life, which can result in individuals living out their lives in isolation. During this time, family members are typically the primary social support system, chiefly spouses, children, and siblings. The shift of social support networks toward family members is due to many factors such as retirement, death of those in individual's life, mobility restrictions, or caregiving of a significant other. Carstensen's socioemotional selectivity theory, perhaps the most noted theory of later life, specifies that the support systems of older adults shrink due to time spent fulfilling immediate emotional needs (Carstensen, Isaacowitz, & Charles, 1999). Specifically, the perspective of time remaining of one's life significantly contributes to the engagement of social activities.

The need for an extensive social support network provides evidence of direct positive influence of the family at later life. Positive interactions with the adult children promote the concept of living on through their pedigrees that promotes experiential transcendence (Newman, 2014). Perceptions of uselessness to others were found to be a significant risk factor for disability and mortality (Gruenewald, Karlamangla, Greendale, Singer, & Seeman, 2007). Social relationships also have a significant correlation with health (Bosworth & Schaie, 1997; Vaillant, Meyer, Mukamal, & Soldx, 1998), whereas social isolation could lead to an increased progression with physical and cognitive decline (Hawkley & Cacioppo, 2007). Social support has also been found to lower risk of death within this population (Eng, Rimm, Fitzmaurice, & Kawachi, 2002; Obisesan & Gillum, 2009).

This sets the background for the sociological factors of the aging family. We start with the aging couple. Orathinkal and Vansteenwegen (2007) found couples that remained together in late adulthood were more likely to have higher satisfaction and fewer adjustment difficulties in their marriage when compared to middle-aged couples. Close marital relationships can foster self-esteem and decrease anxiety, which has been shown to moderate negative psychological ramifications of disabilities (Mancini & Bonanno, 2006). However, as we see below, health and stress significantly contribute to quality of marital satisfaction over time and into later life (Silverstein & Giarrusso, 2010). The added strain of caregiving for a significant other can foster feelings of ambivalence and strain the marriage. This can lead to aggravation of an illness of the caregiver, and cause feelings of loneliness and burnout (Papalia, 2012). Divorce is rare in this population; currently 11% of adults' ages 65 and older who divorced were not remarried (Social Security Administration, 2010). Interestingly, remarriage in later life can expand social networks, and remarried elders are less likely than elderly living alone to require assistance from the community (Papalia, 2012). As in many cases, however, one problem can create a cascade of others.

A Medicare study demonstrated that when a spouse was hospitalized, the other spouse's mortality increased (Christakis & Allison, 2006). The Federal Interagency Forum on Aging-Related Statistic (2010) found that women are four times more likely than men to be widowed by the age of 65. Mostofsky et al. (2012) even found that the loss of a significant other increased the risk of a heart attack by sixfold within the first week after death. Widowhood is one of the most difficult transitions in later life, which can cause the family structure to radically change. In 2011, older women outnumbered older men 23.4 million to 17.9 million (Greenberg, 2012). When elderly parents lose their significant other, they are more likely to rely on their adult children and the adult children rely less on their parents (Ha, Carr, Utz, & Nesse, 2006).

Intergenerational cohabitation between adult children and their parents has become more common within the past several decades. Brown, Bulanda, and Lee (2005) demonstrated that married elder and middle-age cohabitants have higher psychological well-being and quality of partner relationships than their non-married counterparts. Cohabitation is not restricted to adult children and their parents, however. Multigenerational households have slightly increased to 4% in 2010 from 3.7% in 2000 (Lofquist, 2012). There has been a 30% increase, too, of grandparents raising or helping raise grandchildren in the past 15 years, totaling to 6.2 million children (Benokraitis, 2011). The bond between grandparent and grandchild is highly sensitive to familial configuration changes as well as fluctuating circumstances (Silverstein & Marenco, 2001). For example, conflict between parent and grandchild (Monserud, 2008), as well as marital disputes of the parents, can negatively impact the grandparent and grandchild relationship (Amato & Cheadle, 2005). Grandparents are often perceived as the bonding force within a family system and serve as mediators within the unit (Benokraitis, 2011). Grandparents of children with single mothers actually provide more achievement in increasing the child's language skills and academic attainment (Benokraitis, 2011). Therefore, when an aging grandparent declines and is in need of assistance, the outcome can have negative effects on the family system.

10.1.3 Chronic Illness in Families

It has become common that at least one member of a family has lived long enough to have one or more chronic illnesses that can cause emotional and physical depletion for the other family members. Now that the fastest-growing segment of the population is age 85 and over, many people in their late sixties or beyond, whose own health and energy may be faltering, find themselves serving as caregivers. Chronic illness can have ripple effects throughout a family system, especially the latter stages of the disease or disorder in later life. Typical onset of chronic illness is a gradual development of symptoms earlier in life, such as with HIV or cancer. The progression of chronic illness has different phases that require different familial changes (Rolland, 1984). Chronic illness at later life is often stressful and expensive for those of the family (Lynn & Adamson, 2003).

Despite the increase of elderly individuals with chronic illnesses, many are still fully functional. Freedman et al. (2014) analyzed 2011 National Health and Aging Trends of 8077 adults ages 65 years and older. Results revealed that 31% were fully capable of mobile activities and self-care. In comparison, 25% of adults were able to be successful with these activities with assistance of devices, 5% had reduced activities, 18% remained to have difficulties despite assistant devices, and 21% of adults received help. For the population over age 90, about 50% required significant assistance. Appropriate accommodations to assist with disabilities with functioning were found to be associated with maintaining participation in perceived valued activities and well-being. However, there were high disparities within race, ethnicity, and income.

Chronic illness is the norm at late life, resulting in outcomes mostly for the worse. Immediately after a near fatal episode occurs, many families become more cohesive (Steinglass, Temple, Lisman, & Reiss, 1982). However, these families also find the adjustment to the chronic illness difficult. Families may need redefined roles to assist with the care of the individual, whether the illness is progressive, relapsing, or constant. Medicare analyses demonstrated that only one-fifth of people suffered from a short period of decline that lead to death; most lingered or showed a slow trajectory (Lunney, Lynn, & Hogan, 2002). Given that approximately 36% of Social Security recipients relied almost solely on this income, and 3.6 million elderly adults live below poverty (Greenberg, 2012), many families may need to reconfigure finances in order to accommodate expensive medical necessities. This can add burden to the family system in addition to role changes that can necessitate systemic interventions. One meta-analysis (Martire, Lustig, Schulz, Miller, &

Helgeson, 2004) found that psychosocial inventions for family members caring for an elderly adult with chronic illness had an impact on decreased mortality rates among elders with chronic illnesses, excluding dementia.

Chronic illness can impact a relationship as much as abuse, addiction, and infidelity. One person in the couple will outlive the other. Additionally, the majority of couples will face illness or loss of at least one parent. Given varying expectations and resources available for the care of older adults, chronic illness can become a serious point of concern for all within a family. Specifically, family members' responsibilities and emotional strain can have a detrimental impact. Issues such as role strain, role conflict, and reemergence of parent-child problems are typically seen. This role transition of taking care of ailing parents generally occurs when couples have raised their children and are renewing the relationship. Adults who may be older or are newly wed who are taking care of aging or ailing parents present with different issues, including lack of a sense of obligation or lack of empathy toward their significant other.

A modal concern is the potential deleterious psychological and medical effects of long-term family caregiving. Women have a higher risk of developing these adverse consequences when they serve as the sole caretaker. These effects are also aggregated when the caretaker is also employed. As a result, caregivers experience increased rates of isolation and loneliness. Therefore, each of these components needs to be considered in the assessment and treatment of those dealing with chronic illness. For an extensive review of these interventions and treatment considerations of medical family therapy, please refer to McDaniel, Doherty, and Hepworth (2014).

10.1.4 Psychotherapy at Late Life

Psychotherapy works, even at later life. A number of older general reviews are available for the treatment of depression in older adults, the core problem at later life (but the same conclusions apply to anxiety). Reviews of psychotherapy (e.g., Gallagher-Thompson & Thompson, 1995; Hyer, 2014; Scogin & Shah, 2012; Scogin, Welsh, Hanson, Stump, & Coates, 2005; Teri, Curtis, Gallagher-Thompson, & Thompson, 1994) are universally favorable. The American Psychological Association Division 12 task force on depression at later life identified six different psychological treatments as evidence-based: behavioral therapy, cognitive behavioral therapy (CBT), problem (group) solving, IPT, cognitive bibliotherapy, and (group) reminiscence (Hartman-Stein & LaRue, 2011). And the net for psychosocial problems is wide (see Hyer, 2014). The effect sizes are generally moderate to good, but do not generally surpass many medication studies. Most new studies now tend to be done in primary care (e.g., Serfaty et al., 2009).

There is very little in the way of empirically supported data for family therapy at later life except for caregiving (covered below). Like those of individual patients, the symptoms of older families respond but do not remit. The challenge of getting older is to strike a balance between fighting disabilities/diseases and coming to terms with the limitations they impose in the context of supports and challenges. This battle will change again and again, and unfold in families as power shifts. Importantly, older adults come to therapy (modally) as a couple or family when one partner/parent is in decline. The actual unmet needs of older adults are plentiful and often require an expansive, out of the box listing of help agents—home care, bibliotherapy, telephone therapy, pre-therapy, and booster sessions. All programs have a connection to the family, the necessary base of curative dynamics.

10.2 Implications

10.2.1 Implications for Practice

10.2.1.1 Watch and Wait Model

We now provide an overall model that allows therapy to take hold, the Watch and Wait Model. Academics have been trained to discern the nuanced differences in treatment (one antidepressant vs. another, one psychotherapy vs. another, medication vs. psychotherapy). At later life, these issues help providers very little. Published reports suggest that attending to novel "significantly better," or "evidenced-based," will result in better patient outcomes, but doing so with older adults often diverts attention from the real world issues, and has only marginal evidence of benefit. Instead of presenting a comprehensive algorithm for treating depression in older adults, or offering a canonical framework for describing or incorporating the complex interplay of medical, psychological, and social services into treatment planning, perhaps attention to the basics is more important (Thielke, Vannoy, & Unützer, 2007). Something needs to change in the world of psychotherapy for older adults, especially with family-laden problems.

We have argued for the "Watch and Wait" model; that is, people are assessed and a careful monitoring is instituted where the patient is given hope, psychoeducation, support, and a belief that change will occur with careful preparation (Hyer, 2014). This is a clear case-based, person- and family-centered care that leads to the application of the evidence-based treatments. This is an improved method of a stepped care model. In this effort, the family is highlighted, teams are used, and the monitoring of core problems unfolded. In our system, five areas are targets. They are: depression, anxiety, cognition, health and lifestyle, and general living and adjustment. Each person has a profile representing each issue. Interventions from lectures to support to caregiver therapies and environmental interventions are espoused In effect, the psychotherapist becomes a psychosocial care manager.

In this model, the identified patient is the target, but the family is the core player. Watch and Wait holds that the context is critical, the "problem" is an epigenetic phenomenon of the system. Knowledge of the drilling-down process is important, but only as it is subserved by the family and context. While symptom-based modules are applied and important, a symptom oriented diagnosis is the foot in the door (the necessary CPT code) for the whole system process. Watch and Wait highlights the obvious: During the opening 2–4 weeks before the formal treatment plan is initiated, a profile is outlined for the patient, and the interventions are cooperative endeavors with family and context.

> **Setting the Stage for Treatment**
> "Your treatment is important and we will address all aspects of care. We need to assess your particular problem and rule out others. We will involve family members at times because they are always an influence. We need to see what else is involved with your unique problem. I have several things in mind; we will target your problems but will manage your case slowly using many treatments, perhaps medication, lifestyle changes, as well as some cognitive training. We will have more to say on all of these in the next weeks. We will monitor you carefully over the months also. Remember that your family/spouse will be part of this process. Overall, this therapy is likely to work but it may take longer and it may have to be added to or adjusted. We start with some assessment as we are doing now."

We then provide treatment factors for Watch and Wait. Table 10.1 provides the necessary features of the care process. The problem is validated and alliance is fostered. The value of the alliance in couples and family therapy has no less an effect size or efficacy than individual therapy (Friedlander, Escudero, Heatherington, & Diamond, 2011). Families at a group level want to feel safe, have a within sense of purpose and goals, and feel a sense of balance in the conversation and actions. There is no therapy without this alliance. Much time is spent on psychoeducation on the nature of the problem and necessary input. Empirical validation is emphasized. The assessment process runs in parallel and outlines the core profile and a hierarchy is established for the interventions.

An important part of the model involves the target areas. This involves the profile of the five core problems and the projected input of the family. The five components include depression, anxiety, cognition, medical/somatic status, and practical life issues. In the figure below, Person A has more depression and somatization; Person B has more anxiety and cognition problems; Person C has many problems, less for life adjustment issues; Person D has cognition and life issues; and Person E has somatic issues and life issues. Even though all are different in target issues, all components are relevant all the time.

Table 10.1 Necessary Watch and Wait categories

1. Validate problem, build alliance
2. Psychoeducation of model: Family commitment
3. Assessment: Core areas profiled
4. Monitoring
5. Modules
6. Follow-up/boosters

MODEL FOR THERAPIES FOR OLDER ADLTS

[Bar chart showing symptom levels (0-100) for Patient A through Patient E across five categories: Depress, Anxiety, Cognition, Som/Sleep, Adjustment]

While the degree of symptomatology varies between patients, it is critical that every component is included in each patient profile.

Watch and Wait is a true corrective emotional experience in the confines of the family. Therapy is most about the rough and tumble of life, setting a perspective and remaining engaged in a raucous world: Family members really committed for the hard work of living. With this model as backdrop we can apply family therapies or interventions. Now we discuss psychotherapy at later life and emphasize a model (IPT) that has been applied to family issues.

10.2.1.2 IPT as Model for Family Treatment

IPT is a type of therapy that applies many of these ideas, and has been applied to later life issues. It is family therapy for late life issues. The core features of IPT articulate the importance for families in therapy at later life. Interpersonally relevant problems increase risk for depression; depression damages interpersonal relationships, and interpersonal relationships play an important role in the clinical course of depression (Hinrichsen & Emery, 2005). IPT is typically delivered weekly for a duration of 16 weeks, in three phases of treatment: initial sessions, intermediate sessions, and termination (see Weissman, Markowitz, & Klerman, 2000). The overall focus of IPT is on one or two of four interpersonally relevant problem areas: grief (complicated bereavement), interpersonal role disputes (conflict with a significant other), role transitions (life change), and interpersonal deficits (problems in initiating and sustaining relationships). In the initial sessions (Weeks 1–3), the therapist diagnoses the problem (usually depression), educates the client about depression, reviews current and past significant relationships ("the interpersonal inventory"), determines the problem area(s) that will be the focus of treatment, and outlines therapy goals. In the intermediate sessions (Weeks 4–13), the therapist implements strategies associated with each of the four problem areas, as well as uses different therapeutic techniques, to achieve IPT problem-specific goals in tandem with reduction in depressive symptoms. In the termination phase (Weeks 14–16), the end of treatment is discussed, feelings the client has about ending are explored, treatment progress (or lack of progress) is reviewed, and the possible need for additional treatment is ascertained.

IPT has been shown to be effective with older adults (Miller, 2009). Distinguishing features include a focus on current interpersonally relevant problems; collaborative, supportive, and optimistic stance of the therapist; psychoeducation about depression; and a regular review of options that the client has to deal with life problems. IPT's therapeutic mantras are: "That's your depression speaking" (i.e., clients feel, think, and act differently when they are depressed but are not always cognizant of the pervasive effects of the disorder); "There are always options" (i.e., depression is disempowering and limits perspective on options to deal with life problems related to the depression); "you are not to blame" (as the patient is the victim of a disease); and "your family are part of our dialogue and solution."

Finally, the IPT format is akin to Watch and Wait (our model) as it is step based, provides considerable psychoeducation, prepares the patient, and allows for considerable family involvement. It considers the three forms of interpersonal problems at late life routinely (see Table 10.2). The most common problem area among older adults treated with IPT is role transitions (Hinrichsen & Clougherty, 2006; Reynolds et al., 1999). The modal late-life role transition is acquisition of responsibility for care of a spouse with physical health problems and/or dementia. Other late-life role transitions include onset of health problems (i.e., transition into the patient role), residential move (e.g., to new community, assisted living, long-term care), retirement or late-life job loss, and care for a grandchild (i.e., acquisition of parenting role). The other problem commonly encountered is interpersonal role disputes. Among older adults, disputes typically involve spouse/partner and adult children. Others involve siblings and friends. Usually, grief is a problem area. It can be seen then that the steps in the IPT apply to older adults in a family. Everything here also applies to the caregiver.

Table 10.2 IPT model for family therapy

Role transition
I miss what I used to do
Limited ability to accept reality now
Mourning loss of a cognitive/physical skill
Role dispute
I do not like being told I lose my temper
I cannot recall things and ask my spouse
I am losing my sense of independence
Grief
Mourning the loss of a death
Deficits now exposed after the death of a spouse who did everything
Depression that follows grief

10.3 Implications for Understanding Family Resilience

10.3.1 Caregiving and Dementia as Model for Later Life Family Issues

The best data about older adult families comes from work in caregiving and dementias (Mittelman, Epstein, & Piezchala, 2003). In fact, over the years the crescendo for caregiving has increased measurably. For many, this is the only therapy game in town. Unfortunately, when you have worked with one family of an older adult who is in decline, you have only worked with one family of an older adult. No sure-fire model exists that is empirically supported for families of older adults. Some families, for example, fear a dementia diagnosis; others welcome it. Families need something, support in the loose sense, to keep quality of life alive for all concerned. How this is done is the therapeutic issue. This "non-family" therapy that involves only the family is the therapy.

The National Alliance for Caregiving in collaboration with the American Association of Retired Persons surveyed 1480 family caregivers age 18 and over (Gaines, 2010). The report estimated some 65.7 million Americans served as caregivers to a family member in the past year. That figure represents 28% of the US population; nearly 1/3 of the American households reported at least one person serving in an unpaid caregiving role. More than 1/3 report taking care of two or more people. Just under 90% are taking care of a relative. The typical person providing help is a female, 61 years old, providing 20.4 h/week. Caregivers report medium or high burden at a 51% level. On average, caregivers have been at the task for 4.6 years and 33% have been involved for more than 5 years. Just being a caregiver puts the person at risk for depression and anxiety; with more care comes more problems (Hyer, 2014).

This older family drama most often plays out in health (often neurodegenerative) issues, principally dementia. Over the years it has been observed that later life families and their challenge with degenerative diseases have certain commonalities. Family solidarity is maintained between generations (Bengtson & Treas, 1980). Families also tend to keep their identified patient (IP) as long as possible (Brody, Poulshock, & Masciocchi, 1978), but there is a cost (Niederehe & Frugé, 1984). It is also common for one single person to take on this role of caregiver, usually a female spouse or daughter (Johnson, 1983). Some sharing of course does occur. In fact, filial responsibility is normative (Seelbach, 1977). Regardless of a patient's core event, the specific stressors are mediated by the social context, the family (Hinrichsen & Niederehe, 1994).

10.3.2 Caregiver Family Treatment Overview

Caregiving is about the family. It is the model for later life family therapy (Schulz & Beach, 1999). There are three categories of Empirically Based Treatments (EBT) for families who are caregivers. They include psychoeducational programs (behavioral management, depression management, anger management, progressively lower stress); psychotherapy, involving CBT especially; and multicomponent programs using a combination of two or more approaches (counseling, support group attendance) (Gaughler, 2010). Data from the Resources for Enhancing Alzheimer's Health (REACH: Harrow et al., 2004) caregiver project has shown that the caregiver spouse and family can receive valuable help from the patient in any of these areas. When the patient is responding well, the system thrives. Similarly, when caregivers are distressed, the patient almost invariably does poorly, so adjunctive care for the caregiver is beneficial to both. Unfortunately, interventions with families are helpful but meta-analyses show that the effects are small and domain-specific rather than global.

For some time now treatment of the caregiving family has expanded. It is present in the home with telephone support (Smith & Toseland, 2006) and Adult Day Services (ADS-Plus, Gitlin, Reever, Dennis, Mathieu, & Hauck, 2006), among others. The primary target is behavioral problems of the care recipient, and the physical, mental, and social health of the system targeting the caregiver. Family caregivers initially meet face-to-face with the service director in order to: (1) identify areas of concerns and needs; (2) develop a care plan to minimize identified areas of difficulty; and (3) implement an agreed upon care plan that involves four components (counseling, education, referral, and periodic supportive contact with the site family service director).

Other family therapy interventions may address self-care, knowledge (resources, normal aging), role adjustment (meaning, impact, transitions), competence (manage behaviors, feelings), depression (pleasant activities, feelings), distress tolerance, burnout for caregiver, loss of self (boundaries, roles), family communication, as well as social support (roles, skill building) (see Foster, Layton, Qualls, & Klebe, 2009). Teri et al. (1997) optimized validation and pleasant events; Mittelman et al. (2003) treated couples to good effect.

10.3.3 Resilience

We have stressed that family therapy at later life is deficit focused. At later life, decline and debility are the issues. Family care ideas then require a basic "psychophilosophy" of data-based ideas for the family. Positivity can be applied. The family needs to know the scope and depth, as well as the normative features, of their plight. The family is not the problem. The family will have conflict and will make mistakes; few incentives will make an unwilling family motivated, and a family is rarely one voice. The divisions in the family are normative. Additionally, most families delay care until well into a dementia.

Psychological resilience training occurs all the time in dementia care. It is defined as an individual's ability to properly adapt to stress and adversity. Stress and adversity can mean anything from family or relationship problems, health problems, or workplace and financial stressors. Families or individuals demonstrate resilience when they can face difficult experiences and rise above them with ease. Resilience is not a rare ability; in reality, it is found in the average individual and it can be learned and developed by virtually anyone. Resilience should be considered a process, rather than a trait to be had. The primary factor in resilience is having positive relationships inside or outside one's family. It is the single most critical means of handling both ordinary and extraordinary levels of stress (see Henry, Morris, & Harrist, 2015). Changes in one family member (e.g., a dementia), a subsystem (e.g., moving in with adult children), or the overall system (e.g., home destroyed by a tornado) reverberate across the family system. Resilient families show family cohesion, family adaptability, family coherence, family hardiness, and valuing of family time and routines. Small changes result in big concerns.

There is no family therapy at later life that highlights resilience. All, however, apply resilience in the training of the caregiver for problems. The American Psychological Association suggests "10 Ways to Build Resilience," including advice to "(1) maintain good relationships with close family members, friends and others, (2) avoid seeing crises or stressful events as unbearable problems, (3) accept circumstances that cannot be changed, (4) develop realistic goal and move towards them, (5) take decisive actions in adverse situations, (6) look for opportunities of self-discovery after a struggle with loss, (7) develop self-confidence, (8) keep a long-term perspective and consider the stressful event in a broader context, (9) maintain a hopeful outlook, expecting good things and visualizing what is wished, (10) take care of one's mind and body, exercising regularly, paying attention to one's own" (http://en.wikipedia.org/wiki/Psychological_resilience). These APA resilience components emphasize positive coping in the context of family/caregiver interventions for a dementia. Henry, Morris, and Harrist (2015) provide examples of such qualities in a family setting include a positive outlook, spirituality, family member accord, flexibility, communication, financial management, time together, mutual recreational interests, routines and rituals, and social support. Also included are building new strengths, such as family belief systems (making meaning of adversity, positive outlook, transcendence and spirituality), family organizational patterns (flexibility, connectedness, social and economic resources), and family communication patterns (clarity, open emotional sharing, collaborative problem solving). Family emotion-related processes are also evident (see Henry et al., 2015).

Table 10.3 lists common messages of resilience for families (Gwyther, 2000). Goals of families with older adults with a degree of impairment involve the normalization of variability, attention to safety, the mobilization of family support, the facilitation of decision making, and the necessity for families to accept help. It is best to tailor information to the family's tolerance and capacity to accept and understand as well as current need to know.

We embellish on these ideas in Table 10.4, and assert that resilience can take other forms (Fishman et al., 2012). Again, it is important to note that the interventions which work best are multimodal and bring all sources on-board. Typical treatment includes a focus on the target issue, like agitation with medications, but also support groups and skills training for caregivers, structured exercise for both, and family therapy for all. Best care involves a team: psychiatry, social work, nurses,

Table 10.3 Common messages for families including older impaired member

- You will have good and bad days
- You are not to blame. You did not create this
- Tell people whom you trust about your situation. Do not try to hide
- Regular medical care, good nutrition, exercise, structure help
- Your relative has a brain disorder. We will help you
- Be willing to listen to the IP
- You have limited choices
- You can only do what seems best at the moment. No second regrets
- Solving problems is easier than living with solutions
- Comparisons are fallible and pointless
- Your IP is not unhappy for what you did. Frustration is directed to you

Table 10.4 Resilience components for successful treatment

1. Overall caregiver tasks
    (a) Acknowledge the disease
    (b) Make a cognitive shift
    (c) Develop emotional tolerance
    (d) Take control
    (e) Establish a realistic goal
    (f) Gauge the recipient's capacities
    (g) Design opportunities for satisfying work
    (h) Become a sleuth
2. Patient skills
    (a) Self-efficacy
        - I believe that I have good skills when it comes to my care situation
    (b) Relational coping with caregivers
        - I often tell my caregiver that I appreciate her/him
    (c) Perceptions of dependence
        - People tend to think I cannot do things that I can do
    (d) Performance related quality of life
        - I can still do a number of things that I enjoyed all my life
    (e) Accepting help
        - I just accept the fact that that I need help
3. Relationship
    (a) Current relationship
        - He/she shows me that he/she loves me
        - We like each other
        - Our lives are better because of our relationship
        - He/she is important to me
        - We care about each other's well-being
        - I feel sure about our relationship

(continued)

Table 10.4 (continued)

	(b) Past relationship
	• We have accepted each other's gentle criticism
	• He/She has made some real sacrifices for me in past
4.	Compassion fatigue. *Do you ever feel...*
	(a) That you care for others more than yourself?
	(b) Compelled to "make it all better, fix it or solve problems?
	(c) You must watch/do for your CR all day/everyday?
	(d) Like a failure when you can't?
	(e) You have cared for others more than yourself?
	(f) You exaggerate your sense of responsibility to others?
5.	Cope with willingness
	(a) Will you feel what you feel when you feel it?
	(b) Are you willing to think the thoughts you are already thinking?
	(c) Are you willing to engage in the experience in which you are already in?
	(d) Remember that willingness is not about a belief of whether or not you are able to do something but rather are you willing in the moment
	(e) Do not use "if" statements or self-deception.
	(f) Never ask someone "if" they would enter an anxiety-provoking situation
6.	Basic strategies for caregivers
	(a) Keep it simple
	(b) Search for strategies that enhance self esteem in identified patient
	(c) Praise ID for attempts
	(d) De-emphasize the negative
	(e) Offer choices and de-emphasize micromanaging
	(f) Structure time for caregiver to change
	(g) Give the patient the "sick role."
	(h) Integrate information from all sources
7.	Keep upbeat
	(a) What is best is always a compromise among competing needs, loyalties and commitments
	(b) Find ways to have the IP help you
	(c) Celebrate victories
	(d) Keep to your cherished activities
	(e) Develop affirmations for self: "I am doing the best I can and it is working mostly."
8.	Practical problems
	(a) Shifting of power and renegotiation of roles
	(b) Financial and legal concerns
	(c) Palliative care
	(d) The question of institutionalization
	(e) Amount of time spent caring for the patient
	(f) Loss of own and CR identity
	(g) Patient misidentifications and clinical fluctuations
	(h) Nocturnal deterioration of patient

and psychologists. The individual and the conjoint/disjoint nature of the treatment is pliable and based on the needs of the family. Treatment starts with overall caregiving tasks, what needs to be done, and what can be done. It builds on the core relationship that the identified patient has, and begs the question, "Is this relationship a good one?" It extends to aspects of exemplary care: Is the relationship one of love and respect worthy of special consideration? (Dooley & Hinojosa, 2004). Exemplary behavior mediates the relations between subjective appraisals (daily bother, burden, and behavioral bother) and emotional outcomes (depression and positive aspects of caregiving). Willingness is also a feature as the caregiver can accept and be willing to undergo difficult tasks. Finally, practical issues and basic strategies for caregivers are never far from the mix.

10.4 Important Variables

We discuss three of variables that play a key role in all family problems. Their presence is more than just relevant: They influence and alter interventions.

10.4.1 Cultural Issues

The importance of the impact of culture is critical at later life. Culture contributes to how adults make meaning in their lives as they age, how they adjust to changing demands, and beliefs on aging. How families interact and manage caregiving roles also functions within cultural bounds (Waid & Frazier, 2003). Simply put, culture matters.

Cultural differences may also exist in the amount and type of support the family provides. In Western culture, many elderly do not live with a family member (specifically children), but the family may live close by. Comparing the elderly living in Shanghai and Canada, those in Shanghai were more likely to live with someone outside the family than in Canada. They were also more likely to have a paid caregiver. It may be that modern collectivistic cultures such as this reward living situations stemming from financial or cultural motives. Regardless, researchers find that, independent of culture, those with more social support had increased life satisfaction (Chappell, 2003). Those families in a Western culture may have more caregiving burden even if they don't live with the older family member. In the Eastern culture, the children were the ones typically paying for the caregiving by a non-family member, but the spouse was typically the one who lived in the home taking on the caregiving burden.

So let's take another look at Joe and his family presented at the beginning. This time, Joe is Asian American and coming in with his eldest son and wife. For this family, an intervention may be formulated around how the son wants treatment. The therapist will acknowledge his role in the family dynamic based on their possible cultural expectations. There is also a tacit understanding that clinical decisions are influenced by the best interests of the family which are a function of the culture of the patient, in this case the filial responsibility of the son.

Another study (Dilworth-Anderson, Williams, & Gibson, 2002) examined research over the last 20 years to see how race, ethnicity, and culture played a role in caregiving. Minority families tended to have more extended help, but they also reported needing more formalized support. Culture also played a role in the gender of the caregiving family member as well as the support provided to that caregiver. The perception of social support was also important for positive outcomes across cultures. As the level of need increased with elderly family member, the level of informal social support increased across cultures. When considering formal support systems, minority families may be utilizing them less, and yet experiencing more disatisfaction with them.

For families, culture may be associated with differing levels of caregiver stress, burden, and coping. Although research is conflicting, most studies have found that for White Americans, burden and depression were higher than for African American families. White families and Hispanic families shared similar levels of depression, while Hispanic families and African American families shared similar levels of burden. Coping strategies differed then between culturally different populations (American Indian, White, African American), but interestingly also between culturally similar populations in rural versus urban settings (Dilworth-Anderson, Williams, & Gibson, 2002). This implies that cultural aspects are an important consideration, but the extent to which acculturation is influential needs clarification.

When working with older adults, it is important to acknowledge the family culture, the family perceptions of the older family member and aging in general. These perceptions will influence the amount and quality of care given. It may also influence whether the family provides care at home or in an institution, as well as who in the family will take on that responsibility.

10.4.2 End of Life

We start with the grief before the grief. Anticipatory grief is often a necessary prelude to decline in the degenerative process. This is the experience of the pangs of anticipatory loss before the fact (of a death). Sadness starts early in the caregiving process. Data on 948 older people who were classified as demented, frail, or healthy revealed that treatments that slowed the progression of dementia did not necessarily relieve caregiver strain as 2/3 of caregivers reported grief before death resulting from ambiguity about the relationship, loss of previously established roles, loss of intimacy, and loss of control (Holley et al., 2006). Meuser, Marwit, and Sanders (2004) noted that anticipatory grief explained an additional 12–21% of the variance of burden beyond background characteristics, primary stressors, and depressive symptoms.

Families, not patients, are the ones having the difficult conversations with physicians about end-of life decisions (Haley et al., 2002). Even though death is inevitable, and in many cases expected, many families and practitioners still avoid discussion about this topic (Benokraitis, 2011). Research has suggested that the family's end-of-life wishes for the patient may conflict with the patient's wishes (Haley et al., 2002). It is important to provide encouragement and resources for the families to act proactively, as well as assist with the pain of the loss itself. In the authors' medical setting, protective services is asked to be present at hospice more than any other hospital setting. Loss brings on intense emotions. As noted above, culture also plays a role in the types of decisions that families make with end-of-life care decisions. For example, African American and Hispanic families may tend to use more life-sustaining means and be skeptical of how physicians view advance directives (Haley et al., 2002). Cultural meanings do play a large role in how families deal with death itself. Pre-death interventions meant to provide relief for caregiving can also help post-death (Bass & Bowman, 1990).

After death, families or spouses with anticipatory grief have additional problems regarding the after-death grief process itself. Issues of ambivalence, excessive attachment, separation fears, and practical life adjustment can influence the grief process. One way to acknowledge a death is by incorporating personal or spiritual values into rituals. Rituals can be a cherished means for comfort and connection to the deceased family member. These can be religious customs, conventional practices, or the family can be encouraged to create their own ritual in a way that is meaningful for that family (McDaniel, Doherty, & Hepworth, 2014).

Handling the pain of death has many models. Family members are always involved. Many may even find relief after the death of a loved one who has suffered a chronic illness like dementia (Benokraitis, 2011). Studies have found that families faced with increased stress during caregiving showed improved health after the loved one's death. On the other hand, arguments have been made that families with increased caregiving strain face increased difficulty with the death of the loved one. To this end, it is important to consider the family's reactions in whole both pre-death and post-death.

10.4.3 Elder Abuse

While not related to grief specifically, elder abuse is a hidden public health problem and is more likely to occur in extended caregiving. Often the distinction is made between abuse and neglect, the latter occurring more passively. Both result in increased mortality rates, injury pain, and decreased quality of life. It is under-recognized, underreported, and under-prosecuted. Roughly 5% of older adults appear to be victims (Bomba, 2006). Financial exploitation is the most common reason; however, physical abuse, psychological abuse, domestic violence, and sexual abuse also occur. Unfortunately, perpetrators are most often family members. Abuse is also more likely to occur when assets are in play, the patient is alone and confused, and psychiatric issues are involved. Nonetheless, elder abuse also occurs rather simply, as the result of a poor understanding of the needs of caregiving. Minimal safety needs, too, may not be understood. Families who feel powerless due to the complexity of psychiatric issues with the identified patient are at some risk of abuse.

Evaluation of elder abuse is difficult and beset with failure pockets; the ethical challenge is to balance safety with self-determination (Bomba, 2006). While there are abuse markers related to patients (e.g., lives alone, bruises, patient has resources, etc.), others are more systemic and relate to the patient's caregiving network. In any case, an evaluation of potential abuse is always necessary, difficult, and best made with a team. At times, the identified patient is perceived as a willing "co-conspirator" in this abuse process as they can willingly "rot with their rights on," causing confusion. Physicians often feel discomforted, impotent, or constrained legally. Regardless, the family is front and center, psychologically and legally.

Virtually any family stress can trigger elder abuse. A multitude of factors, including mental illness, alcohol abuse, job loss, financial losses, and the like, will eventually addle families. The therapist can make a difference with careful listening, strategic validation, reduced moralizing, and practical common clinical sense. Families will take notice as a result of a knowing and caring therapist. It was Frank Pittman, the noted family therapist, who insisted that therapy is an expression of the therapist's character, about the problem solving of right and wrong. This is needed here. As with most problems at later life, the Watch and Wait model is most helpful

Box 10.1. Focus on Practice, Gerontology
As a practicing gerontologist, I concur that greater attention must be given to the mental health needs of older adults. In particular, the need to implement effective evidence-based clinical and therapeutic treatment options for aging families is long overdue. Continued population growth among the older adult population, age 65 and older, has given rise to a complex maze of health-related systems that families must navigate. Many family members caring for older loved ones can struggle to comprehend and understand the origin, progression, and short- and long-term changes that occur with age-associated psychopathologies (e.g., depression, anxiety, dementia). It is not uncommon for age-associated changes in mental health to co-occur with other on-going physical and functional health declines. Family caregivers may further feel they lack the necessary social or financial support resources to seek professional advice and consultation, navigate the aging service network, or acquire appropriate clinical intervention for their aging family member. As a result, this often translates into feelings of mental depletion and stress among family caregivers. Step-based family psychotherapy interventions, such as the

(continued)

> "Watch and Wait" model, represent evidenced-based alternatives within family psychotherapy that have promising implications for clinical gerontological practice. Such treatment models therapeutically integrate education, support, and guidance applicable to the older care recipient as well as family care providers. In effect, this gives clinical gerontologists a new treatment tool by which to build and strengthen family resilience and improve individual quality-of-life.
>
> —Alex J. Bishop, Ph.D., Oklahoma State University

as it optimizes the possibility for a better deliberative therapy response and a fairer hearing and fuller understanding of the problems.

10.5 Conclusion and Future Directions

We have emphasized that treatment at later life is best done in the context of the family. The time is later life, the place most often is primary care, and the patient is the family. At late life, more than any other time, the family is front and center. Psychotherapy or psychosocial interventions work, but not as medicine; at late life medicine needs, however, to work as psychotherapy. Very importantly, the overall model for us is the friendly Watch and Wait structure. Given this, the therapy strategies of IPT or resilience can be applied.

In reality, situations resolve or not through the puzzling vagaries of the sloppy-known main effects of psychotherapy; more likely at late life, change occurs through spontaneous recovery, self-generated change, placebo effects, activation of resilience, post-traumatic growth, corrective effects of disclosure and feedback, or accepting family input. Other reality constraints are also aplenty: The client/family's readiness to change; acceptability of the treatment and preferences of the client; caregiver acceptance; availability of desired or needed services; probability of 3rd party payer approval; tolerance of incongruous recommendations; prior treatment failures or successes; and side effects. These all play out in the family.

With older adults, the core targets of therapy (depression, anxiety, cognition, somatic/health issues, and life adjustment/function) emerge against these factors as background. Again, the family is the player in the room. We have tried to walk a tightrope between empirically supported suggestions and the real world of later life psychotherapy. At a simple level there is the essential tension between the practical concerns of living, now with more demands, and the psychotherapy rubrics of empirically supported treatments. Does the clinician behaviorally activate, socially or structurally intervene, or finesse the situation? At late life, then, the melding of a commitment to practical person-centered care and the use of evidence-based practice is always at issue.

The ultimate demonstration of evidence is the fit between the individual at a particular point in time as judged by the participation and response of that person. To date, there are really little data articulating the exact sequential road map of using evidence based practice for older adults, especially those in decline. There are also many features at late life where the realities of practice trump science, such as SES, medical comorbidities, and patient attitudes. Often clinical experience and science butt heads with later life issues. In this place and with these older adult issues, psychotherapy is as much art as science.

Family therapy at late life thrives with a Watch and Wait scaffold. Marital, family, and intergenerational support is never simple, especially when a decline process is in effect, but at least there are more people in the room. The presence of the family, the use of system interventions, and the logistical management of struggle in a degenerative target are monumental. Emotional and instrumental support bubble up in complex ways at later life. It has been found that receiving emotional support is more empowering and associated with the well-being of older adults than receiving instrumental support, presumably because emotional support is more associated with empathy, affection, and emotional commitment within the relationship than with an increased dependency on the caregiver's side (Merz, Schuengel, & Schulze, 2009). As one example then, just decreasing relationship quality is a greater threat to the well-being of caregiving children than increased support and care tasks; meaningful and long-lasting relations between family members in all phases of the life span cannot be taken for granted.

Apply this, writ large. The presence of the family is necessary and can be for the better or worse. It is a necessary deliberation that can turn practical or psychodynamic, both necessary for change. And we believe it is also the only meaningful game in town.

Discussion Questions

1. What are the two most prevalent psychiatric difficulties that older adults struggle with? How do they affect quality of life? What other areas of life are affected by these psychiatric problems?
2. How does aging impact families? How do social support systems change? How can individuals improve social support systems?
3. How does family structure change once a parent is no longer able to take care of him/herself? How does this strain the family unit?
4. What does the typical family consist of? How does this change through the life cycle? What transitions must adult children make to accommodate for their dependent parents?
5. How does chronic illness impact the family? How does chronic illness impact quality of life? How does this impact the role of a caregiver?

6. In what ways is culture an important component in elder care? How does it play a role in end of life decisions?
7. What problem should clinicians screen for in elderly who are dependent on caregivers? What types of stressors make families more susceptible to this problem?
8. What types of therapeutic interventions may be useful later in life?
9. Describe the Watch and Wait Model. Why is it effective?
10. What is resilience? Why is it important in treatment? What are some ways to build resilience?

References

Amato, P. R., & Cheadle, J. (2005). The long reach of divorce: Divorce and child well-being across three generations. *Journal of Marriage and Family, 67*, 191–206. doi:10.1111/j.0022-2445.2005.00014.x

Bass, D. M., & Bowman, K. (1990). The transition from caregiving to bereavement: The relationship of care-related strain and adjustment to death. *The Gerontological Society of America, 30*, 35–42. doi:10.1093/geront/30.1.35

Bengtson, V. L., & Treas, J. (1980). The changing family context of mental health and aging. In J. E. Birren & R. B. Sloan (Eds.), *Handbook of mental health and aging* (pp. 400–428). Englewood Cliffs, NJ: Prentice Hall.

Benokraitis, N. V. (2011). *Marriages and families: Changes, choices, and constraints* (7th ed.). Boston, MA: Prentice Hall.

Binstock, R. H., George, L. K., Cutler, S. J., Hendricks, J., & Schulz, J. H. (Eds.). (2006). *Handbook of aging and the social sciences* (6th ed.). Boston, MA: Academic.

Bodenheimer, T., Chen, E., & Bennett, H. D. (2009). Confronting the growing burden of chronic disease: Can the U.S. Health Care workforce do the job? *Health Affairs, 28*, 64–74. doi:10.1377/hlthaff.28.1.64

Bomba, P. A. (2006). Elder abuse: "It Shouldn't Hurt To Be Old.". In T. C. Rosenthal, M. E. Williams, & B. J. Naughton (Eds.), *Office care geriatrics*. Philadelphia: Lippincott, Williams & Wilkins.

Bosworth, H. B., & Schaie, K. W. (1997). The relationship of social environment, social networks, and health outcomes in the Seattle Longitudinal Study: Two analytical approaches. *The Journals of Gerontology. Series B, Psychological Sciences and Social Sciences, 52*, 197–205.

Brody, S. J., Poulschock, S. W., & Masciocchi, C. F. (1978). The family caring unit: A major consideration in the long-term support system. *The Gerontologist, 21*, 471–480.

Brown, S. L., Bulanda, J. R., & Lee, G. R. (2005). The significance of nonmarital cohabitation: Marital status and mental health benefits among middle-aged and older adults. *The Journals of Gerontology. Series B, Psychological Sciences and Social Sciences, 60*, S21–29.

Carstensen, L. L., Isaacowitz, D. M., & Charles, S. T. (1999). Taking time seriously: A theory of socioemotional selectivity. *American Psychologist, 54*, 165–181. doi:10.1037/0003-066X.54.3.165

Chappell, N. L. (2003). Correcting cross-cultural stereotypes: Aging in Shanghai and Canada. *Journal of Cross-Cultural Gerontology, 18*, 127–147. Retrieved from http://dx.doi.org.medlibproxy.mercer.edu/10.1023/A:1025156501588

Christakis, N. A., & Allison, P. D. (2006). Mortality after the hospitalization of a spouse. *The New England Journal of Medicine, 354*, 719–730. doi:10.1056/NEJMsa050196

Dilworth-Anderson, P., Williams, P., & Gibson, B. (2002). Issues of race, ethnicity, and culture in caregiving research: A 20-year review (1980–2000). *The Gerontologist, 42*, 237–272. Retrieved from http://gerontologist.oxfordjournals.org/

Dooley, N. R., & Hinojosa, J. (2004). Improving quality of life for persons with Alzheimer's disease and their family caregivers: Brief occupational therapy intervention. *American Journal of Occupational Therapy, 58*, 561–569.

Eng, P. M., Rimm, E. B., Fitzmaurice, G., & Kawachi, I. (2002). Social ties and change in social ties in relation to subsequent total and cause-specific mortality and coronary heart disease incidence in men. *American Journal of Epidemiology, 155*, 700–709.

Fishman, P. A., Johnson, E. A., Coleman, K., Larson, E. B., Hsu, C., Ross, T. R., et al. (2012). Impact on seniors of the patient-centered medical home: Evidence from a pilot study. *The Gerontologist, 52*, 703–711. doi:10.1093/geront/gnr158

Foster, S. M., Layton, H. S., Qualls, S. H., & Klebe, K. J. (2009). Tailored caregiver therapy: Consumer response to intervention. *Clinical Gerontologist, 32*(2), 177–197. doi:10.1030/07317110802677237

Freedman, V. A., Kasper, J. D., Spillman, B. C., Agree, E. M., Mor, V., Wallace, R. B., et al. (2014). Behavioral adaptation and late-life disability: A new spectrum for assessing public health impacts. *American Journal of Public Health, 104*(2), e88–94. doi:10.2105/AJPH.2013.301687

Federal Interagency Forum on Aging-Related Statistics. (2010). *Older Americans 2010: Key indicators of well-being*. Washington, DC: GPO.

Friedlander, M. L., Escudero, V., Heatherington, L., & Diamond, G. M. (2011). Alliance in couple and family therapy. *Psychotherapy, 48*, 25–33. doi:10.1037/a0022060

Gaines, S. (2010). Caregivers: Growing population with growing needs. *Memory: The Magazine of Hope.* Summer, 2010.

Gallagher-Thompson, D., & Thompson, L. W. (1995). Psychotherapy with older adults in theory and practice. In B. M. Bongar & L. E. Beutler (Eds.), *Comprehensive textbook of psychotherapy: Theory and practice* (pp. 359–379). New York, NY: Oxford University Press.

Gaughler, J. (2010). *Doing the best we can: An overview of online and clinical resources for care providers of families struggling with dementia.* Presentation on line from University of Minnesota, Minneapolis MN.

Gitlin, L. N., Reever, K., Dennis, M. P., Mathieu, E., & Hauck, W. W. (2006). Enhancing quality of life of families who use adult day services: Short- and long-term effects of the Adult Day Services Plus Program. *The Gerontologist, 46*(5), 630–639. doi:10.1093/geront/46.5.630

Greenberg, S. (2012). *A profile of older Americans: 2012.* Washington, DC: U.S. Department of Health and Human Development, Administration on Aging.

Gruenewald, T. L., Karlamangla, A. S., Greendale, G. A., Singer, B. H., & Seeman, T. E. (2007). Feelings of usefulness to others, disability, and mortality in older adults: The MacArthur Study of Successful Aging. *The Journals of Gerontology. Series B, Psychological Sciences and Social Sciences, 62*(1), 28–37.

Gwyther, L. P. (2000). Family issues in dementia: Finding a new normal. *Neurologic Clinics, 18*, 993–1010.

Ha, J.-H., Carr, D., Utz, R., & Nesse, R. (2006). Older adults' perceptions of intergenerational support after widowhood: How do men and women differ? *Journal of Family Issues, 27*(1), 3–30. doi:10.1177/0192513X05277810

Haber, D. (2013). *Health promotion and aging: Practical applications for health professionals* (6th ed.). New York, NY: Springer.

Haley, W. E., Allen, R. S., Reynolds, S., Chen, H., Burton, A., & Gallagher-Thompson, D. (2002). Family issues in end-of-life decision making and end-of-life care. *American Behavioral Scientist, 46*, 284–298. doi:10.1177/000276402236680

Harrow, B. S., Mahoney, D. F., Mendelsohn, A. B., Ory, M. G., Coon, D. W., Belle, S. H., et al. (2004). Variation in cost of informal caregiving and formal-service use for people with Alzheimer's disease. *American Journal of Alzheimer's Disease and Other Dementias, 19*, 299–308. doi:10.1177/153331750401900507

Hartman-Stein, P., & LaRue, A. (2011). *Enhancing cognitive fitness in adults: A guide to the use and development of community-based programs.* New York: Springer Science & Business Media.

Hawkley, L. C., & Cacioppo, J. T. (2007). Aging and loneliness: Downhill quickly? *Current Directions in Psychological Science, 16*, 187–191. doi:10.1111/j.1467-8721.2007.00501.x

Henry, C. S., Sheffield Morris, A., & Harrist, A. W. (2015). Family resilience: Moving into the third wave. *Family Relations, 64*(1), 22–43.

Hinrichsen, G. A., & Clougherty, K. F. (2006). *Interpersonal psychotherapy for depressed older adults (Vol. xvii)*. Washington, DC: American Psychological Association.

Hinrichsen, G. A., & Emery, E. E. (2005). Interpersonal factors and late-life depression. *Clinical Psychology: Science and Practice, 12*, 264–275. doi:10.1093/clipsy.bpi027

Hinrichsen, G. A., & Niederehe, G. (1994). Dementia management strategies and adjustment of family members of older patients. *The Gerontologist, 34*, 95–102. doi:10.1093/geront/34.1.95

Holley, C., Murrell, S. A., & Mast, B. T. (2006). Psychosocial and vascular risk factors for depression in the elderly. *The American Journal of Geriatric Psychiatry, 14*, 84–90. doi:10.1097/01.JGP.0000192504.48810.cb

Hyer, L. (2014). *Psychological treatment of older adults: A holistic model*. New York, NY: Springer.

Jeste, D. V., & Palmer, B. W. (2013). A call for a new positive psychiatry of ageing. *The British Journal of Psychiatry, 202*(2), 81–83. doi:10.1192/bjp.bp.112.110643

Johnson, C. L. (1983). Dyadic family relations and social support. *The Gerontologist, 23*, 377–383. doi:10.1093/geront/23.4.377

Kessler, R. C., Chiu, W. T., Demler, O., & Walters, E. E. (2005). Prevalence, severity, and comorbidity of 12-month DSM-IV disorders in the National Comorbidity Survey Replication. *Archives of General Psychiatry, 62*, 617. doi:10.1001/archpsyc.62.6.617

Lofquist, D. A. (2012). Multigenerational households: 2009-2011: American Community Survey Briefs. U.S. Census Bureau. *U.S. Department of Commerce: Economics and Statistics Administration*. http://www.census.gov/prod/2012pubs/acsbr11-03.pdf

Lunney, J. R., Lynn, J., & Hogan, C. (2002). Profiles of older Medicare decedents. *Journal of American Geriatric Society, 50*, 1108–1112. doi:10.1046/j.1532-5415.2002.50268.x

Lynn, J., & Adamson, D. M. (2003). *Living well at the end of life. Adapting health care to serious chronic illness in old age*. Santa Monica, CA: Rand.

Lynn, J., Blanchard, J., Campbell, D., Jayes, R. L., & Lunney, J. (2001). *The last three years of life through Medicare claims*. Society for General Internal Medicine abstract, June 2001.

Mancini, A. D., & Bonanno, G. A. (2006). Marital closeness, functional disability, and adjustment in late life. *Psychology and Aging, 21*, 600–610. doi:10.1037/0882-7974.21.3.600

Martire, L. M., Lustig, A. P., Schulz, R., Miller, G. E., & Helgeson, V. S. (2004). Is it beneficial to involve a family member? A meta-analysis of psychosocial interventions for chronic illness. *Health Psychology, 23*, 599–611. doi:10.1037/0278-6133.23.6.599

McDaniel, S. H., Doherty, W. J., & Hepworth, J. (2014). *Medical family therapy and integrated care* (2nd ed.). Washington, DC: American Psychological Association.

Merz, E.-M., Schuengel, C., & Schulze, H.-J. (2009). Intergenerational relations across 4 years: Well-being is affected by quality, not by support exchange. *The Gerontologist*, gnp043. doi:10.1093/geront/gnp043

Meuser, T. M., Marwit, S. J., Sanders, S., et al. (2004). Assessing grief in family caregivers. *Living with Grief: Alzheimer's Disease*, 170–195.

Miller, M. (2009). *Clinician's guide to interpersonal psychotherapy in late life: Helping cognitively impaired or depressed elders and their caregivers*. New York, NY: Oxford Press.

Mittelman, M. S., Epstein, C., & Pierzchala, A. (2003). *Counseling the Alzheimer's caregiver: A resource for health care professionals*. Chicago: American Medical Association.

Monserud, M. A. (2008). Intergenerational relationships and affectual solidarity between grandparents and young adults. *Journal of Marriage and Family, 70*, 182–195. doi:10.1111/j.1741-3737.2007.00470.x

Mostofsky, E., Maclure, M., Sherwood, J. B., Tofler, G. H., Muller, J. E., & Mittleman, M. A. (2012). Risk of acute myocardial infarction after the death of a significant person in one's life:

The determinants of myocardial infarction onset study. *Circulation, 125*, 491–496. doi:10.1161/CIRCULATIONAHA.111.061770

Newman, B. M. (2014). *Development through life: A psychosocial approach* (12th ed.). Stamford, CT: Cengage Learning.

Niederehe, G., & Frugé, E. (1984). Dementia and family dynamics: Clinical research issues. *Journal of Geriatric Psychiatry, 17*, 21–56.

Obisesan, T. O., & Gillum, R. F. (2009). Cognitive function, social integration and mortality in a U.S. national cohort study of older adults. *BMC Geriatrics, 9*, 33. doi:10.1186/1471-2318-9-33

Orathinkal, J., & Vansteenwegen, A. (2007). Do demographics affect marital satisfaction? *Journal of Sex and Marital Therapy, 33*, 73–85. doi:10.1080/00926230600998573

Paez, K. A., Zhao, L., & Hwang, W. (2009). Rising out-of-pocket spending for chronic conditions: A ten-year trend. *Health Affairs, 28*, 15–25. doi:10.1377/hlthaff.28.1.15

Papalia, D. E. (2012). *Experience human development* (12th ed.). New York, NY: McGraw-Hill.

Peck, B. M., Hurwicz, M. L., Ory, M., Yuma, P., & Cook, M. A. (2010). Race, gender, and lifestyle discussions in geriatric primary care medical visits. *Health, 2*, 1150–1155.

Porensky, E. K., Dew, M. A., Karp, J. F., Skidmore, E., Rollman, B. L., Shear, M. K., et al. (2009). The burden of late-life generalized anxiety disorder: Effects on disability, health-related quality of life, and healthcare utilization. *The American Journal of Geriatric Psychiatry, 17*, 473–482. doi:10.1097/JGP.0b013e31819b87b2

Reynolds, C. F., Frank, E., Perel, J. M., Imber, S. D., Cornes, C., Miller, M. D., et al. (1999). Nortriptyline and interpersonal psychotherapy as maintenance therapies for recurrent major depression: A randomized controlled trial in patients older than 59 years. *Journal of the American Medical Associate, 281*, 39–45. doi:10.1001/jama.281.1.39

Rolland, J. (1984). Toward a psychosocial typology of chronic and life-threatening illness. *Family Systems Medicine, 2*, 245–262.

Royall, D. R., Chiodo, L. K., Mouton, C., & Polk, M. J. (2007). Cognitive predictors of mortality in elderly retirees: Results from the Freedom House Study. *The American Journal of Geriatric Psychiatry, 15*, 243–251. doi:10.1097/01.JGP.0000240824.84867.02

Rowe, J. W., & Kahn, R. L. (1997). Successful aging. *The Gerontologist, 37*, 433–440. doi:10.1093/geront/37.4.433

Schulz, R., & Beach, S. R. (1999). Caregiving as a risk factor for mortality: The caregiver health effects study. *JAMA, 282*(23), 2215–2219.

Scogin, F., & Shah, A. (2012). Introduction to evidence-based psychological treatments for older adults. In F. Scogin & A. Shah (Eds.), *Making evidence-based psychological treatments work with older adults* (pp. 3–8). Washington, DC: American Psychological Association.

Scogin, F., Welsh, D., Hanson, A., Stump, J., & Coates, A. (2005). Evidence-based psychotherapies for depression in older adults. *Clinical Psychology: Science and Practice, 12*, 222–237. doi:10.1093/clipsy.bpi033

Seelbach, W. C. (1977). Gender differences in expectations for filial responsibility. *The Gerontologist, 17*, 421–425. doi:10.1093/geront/17.5_Part_1.421

Serfaty, M., Haworth, D., Blanchard, M., Buszewicz, M., Murad, S., & King, M. (2009). Clinical effectiveness of individual cognitive behavioral therapy for depressed older people in primary care: A randomized controlled trial. *Archives of General Psychiatry, 66*, 1332–1340. doi:10.1001/archgenpsychiatry.2009.165

Silverstein, M., & Giarrusso, R. (2010). Aging and family life: A decade review. *Journal of Marriage and Family, 72*(5), 1039–1058. doi:10.1111/j.1741-3737.2010.00749.x

Silverstein, M., & Marenco, A. (2001). How Americans enact the grandparent role across the family life course. *Journal of Family Issues, 22*(4), 493–522.

Social Security Administration (SSA). (2010). *Income of the population 55 or older, 2008*. Washington, DC: SSA.

Smith, T. L., & Toseland, R. W. (2006). The effectiveness of a telephone support program for caregivers of frail older adults. *The Gerontologist, 46*, 620–629. doi:10.1093/geront/46.5.620

Steinglass, P., Temple, S., Lisman, S., & Reiss, D. (1982). Coping with spinal cord injury: The family perspective. *General Hospital Psychiatry, 4*, 259–264.
Suthers, K. (2008). *Evaluating the economic causes and consequences of racial and ethical health disparities*. Washington, DC: American Public Health Association.
Teri, L., Curtis, J., Gallagher-Thompson, D., & Thompson, L. (1994). Cognitive–behavioral therapy with depressed older adults. In L. S. Schneider, C. F. Reynolds, B. D. Lebowitz, & A. J. Friedhoff (Eds.), *Diagnosis and treatment of depression in late life: Results of the NIH Consensus Development Conference* (pp. 279–291). Washington, DC: American Psychiatric Press.
Teri, L., Logsdon, R. G., Uomoto, J., & McCurry, S. M. (1997). Behavioral treatment of depression in dementia patients: A controlled clinical trial. *The Journals of Gerontology Series B: Psychological Sciences and Social Sciences, 52*(4), 159–166.
Thielke, S., Vannoy, S., & Unützer, J. (2007). Integrating mental health and primary care. *Primary Care; Clinics in Office Practice, 34*, 571–592. doi:10.1016/j.pop.2007.05.007
Thorpe, K. E., & Howard, D. H. (2006). The rise in spending among Medicare beneficiaries: The role of chronic disease prevalence and changes in treatment intensity. *Health Affairs, 25*, w378–w388. doi:10.1377/hlthaff.25.w378
Vaillant, G. E., Meyer, S. E., Mukamal, K., & Soldz, S. (1998). Are social supports in late midlife a cause or a result of successful physical ageing? *Psychological Medicine, 28*(5), 1159–1168.
Waid, L. D., & Frazier, L. D. (2003). Cultural differences in possible selves during later life. *Journal of Aging Studies, 17*, 251–268. doi:10.1016/S0890-4065(03000031-8
Weissman, M. M., Markowitz, J. C., & Klerman, G. (2000). *Comprehensive guide to interpersonal psychotherapy*. New York, NY: Basic Books.

Index

A
Acute, 40, 115, 136, 138, 139, 185, 187
Acute Chest Syndrome (ACS), 40–42
Activities of daily living (ADLs), 187
Adherence, 35, 47, 49–51, 53–55, 57, 64–70, 74, 76–78, 80, 81, 83, 84, 92, 96, 98–100, 102–104, 107, 108, 122, 124, 125, 127
Aerosolized medication, 68
Age-matched, 67, 82
Aging, 170, 180, 187, 190, 197, 201–204, 210, 214, 215, 217, 219
Airway clearance, 64, 65, 68
Alzheimer's disease, 210
Ambiguous loss, 215
Analgesic, 40, 41, 46, 48, 57, 185, 187
Antidepressants, 199
Anxiety, 20–22, 44, 45, 48–50, 57, 63, 70–73, 75, 77, 80, 82, 84, 121, 124, 128, 138, 146, 147, 156, 158, 159, 166, 168, 170, 172, 191, 198, 201, 202, 204–206, 209, 213, 217, 218
Assessment, 27, 28, 30, 33, 35, 42, 81, 92, 93, 95, 97, 98, 100, 104, 121, 124, 125, 199, 204, 206
Attachment, 23–26, 35, 137, 138, 144, 216
Authoritative feeding style, 96
Avascular necrosis, 41
Azoospermia, 82

B
Biomarkers, 197
Body mass index (BMI), 66, 67, 92, 93, 96, 97, 99, 101, 108, 138
percentile, 66, 97, 98

C
Caregiving burden, 31–32, 51, 155–157, 214
Cerebral vascular accidents, 42, 43
CFfone, 77
Chemotherapy, 157, 162–163, 172
Child development, 29, 31, 33, 35
Child maltreatment, risk for, 31, 32, 134
Child obesity, 96, 102, 106–109
Child overweight, 92, 95
Children with Medical Complexity (CMC), 34, 35
Chronic, 1, 2, 4, 6–14, 16, 27, 31, 32, 34–35, 40, 41, 43–45, 47, 48, 51, 52, 55–57, 63, 64, 70, 72, 75, 94, 95, 105, 106, 108, 115, 116, 118–121, 124, 125, 136, 138, 140, 141, 153, 179–181, 185–187, 189–192, 197–199, 201, 203–204, 216, 219
Chronic lung disease (CLD), 20, 21
Cognitive behavioral therapy (CBT), 147, 158, 204, 210
Community health centers (CHCs), 31
Complementary remedy, 170

D
Dementia, 5, 6, 12–13, 186, 197–199, 203, 208–211, 215–217
Depression, 30, 45, 46, 48, 57, 63, 65, 70–73, 75, 80, 83, 94, 101, 105, 138, 140, 141, 146, 147, 162, 163, 191, 198, 199, 204–210, 214, 215, 217, 218
Dornase alfa (pulmozyme), 79
Ductal carcinoma in situ, 155

E
Early intervention services, 34
Emotional eating, 96
Epigenetic, 136, 205
Executive functioning, 20, 24, 43
Explicit weight bias, 101, 104
External eating, 96

F
Facebook, 27
Family adaptive systems (FAS), 84, 106
Family cohesion, 69, 96, 104, 107, 211
Family maintenance systems, 190
Family meaning systems, 189, 190
Feeding and growth, difficulties with, 20
Foster care, 133–149

G
Generalized Anxiety Disorder (GAD), 198
Generalized Anxiety Disorder Questionnaire (GAD-7), 71, 75
Graft, 116, 120–123, 126, 128
Grief, 13, 14, 197, 207, 208, 215, 216

H
Hb SC, 39, 41, 42
Hb SS, 39–42
Hb Sβ+ thalassemia, 39
Hb Sβ° thalassemia, 39
Health-related quality of life (HRQOL), 45, 46, 49, 50
Herrick, James, 39
Home visitation, 30
Hope theory, 50
Hydroxyurea, 41, 42, 57

I
Immunosuppressant, 115–117, 122
Implicit weight bias, 104

Infant mental health, 26, 29, 31, 32, 34, 35
Infarcts/microbleeds, 201
Infection, 20, 28, 40, 41, 65, 67, 70, 75–77, 82–84, 138, 162, 187
Instrumental activities of daily living (IADLs), 199
Insurance, problems with, 124
Interpersonal therapy, 50, 74, 79, 94, 207, 208
Invasive breast cancer, 155
Ischemic heart disease, 141
Ivacaftorm, aka Kalydeco, 64, 83

K
Kangaroo care, 25

M
Magnetic resonance imaging (MRI), 45
Major depressive disorder (MDD), 198
Marriage, 80, 154, 162, 166, 167, 170, 171, 202
Mastectomy, 159–160, 172
Medicaid, 31, 119, 123, 143, 188
Medical home, 21, 30–32, 35, 144, 146, 147
Medical mistrust, 165
Menarche, 82
Mild Cognitive Impairment (MCI)/Mild Neurocognitive Disorder
Motivational interviewing (MI), 100, 101, 105
Mucolytic, 79

N
National Institutes of Health (NIH), 39–41, 77
Nebulized medications, 64, 78
Nebulizer
Needs assessment, psychosocial, 120, 124
Neglect, 30, 31, 34, 133–135, 138, 140–142, 146, 148, 216
Neonatal Intensive Care Unit (NICU), 19–36
Neurocognitive functioning, 43, 45
Newborn Individualized Developmental Care and Assessment Program (NIDCAP), 24
Newborn screening, 40, 42, 56, 63, 64

O
Obesity prevention, 93–95, 97, 99–100, 106, 107
Obesogenic environment, 92, 105
Oncology, 154
Oppositional Defiant Disorder, 138
Optimistic acceptance, 73, 74
Outcome expectancy, 99

Index

P
Palliative treatment, 64, 164
Pathogens, 75, 76
Pathology/pathological, 138, 181–183
Patient Health Questionnaire (PHQ-9), 71, 75
Priapism, 41
Primary care clinics (PCC), 199
Primary care providers (PCP), 28–30, 35, 97, 125, 144
Problem solving therapy (PST), 217
Psychotropic, 146–147
Pulmonary exacerbations, 63–65, 82

R
Radiation
    therapy, 157, 161, 162
    treatment, 157
Reconstructive surgery, 160
Recurrence, 157, 163, 169
Respiratory system, problems with, 20
Restrictive feeding practices, 96
Retinopathy of prematurity (ROP), 20, 21
Reunification, 135, 141
Rhinitis, 138
Rooming in, NICU, 28

S
Scabies, 137
Screening, developmental, 33
Sensory deprivation, 137
Severe child obesity, 52
Sickle cell trait, 39
Skin to skin contact, 24, 25
Socioemotional selectivity theory, 201
Solid organ transplant, 115–129
Stage four tertiary care, 98
Stage one treatment (prevention plus), 98

Stage three treatment (comprehensive multidisciplinary intervention), 98, 104, 108
Stage two treatment (structured weight management), 98
Stem cell transplantation, 42
Stressors, 32, 35, 44, 45, 50–53, 56, 94, 115, 121, 122, 124, 138, 139, 142, 144, 147, 154, 189, 190, 199, 209, 210, 215, 219
Stroke, 41–43, 45, 55, 186

T
Terminal stages, 156
Toxic stressors, 139, 140
Transcranial Doppler (TCD), 41, 43, 57
Transfer of care, 81, 124–126
Transfusion, 41–43, 57
Transition
    from NICU, 28, 29
    from pediatric care, 28, 80
    responsibility, 77–81
Trauma, 30, 117, 133, 136, 138, 140, 145–148

U
United Network of Organ Sharing (UNOS), 116

V
Vasoocclusion, 40–42

W
Watch and Wait model, 205, 217, 219
Wave one family resilience, 106
Wave three family resilience, 106
Wave two family resilience, 106
Weight cycling, 101

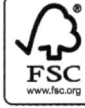

MIX
Papier aus verantwortungsvollen Quellen
Paper from responsible sources
FSC® C105338

If you have any concerns about our products,
you can contact us on
ProductSafety@springernature.com

In case Publisher is established outside the EU,
the EU authorized representative is:
**Springer Nature Customer Service Center GmbH
Europaplatz 3, 69115 Heidelberg, Germany**

Printed by Libri Plureos GmbH
in Hamburg, Germany